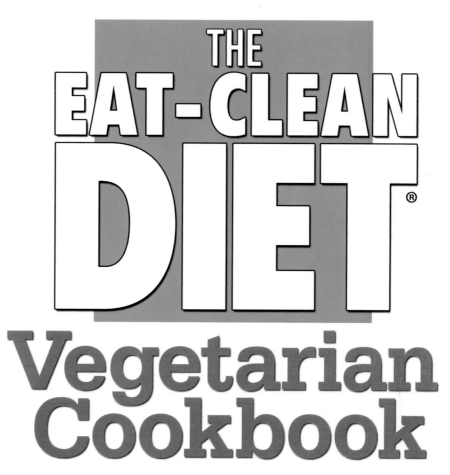

THE EAT-CLEAN DIET®

Vegetarian Cookbook

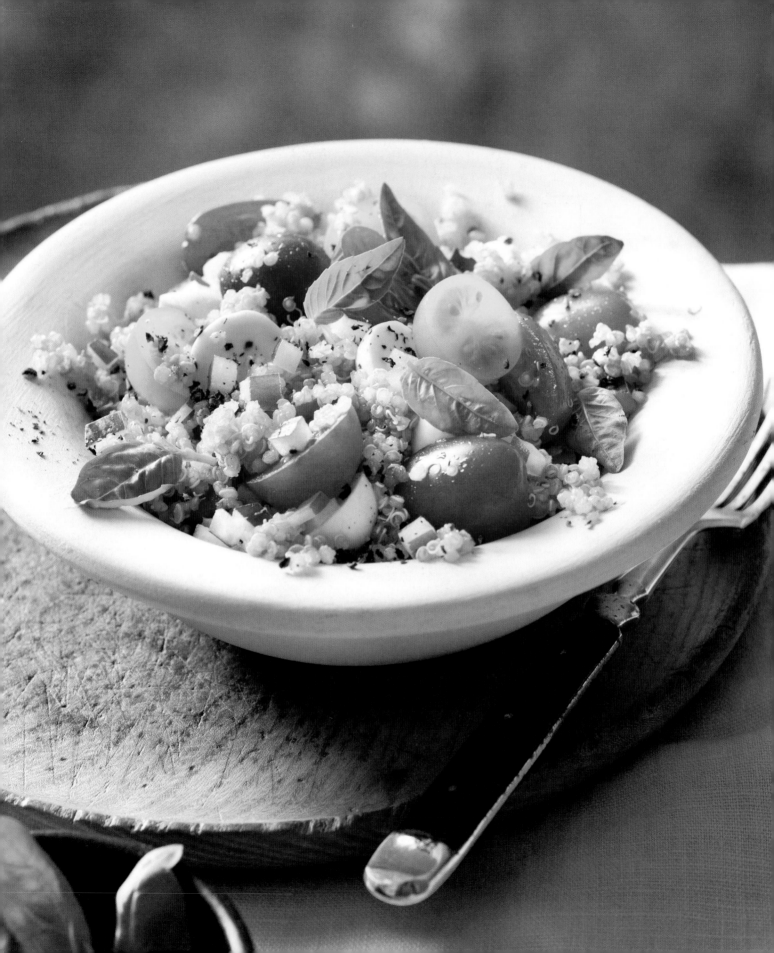

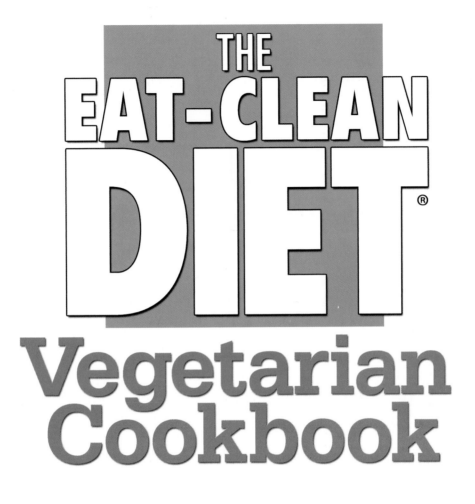

THE EAT-CLEAN DIET®
Vegetarian Cookbook

**Lose weight – get healthy –
one mouthwatering meal at a time!**

FROM *NEW YORK TIMES* BEST-SELLING AUTHOR

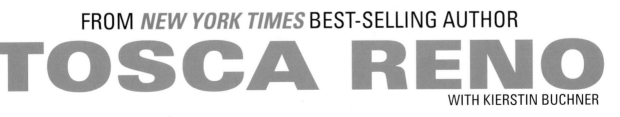

TOSCA RENO

with KIERSTIN BUCHNER

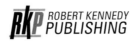

RKP ROBERT KENNEDY
PUBLISHING

Published by Robert Kennedy Publishing
400 Matheson Blvd. West
Mississauga, ON
L5R 3M1 Canada
Visit us at **www.rkpubs.com**, **www.toscareno.com**
and **www.eatcleandiet.com**

Library and Archives Canada Cataloguing in Publication

Reno, Tosca, 1959-
      The eat-clean diet vegetarian cookbook : lose
weight and get
healthy - one mouthwatering meatless meal at a time! /
Tosca Reno.

Includes index.
ISBN 978-1-55210-106-3

      1. Weight loss. 2. Reducing diets--Recipes.
3. Vegetarian cooking. 4. Cookbooks. I. Title.

 RM222.2.R4649 2012   613.2'5
C2011-906173-2

10 9 8 7 6 5 4 3 2 1

Distributed in Canada by
NBN (National Book Network)
67 Mowat Avenue, Suite 241
Toronto, ON
M6K 3E3

Distributed in USA by
NBN (National Book Network)
15200 NBN Way
Blue Ridge Summit, PA
17214

Printed in Canada

Robert Kennedy Publishing
BOOK DEPARTMENT

MANAGING DIRECTOR Wendy Morley	**ART DIRECTOR** Gabriella Caruso Marques
SENIOR EDITOR Amy Land	**ASSISTANT ART DIRECTOR** Jessica Pensabene Hearn
EDITOR, ONLINE AND PRINT Meredith Barrett	**EDITORIAL DESIGNER** Brian Ross
ASSOCIATE EDITOR Rachel Corradetti	**PROP/WARDROBE STYLIST** Kelsey-Lynn Corradetti
ONLINE EDITOR Kiersten Corradetti	**SENIOR WEB DESIGNER** Chris Barnes
EDITORIAL ASSISTANTS Brittany Seki, Chelsea Kennedy	

INDEXING
James De Medeiros

IMPORTANT

The information in this book reflects the author's experiences and opinions and is not intended to replace medical advice.

Before beginning this or any nutritional or exercise regimen, consult your physician to be sure it is appropriate for you. Ask for a physical stress test.

This book is truly dedicated to

Robert Kennedy, my husband, the love and
joy of my life. He is to me like sunshine to
seeds – the life force I needed to discover
myself. He is the finest man. His joy for life
fills me. I love you Robert.

Table of Contents

"I'm so thrilled to be celebrating my love for plant-based foods with you in this book. As we say at my house, the more vegetables the better!"

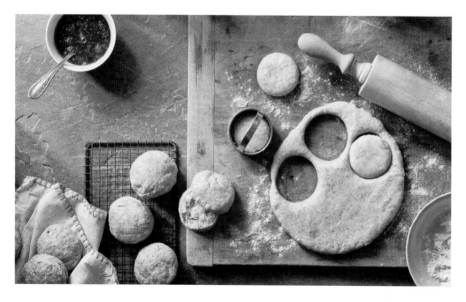

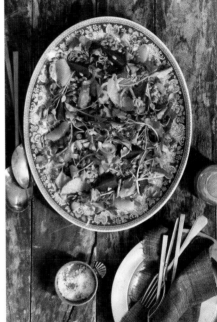

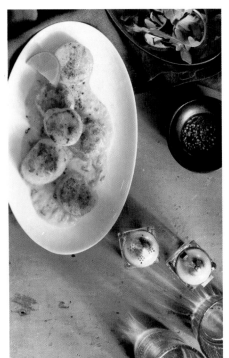

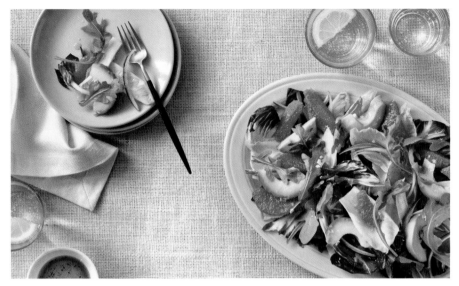

"Some of my favorite foods are oatmeal, kale, sweet potatoes, beans and flaxseed. They are all super-nutritious and delicious – and can be found in the recipes throughout this book!"

"Nothing makes me happier than sitting down to a sexy salad made of sunflower sprouts, radicchio, mesclun greens, blueberries, pumpkin seeds, sauerkraut and pumpkin seed oil dressing. Delicious!"

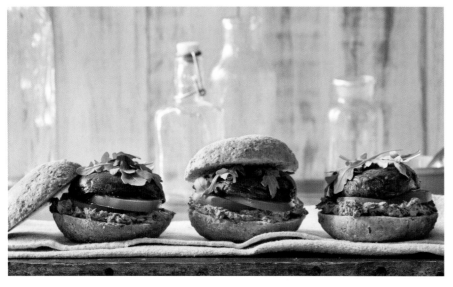

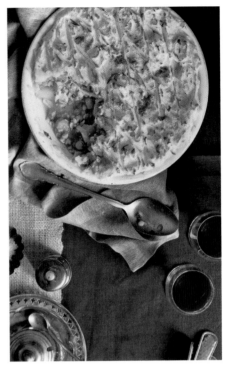

Introduction

I'm going to be straight with you – I'm not a vegetarian. Are you going to put the book down and run away? I hope not, because the principles of a vegetarian lifestyle can easily be incorporated into any diet – vegetarian or not.

If you're an *Eat-Clean Diet®* veteran you know this lifestyle is based on eating a wide variety of fruits, vegetables, whole grains and lean protein sources. But not all of the protein needs to come from animals. In fact, it's more healthful, beneficial and wallet-friendly to limit your intake of meat and stick to a mainly plant-based diet. This is especially true with the plethora of hormone-injected, antibiotic-ridden, unnaturally fed meats currently filling our grocery store shelves, not to mention how expensive good-quality meats can be. In fact, vegetarianism and *The Eat-Clean Diet* make a perfect pair! This must be why so many of my readers asked for it.

After attending countless trade shows and meeting tons of *Eat-Clean Diet* fans I found many were asking the same thing: "When, oh when, Tosca, will you have a vegetarian cookbook?" I decided to bite the bullet and delve into the project. What I learned throughout the process is that vegetarianism can be an extremely healthful lifestyle choice, but it can also be harmful if not followed properly. I was shocked to learn about the countless vegetarians who think that simply cutting out meat makes you healthy. Not so – especially if you are surviving on little but pasta and bread (more common than you might think), thereby avoiding important vitamins and minerals and overloading your blood-sugar handling.

Vegetarianism is a lifestyle choice that needs to be adopted carefully and thoughtfully. I have done my best throughout this book to clarify the most important aspects of a healthy vegetarian lifestyle and discuss how they can be incorporated into your life, all while offering gorgeous, delicious food that satisfy all your needs. Don't forget to talk to your healthcare provider for more information and to make sure you are taking good care of yourself.

There are many different ways to eat vegetarian food, whether you're choosing simply to eat a few vegetarian meals each week (this is what we do in my house) or choosing to avoid all animal products as a vegan. Ultimately, the point is to eat clean, healthy, whole foods.

So, as a non-vegetarian, I present to you *The Eat-Clean Diet Vegetarian Cookbook* entirely dedicated to plant-based *Eat-Clean Diet* meals. It's heavy on vegetables, heavy on love and heavy on helping hands around the kitchen!

Need more? Don't forget to visit my team, tons of other *Eat-Clean Diet* followers and me on Facebook and Twitter, at eatclean-diet.com or toscareno.com, and on the Kitchen Table (our virtual support system) at eatcleandiet.com/kitchentable.

Sincerely,

Tosca Reno

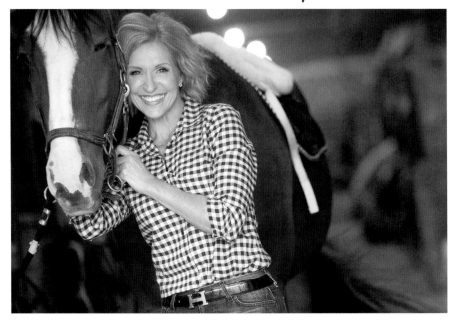

How to Use This Book

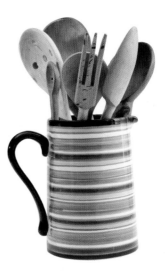

The term "vegetarian" can mean different things to different people. One person will eat no animal products whatsoever, another will consume dairy and another still will eat dairy, eggs and even fish sometimes. Of course we have other concerns when cooking too – do any of our guests keep a gluten-free diet? Do we need something fast to make after a long day of work? Will our kids eat it?

I want to make sure this book is as easy as possible for you to use, and so I've come up with some handy symbols. Simply look at the top of each recipe and you'll be able to tell in seconds whether the dish is right for your needs.

LEGEND

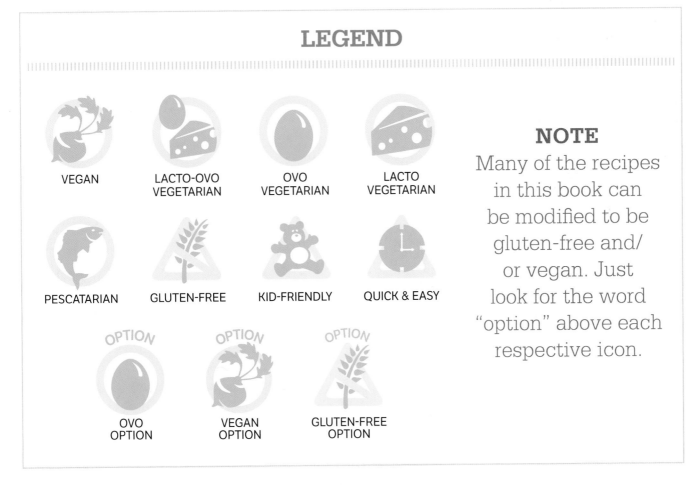

VEGAN

LACTO-OVO VEGETARIAN

OVO VEGETARIAN

LACTO VEGETARIAN

PESCATARIAN

GLUTEN-FREE

KID-FRIENDLY

QUICK & EASY

OPTION
OVO OPTION

OPTION
VEGAN OPTION

OPTION
GLUTEN-FREE OPTION

NOTE

Many of the recipes in this book can be modified to be gluten-free and/ or vegan. Just look for the word "option" above each respective icon.

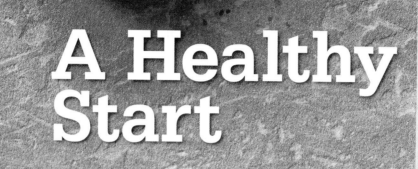

A Healthy Start

Baking Powder Biscuits, p. 16

Baking Powder Biscuits

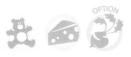

PREP: 10 minutes | **COOK:** 15 minutes | **YIELD:** 8 biscuits

Biscuits are a popular Southern breakfast accompaniment, but they're usually full of fat. These biscuits have been Cleaned up, but you wouldn't know it by biting into one. Y'all try them out now, y'hear?

2 cups (480 ml) whole wheat flour

1 Tbsp (15 ml) baking powder

¼ tsp (1.25 ml) sea salt

1 Tbsp (15 ml) raw virgin coconut oil at room temperature or refrigerated (do not melt)

¾ cup (180 ml) + 2 Tbsp (30 ml) plain, low-fat kefir or a combination of plain soy yogurt and almond, soy, hemp or other milk subsitute

Additional kefir for brushing the tops of the biscuits

Preheat the oven to 450ºF (230ºC).

In a large bowl, whisk together flour, baking powder and sea salt until thoroughly combined. Using your fingers, break coconut oil into very small pieces and work it into the flour. Stir in kefir until dry ingredients are just moistened.

Transfer dough to a floured working surface, keeping some flour handy for additional dusting to prevent sticking, as needed. Use your hands to bring dough together, pressing it into a ball. Knead it once or twice before using a rolling pin to roll it into a disk that is eight inches across and about one inch thick.

Using a round biscuit cutter, cut dough into eight circles. Or, for complete use of the dough, use a chef's knife to cut the dough into eight wedges.

Place biscuits on a baking sheet and brush the tops with kefir. Bake in oven for about 15 minutes or until puffed up and lightly browned. Serve hot with a little pure honey or unsweetened jam, if desired.

NUTRITIONAL VALUE PER BISCUIT:
Calories: 122 | Calories from Fat: 19 | Protein: 5 g | Carbs: 25 g | Total Fat: 2 g | Saturated Fat: 1 g | Trans Fat: 0 g | Fiber: 4 g | Sodium: 127 mg | Cholesterol: 2 mg

Green Energy Whole Food Smoothie

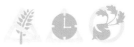

PREP: 10 minutes | **COOK:** 0 minutes | **YIELD:** 4 x 10-oz servings

We all know how important it is to fulfill your fruit and veggie quota, but it can be hard to squeeze enough servings into one day. Why not blend them up and enjoy them all in one delicious drink?

1 kiwi, peel on

½ baby zucchini, peel on

¼ pineapple, peel removed

1 cup (240 ml) green or white grapes

4 kale leaves, stemmed

4 fresh strawberries, including green tops

1 thin slice of lime, peel on

½ peeled orange

½ peeled banana

Small handful wheatgrass

1 Tbsp (15 ml) spirulina

1 Tbsp (15 ml) kelp granules

1 Tbsp (15 ml) flaxseed

1 cup (240 ml) cold water

1 cup (240 ml) ice, or more

To a whole foods blender, add all of the ingredients starting with fruits and vegetables, then spirulina, kelp and flaxseed. Lastly, add water and the ice.

Start the machine on low speed and gradually increase speed until machine is whirring nicely and smoothie ingredients are moving freely. Blend for about 1 minute.

Stop machine to check smoothie temperature and consistency. If not cold, add more ice. If not super smooth, continue to blend for 1 to 2 minutes, adding more ice if necessary to keep smoothie cold as the blender processes. Pour into a glass and serve.

ON THE GO
This smoothie will keep overnight in the fridge. Just seal it in a portable container so you can wake up, grab it and go. Note: The flaxseed might cause the smoothie to thicken slightly as it sits.

EQUIPMENT TIP
If you don't have a whole foods blender, such as a Vitamix® or Omega blender, don't worry! You can still make this recipe by breaking down the ingredients in a food processor and then transferring them to a blender.

PREP TIP
When making a whole foods smoothie, it is best to use organic fruit, since many of the peels will be blended. Remember to wash your fruit thoroughly, too!

NUTRITIONAL VALUE PER SERVING:
Calories: 132 | Calories from Fat: 11 | Protein: 3 g | Carbs: 25 g | Total Fat: 1 g | Saturated Fat: 0.2 g | Trans Fat: 0 g | Fiber: 6 g | Sodium: 39 mg | Cholesterol: 0 mg

Breakfast Eggel Sandwich

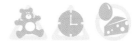

PREP: 15 minutes | **COOK:** 3 minutes | **YIELD:** 1 sandwich

Preparing a delicious and nutritious breakfast is a snap when you have eggs and bagels in the fridge. Simply add some tomato, avocado, mustard and sprouts, and you've got a Clean and colorful meal that's perfect for the whole family.

1 whole wheat bagel, split

1 tsp (5 ml) Dijon mustard

2 Tbsp (30 ml) Yogurt Cheese* (see p. 276)

¼ avocado, slightly mashed

2-3 slices tomato

¼ cup (60 ml) alfalfa sprouts

1 whole egg + 2 egg whites

Pinch sea salt and black pepper

Eat-Clean Cooking Spray (see p. 277)

Place oven rack six inches from top of oven, and turn on broiler. Place bagel on a baking sheet, cut side up, and toast under broiler.

Spread both sides of toasted bagel with Dijon mustard and yogurt cheese. On the top half of the bagel, spread mashed avocado and add the tomato slices and sprouts.

Heat an 8-inch nonstick skillet on medium. Beat eggs and season with a pinch of salt and pepper. Spray skillet lightly with Eat-Clean Cooking Spray and pour in eggs. Allow edges to firm, then lift edges up bit by bit, using a rubber spatula, and let uncooked egg run underneath. Repeat until no more egg will run under.

With confidence, and the assistance of a rubber spatula, flip! Cook for about 30 seconds longer, and then slide out of pan. Fold edges of eggs into the shape of a square and place on the bottom half of bagel. Put the two halves of the bagel together and eat while still warm.

> **NOTE:**
> *Yogurt Cheese must be made ahead of time.

NUTRITIONAL VALUE PER SANDWICH:

Calories: 396 | Calories from Fat: 71 | Protein: 17 g | Carbs: 71 g | Total Fat: 8 g | Saturated Fat: 1.4 g | Trans Fat: 0 g | Fiber: 13 g | Sodium: 727 mg | Cholesterol: 1 mg

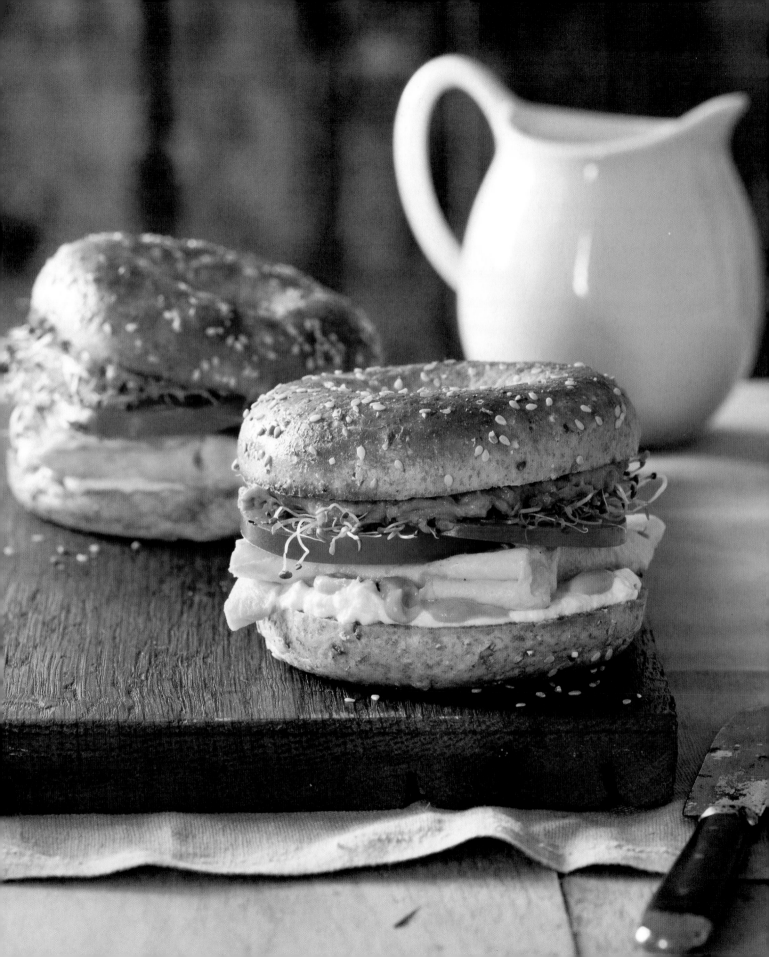

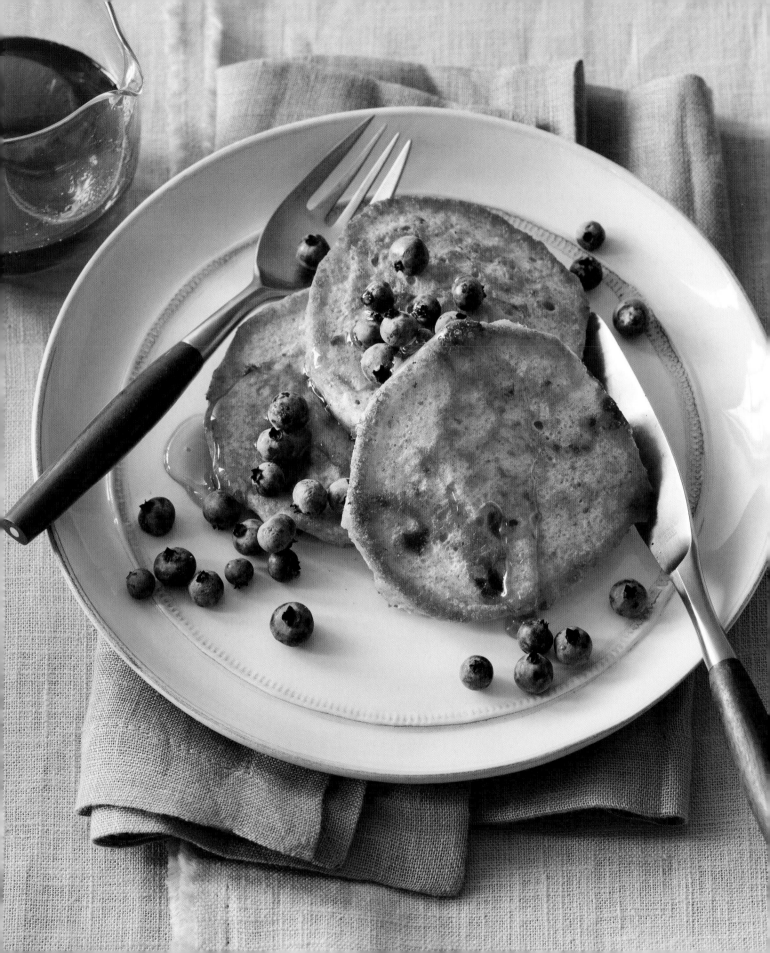

Lemon Cottage Cheese Griddlecakes

PREP: 15 minutes | **COOK:** 20 minutes | **YIELD:** 14 griddlecakes

I used to love it when my dad would fire up the griddle and create the most delicious, fluffy pancakes – a true breakfast treat. I've healthed up the typical griddlecake by adding cottage cheese and whole wheat, but don't worry – not an ounce of fluff or flavor has been lost!

1¼ cups (300 ml) whole wheat flour

2 tsp (10 ml) baking powder

½ tsp (2.5 ml) baking soda

3 Tbsp (45 ml) Sucanat or other unrefined sugar

Pinch freshly grated nutmeg

Pinch sea salt

1 cup (240 ml) low-fat milk

1 cup (240 ml) cultured low-fat cottage cheese
    or regular low-fat, low-salt cottage cheese

1 egg yolk

1 tsp (5 ml) pure vanilla extract

1 tsp (5ml) finely grated lemon zest

3 egg whites

Eat-Clean Cooking Spray (see p. 277) or
    coconut oil

In a large bowl, whisk together flour, baking powder, baking soda, Sucanat, nutmeg and sea salt. In a separate bowl, whisk together milk, cottage cheese, egg yolk, vanilla extract and lemon zest. Add wet ingredients to dry ingredients and mix together until just combined.

Add egg whites to a separate bowl and beat them into stiff peaks. Fold egg whites into batter. It will be thick and lumpy.

Heat a pancake griddle thoroughly on medium low, and spray with Eat-Clean Cooking Spray or use a little coconut oil to prevent griddlecakes from sticking. Scoop about ⅓ cup (80 ml) of batter onto the griddle for each cake, and shape it into a round. Cook until the top is filled with bubbles and holes, and the edges are starting to dry, 4 to 5 minutes. Flip and cook for 1 to 2 minutes longer. Repeat until all of the batter is used. Serve immediately or keep warm in a 200ºF (90ºC) oven.

TRY THIS!
Top these griddlecakes with fresh fruit, yogurt, Blueberry Compote (see p. 227), or for a treat, a drizzle of pure maple syrup.

NUTRITIONAL VALUE PER GRIDDLECAKE:
Calories: 67 | Calories from Fat: 8 | Protein: 4 g | Carbs: 13 g | Total Fat: 1 g |
Saturated Fat: 0.3 g | Trans Fat: 0 g | Fiber: 1 g | Sodium: 137 mg | Cholesterol: 3 mg

Amaranth Oat Waffles

PREP: 15 minutes | **COOK:** 21-28 minutes | **YIELD:** 14 waffles

Waffles – they are a big breakfast favorite. However, they are typically laden with sugar, milk and eggs. Luckily, this vegan version is full of flavor as well as nutritious grains and seeds. Now waffles can be more than a special treat!

DRY INGREDIENTS

1 cup (240 ml) whole grain amaranth flour

½ cup (120 ml) oat flour

½ cup (120 ml) oat bran

½ cup (120 ml) whole soy flour

½ cup (120 ml) whole grain corn flour (not corn starch)

¼ cup (60 ml) whole grain coarse cornmeal

2 Tbsp (30 ml) flax meal or ground flaxseed

2½ tsp (12.5 ml) baking powder

½ tsp (2.5 ml) baking soda

Pinch sea salt

WET INGREDIENTS

2½ cups (600 ml) low-fat buttermilk or a combination of equal parts soy or almond milk and soy yogurt

1 egg + 2 egg whites or equivalent vegan egg replacer

¼ cup (60 ml) Sucanat or other unrefined sugar

1 tsp (5 ml) pure vanilla extract

Eat-Clean Cooking Spray (see p. 277)

Preheat a waffle iron and place a baking sheet underneath to catch any spills.

In a large bowl, whisk together dry ingredients. In a separate bowl, whisk together wet ingredients. Stir wet ingredients into dry ingredients until just moistened.

Spray the inside of a waffle iron with Eat-Clean Cooking Spray and pour enough batter to cover cooking area. Slowly close lid to allow batter to spread out and fill in the spaces. Cook 3 to 4 minutes, or until waffle releases from iron. Slowly open lid and use a fork to gently remove waffle. Repeat with Eat-Clean Cooking Spray and another scoop of batter until all batter is used.

Serve with a smear of natural nut butter, banana slices or a drizzle of pure maple syrup.

CHILL OUT

Waffles will last for up to five days in the refrigerator or up to one month in the freezer. Reheat in the toaster or toaster oven.

NUTRITIONAL VALUE PER SERVING (2 WAFFLES):
Calories: 280 | Calories from Fat: 62 | Protein: 14 g | Carbs: 52 g | Total Fat: 6 g |
Saturated Fat: 2 g | Trans Fat: 0 g | Fiber: 6 g | Sodium: 292 mg | Cholesterol: 4 mg

Blueberry Baked Oatmeal

PREP: 10 minutes | **COOK:** 35-40 minutes | **YIELD:** 5 x 1 cup servings

We all know oatmeal is a healthy way to start the day, but some kids (and adults for that matter) have a problem with the mushiness factor. Fear not, this palate-pleasing recipe calls for the oatmeal to be baked, which lends it an almost cookie-like texture – a great way to sell it to the kids!

Eat-Clean Cooking Spray

1 cup (240 ml) unsweetened soy, rice or almond
milk, or other milk substitute

1 whole egg + 2 egg whites

½ cup (120 ml) unsweetened applesauce

2 Tbsp (30 ml) pure maple syrup

½ tsp (2.5 ml) vanilla extract

1 tsp (5 ml) baking powder

1 tsp (5 ml) ground cinnamon

Pinch freshly grated nutmeg

Pinch sea salt

2½ cups (600 ml) old-fashioned rolled oats

¼ cup (60 ml) oat bran

½ cup (120 ml) chopped pecans

1½ cups (360 ml) frozen or fresh
blueberries, divided

Preheat the oven to 350°F (175°C).

Coat a 3-quart casserole dish or baking pan with Eat-Clean Cooking Spray.

In a large bowl, whisk together milk, egg and egg whites, applesauce, maple syrup, vanilla, baking powder, cinnamon, nutmeg and sea salt. Mix in oats, oat bran and pecans. Gently fold in half of the blueberries. Scatter remaining blueberries across bottom of casserole dish.

Scrape oatmeal mixture into casserole dish and bake, uncovered, for 35 to 40 minutes or until golden brown around the edges.

NUTRITIONAL VALUE PER SERVING:
Calories: 363 | Calories from Fat: 87 | Protein: 13 g | Carbs: 60 g | Total Fat: 10 g |
Saturated Fat: 1 g | Trans Fat: 0 g | Fiber: 9 g | Sodium: 56 mg | Cholesterol: 2 mg

French Toast with Strawberries and Almonds – Heaven for Breakfast

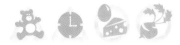

PREP: 20 minutes | **COOK:** 5-7 minutes | **YIELD:** 6 servings

I have fond memories of sitting at a café in the pleasant town of Oakville on the shores of Lake Ontario enjoying delicious strawberries and almonds with sweet toast. I just knew I had to create a Cleaned up version of this yummy meal for all of my readers to enjoy.

BATTER INGREDIENTS

1 x 12-oz (340 g) package organic silken firm tofu

½ cup (120 ml) unsweetened soy, rice or almond milk, or other milk substitute

2 tsp (10 ml) pure maple syrup

1 tsp (5 ml) pure vanilla extract

½ tsp (2.5 ml) almond extract

½ tsp (2.5 ml) ground cinnamon

Pinch sea salt

1-2 Tbsp (15 to 30 ml) raw virgin coconut oil

6 slices rustic whole grain bread

1½ cups (360 ml) sliced fresh strawberries

6 Tbsp (90 ml) sliced almonds

Add all batter ingredients to a blender and blend until combined well. Pour into a bowl big enough to dip a piece of bread into.

Heat a skillet or griddle over medium. Add a little coconut oil and swirl around the surface of the griddle. Dip a slice of bread in batter, then turn it over and dip again until it's completely soaked. Lift out bread, allowing excess batter to drip into the bowl, and place on the griddle. Repeat until griddle is covered with battered bread. Sauté bread until cooked through and browned, 2 or 3 minutes per side.

To serve, top each piece of French toast with ¼ cup (60 ml) sliced strawberries, 1 Tbsp (15 ml) sliced almonds and a drizzle of pure maple syrup, for a treat.

PREP TIP

If you are working in batches, or aren't going to serve the toast right away, place it on a baking sheet and keep it warm in a 200⁰F (90⁰C) oven.

PROTEIN POWER!

Want more protein? Add a smear of natural nut butter to your French toast. Mmm!

NUTRITIONAL VALUE PER SERVING (1 SLICE WITH ¼ CUP STRAWBERRIES AND 1 TBSP SLICED ALMONDS):
Calories: 213 | Calories from Fat: 98 | Protein: 9 g | Carbs: 16 g | Total Fat: 11 g |
Saturated Fat: 4 g | Trans Fat: 0 g | Fiber: 4 g | Sodium: 146 mg | Cholesterol: 0 mg

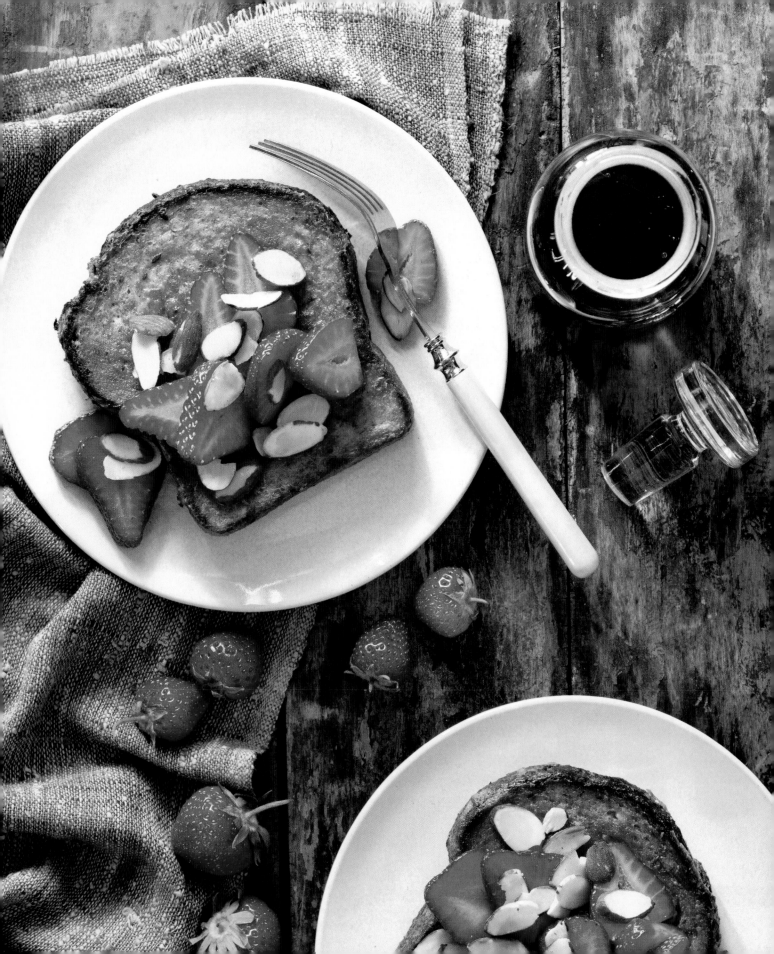

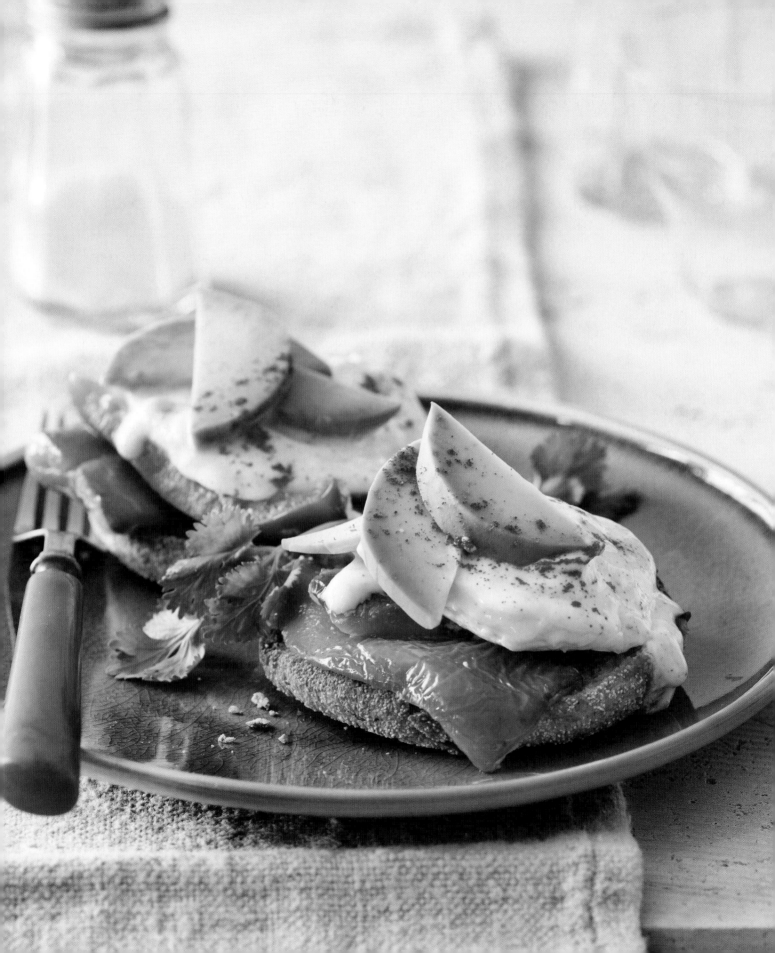

Baja California Eggs Benedict

PREP: 10 minutes | **COOK:** 25 minutes | **YIELD:** 2 servings

This Clean variation of the brunch classic gets a California twist with low-fat yogurt "Hollandaise" sauce, roasted poblano peppers and creamy avocado slices. It's light and fresh – and very satisfying!

SAUCE INGREDIENTS

⅓ cup (80 ml) low-fat Greek yogurt

1 Tbsp (15 ml) lemon juice

1 Tbsp (15 ml) orange juice

Pinch cayenne, plus more for garnish

2 poblano peppers

Eat-Clean Cooking Spray (see p. 277)

2 whole eggs + 4 egg whites

2 whole wheat English muffins, split

½ avocado, pitted, peeled and thinly sliced

Sea salt and freshly ground black pepper, to taste

To make "Hollandaise" sauce: In a small bowl, mix together yogurt, lemon juice, orange juice and cayenne. Set aside.

Place oven rack six inches from top of oven, and turn on broiler. Place peppers on a baking sheet and broil 3 to 5 minutes or until skin is charred and blistered. Turn peppers and repeat until thoroughly blistered. Transfer peppers to a glass bowl, cover with a plate and let sit for about 5 minutes to steam. Peel away blistered skin, using a paper towel to wipe away any remaining blackened bits. Cut peppers in half. Remove stems and seeds.

Fill bottom of an egg poacher with one inch of water and bring to a simmer over medium-high heat. Spray poaching cups with Eat-Clean Cooking Spray, and fill two of the cups with the whole eggs. Divide four egg whites among two remaining cups. Cover and cook whole eggs until whites set and yolks thicken slightly (about 4 minutes). Remove cooked whole eggs, cover and continue cooking egg whites until opaque, another 3 to 4 minutes.

Toast English muffins under broiler, and divide them between two plates. Place half a roasted pepper on each muffin half and top with the poached whole eggs and egg whites. Spoon sauce on eggs and top with avocado slices. Season with a pinch of salt and pepper, and sprinkle with a little cayenne.

NUTRITIONAL VALUE PER SERVING (1 WHOLE ENGLISH MUFFIN,
1 ROASTED POBLANO PEPPER, 1 WHOLE EGG + 2 EGG WHITES, ¼ AVOCADO AND ½ OF SAUCE):
Calories: 353 | Calories from Fat: 118 | Protein: 26 g | Carbs: 40 g | Total Fat: 12 g |
Saturated Fat: 1 g | Trans Fat: 0 g | Fiber: 7 g | Sodium: 479 mg | Cholesterol: 0 mg

Dark and Addictive Bran Muffins

PREP: 25 minutes | **COOK:** 20 minutes | **YIELD:** 15 muffins

I wouldn't normally use the word "addictive" to describe bran muffins, but in this case, it's absolutely true. This recipe is an Eat-Clean vegan version I developed based on my mother's recipe. I grew up eating these muffins for breakfast, snacks and dessert – and I still love them to this day!

Eat-Clean Cooking Spray (see p. 277)
1 cup (240 ml) boiling water
1 cup (240 ml) wheat bran

WET INGREDIENTS

2 Tbsp (30 ml) raw virgin coconut
    oil, melted
¼ cup (60 ml) Sucanat or other unrefined sugar
¼ cup (60 ml) unsulfured blackstrap molasses
½ cup (120 ml) unsweetened applesauce
1 cup + 2 Tbsp (240 ml + 30 ml) soy, rice,
    almond or other milk substitute
1 cup (240 ml) plain soy yogurt
1 Tbsp (15 ml) grated orange zest

DRY INGREDIENTS

2½ cups (600 ml) whole wheat flour
2 Tbsp (30 ml) whole grain soy flour
2 Tbsp (30 ml) flax meal or ground flaxseed
2½ tsp (12.5 ml) baking soda
¼ tsp (1.25 ml) sea salt

2 cups (480 ml) all-natural, whole-grain
    bran flake cereal
Flaxseed for garnish, if desired

Place oven rack in the center of the oven and preheat to 400ºF (200ºC). Prepare muffin tin by lining with paper cups, silicone muffin cup liners or spraying with Eat-Clean Cooking Spray.

Pour boiling water over bran and set aside.

In a large bowl, whisk together wet ingredients until combined thoroughly.

In a medium bowl, whisk together dry ingredients until combined well. Add to the wet ingredients and stir to combine. Add bran flake cereal and bran and water mixture, and stir to combine.

Divide batter among 15 muffin cups and sprinkle the tops with flaxseeds, if desired. Bake for about 20 minutes, or until a toothpick inserted into the center comes out clean. Remove from oven and cool on a wire rack.

NUTRITIONAL VALUE PER MUFFIN:
Calories: 163 | Calories from Fat: 24 | Protein: 3 g | Carbs: 33 g | Total Fat: 3 g | Saturated Fat: 1 g | Trans Fat: 0 g | Fiber: 6 g | Sodium: 159 mg | Cholesterol: 0 mg

Quick Brown Rice Breakfast

PREP: 5 minutes | **COOK:** 0 minutes | **YIELD:** 2 servings

Growing up, my mom made a slightly sweeter version of this for dessert and called it "rice pudding." It's so quick and easy that it works well as an almost-instant breakfast.

2 cups (480 ml) cooked brown rice
(day-old cold rice is best)
2 cups (480 ml) low-fat milk or unsweetened
almond or soy milk
¼ cup (60 ml) sliced, slivered or chopped
raw almonds
1 Tbsp (15 ml) flaxseed
2 tsp (10 ml) pure maple syrup, divided
Healthy pinch freshly grated nutmeg

Divide rice between two bowls and add half of milk and remaining ingredients to each.

ON THE GO
Make this brekkie the night before and place individual servings into portable containers so in the morning you can just grab one as you rush out the door.

NUTRITIONAL VALUE PER SERVING:
Calories: 436 | Calories from Fat: 113 | Protein: 16 g | Carbs: 65 g | Total Fat: 13 g |
Saturated Fat: 2 g | Trans Fat: 0 g | Fiber: 6 g | Sodium: 124 mg | Cholesterol: 15 mg

Smoothie on the Beach

PREP: 10 minutes | **COOK:** 0 minutes | **YIELD:** 3 x 10-oz servings

I developed this smoothie when preparing for a trip to Mexico. It made me feel like I was already on vacation, sipping something delicious while relaxing on the beach. It makes a healthy breakfast or a quick and delicious snack.

2 cups (480 ml) plain organic soy yogurt
2 cups (480 ml) frozen mango, pineapple
chunks, strawberries and peach slices
1 Tbsp (15 ml) hulled hemp seeds
1 Tbsp (15 ml) golden flaxseed
1 Tbsp (15 ml) oat bran
2 Tbsp (30 ml) vegan protein powder
½ tsp (2.5 ml) pure vanilla extract
Juice of 1 lime

Place all ingredients in a blender and blend until smooth. Enjoy immediately.

PROTEIN POWER!
When shopping for vegan protein powders, try to choose ones that are as natural as possible. I don't recommend any flavored powder other than vanilla (if you are using vanilla protein powder, omit the vanilla extract from the recipe).

NUTRITIONAL VALUE PER SERVING:
Calories: 234 | Calories from Fat: 58 | Protein: 13 g | Carbs: 35 g | Total Fat: 6 g |
Saturated Fat: 0.2 g | Trans Fat: 0 g | Fiber: 8 g | Sodium: 110 mg | Cholesterol: 0 mg

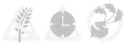

Skillet Eggs in Rustic Tomato Sauce with Butter Beans

PREP: 15 minutes | **COOK:** 30 minutes | **YIELD:** 4 servings

This dish is fantastic for brunch, lunch and even dinner. The sauce can be made ahead of time; just heat it up in the skillet before you add the eggs.

4 cups or 1 x 28-oz (840 ml) BPA-free can
   no-salt-added whole peeled tomatoes,
   drained

1 tsp (5 ml) extra virgin olive oil

½ small yellow or white onion, finely chopped

2 cloves garlic, minced

½ tsp (2.5 ml) smoked paprika

Pinch dried oregano or Italian herbs

¼ cup (60 ml) pitted kalamata olives,
   drained and chopped

2 cups cooked, rinsed and drained, or 1 x 15-oz
   (440 ml) can no-salt-added butter beans,
   drained and rinsed

4 organic eggs, as fresh as possible

Sea salt and freshly ground black pepper,
   to taste

Preheat oven to 350°F (175°C) and place rack in the upper third of oven.

Pour drained tomatoes into a bowl and use your hands to squish them into pieces. Set aside.

Heat olive oil in a 9-inch (or similarly sized) cast-iron skillet on medium low. Add onion and cook until soft, about 3 minutes. Stir in garlic and cook about 1 minute longer. Add squished tomatoes, paprika, oregano, kalamata olives and butter beans and stir to combine. Transfer skillet to oven and cook for about 15 minutes. Remove and set on top of stove. Using a ladle, make 4 indentations and gently crack the eggs into the indentations, keeping yolks intact. Season eggs with a pinch of salt and pepper, and place back in the oven. Bake for 9 to 12 minutes, until whites are set and yolks are slightly thickened. Serve immediately with crusty whole grain bread.

LIGHTEN UP!
This recipe can be made with 4 egg whites instead of whole eggs.

MAKE IT VEGAN!
Simply omit the eggs.

NUTRITIONAL VALUE PER SERVING:
Calories: 245 | Calories from Fat: 53 | Protein: 15 g | Carbs: 32 g | Total Fat: 6 g |
Saturated Fat: 2 g | Trans Fat: 0 g | Fiber: 8 g | Sodium: 486 mg | Cholesterol: 0 mg

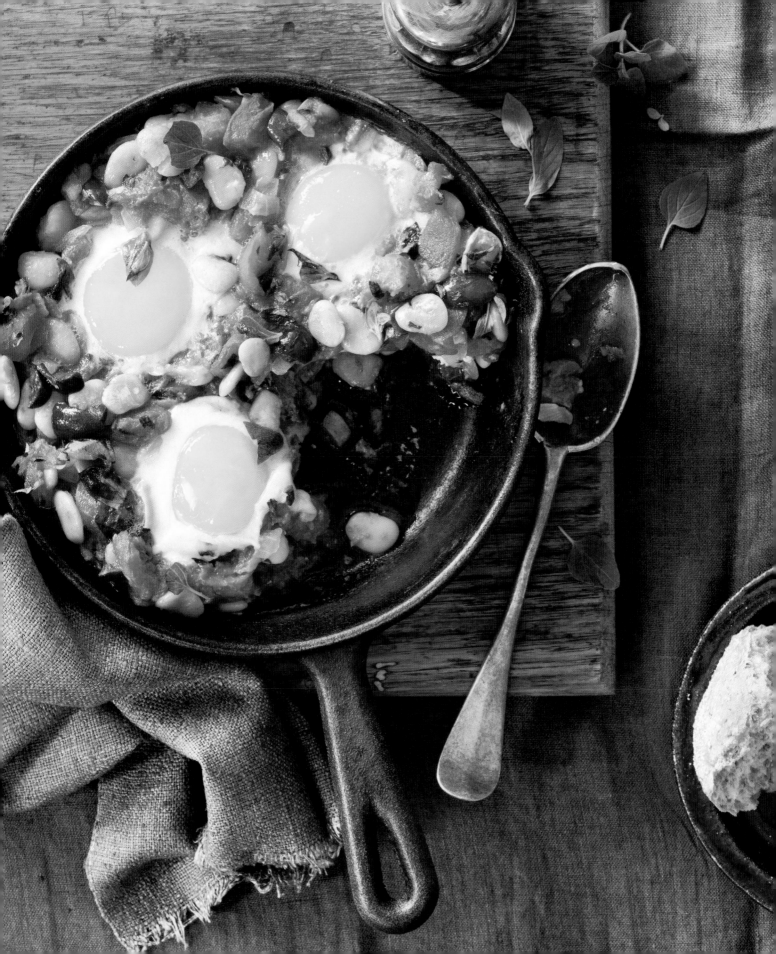

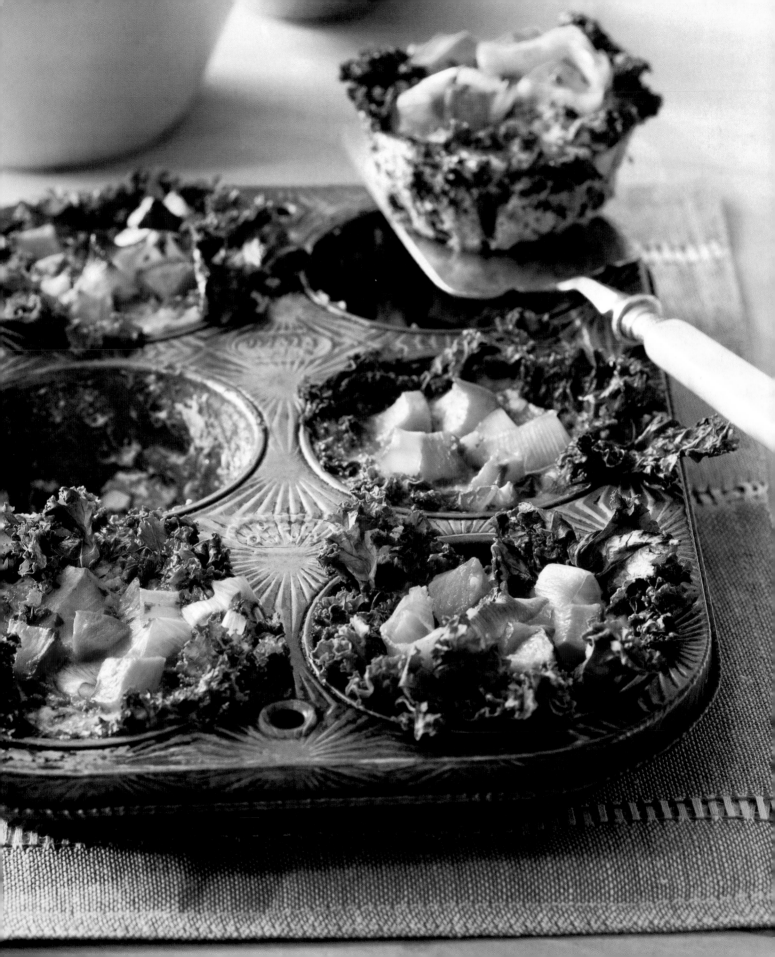

Kale-Wrapped Leek and Sweet Potato Mini Quiches

PREP: 45 minutes | **COOK:** 30 minutes | **YIELD:** 12 mini quiches

Try these for your next brunch or as an hors d'oeuvre at a party. They're adorable, and they're full of kale and sweet potato goodness. They also make a delicious snack!

12 kale leaves, stalk ends trimmed

Eat-Clean Cooking Spray (see p. 277)

1 small or ½ large sweet potato, peeled and diced into ½-inch pieces, about ½ lb (225 g)

1 leek, white and light green parts only, washed well and thinly sliced crosswise

2 tsp (10 ml) extra virgin olive oil

Pinch sea salt and freshly ground black pepper

2 whole eggs + 5 egg whites

2 cups (480 ml) low-fat milk

2 Tbsp (30 ml) Cilantro and Pumpkin Seed Pesto (see p. 52) or any other Clean pesto sauce

Preheat oven to 350°F (175°C). Spread kale leaves in a single layer on two baking sheets and spray with Eat-Clean Cooking Spray. Bake in oven until soft but not crisp, about 10 minutes. Remove from oven, pile kale leaves on one baking sheet and set aside. Increase oven temperature to 400°F (200°C). Add sweet potato and leeks to empty baking sheet. Add olive oil and season with a pinch of salt and pepper. Toss to coat and then spread out in a single layer. Roast in oven until golden brown and soft, stirring once, 15 to 20 minutes.

In a large bowl, whisk together whole eggs and egg whites, milk, pesto and a pinch of salt and pepper.

Line 12 cups of a muffin pan with kale leaves, trimming the stalk ends so kale sticks out no more than 2 inches from the top of the cups. Place muffin pan on a baking sheet and divide leeks and sweet potato among the cups. Pour egg mixture into cups, filling almost to top. Place baking sheet with quiches on it in oven and bake until puffed up and cooked through, about 30 minutes. Remove and allow to cool slightly. Slide a small knife around edges of quiches to loosen them from pan. Gently lift them out while holding onto kale. Transfer to a platter and serve warm or at room temperature.

NUTRITIONAL VALUE PER MINI QUICHE:
Calories: 68 | Calories from Fat: 20 | Protein: 5 g | Carbs: 8 g | Total Fat: 2 g |
Saturated Fat: 0.2 g | Trans Fat: 0 g | Fiber: 0.5 g | Sodium: 53 mg | Cholesterol: 0 mg

Maple Pecan Granola with Raisins

PREP: 15 minutes | **COOK:** 65-70 minutes | **YIELD:** 10 x ½-cup servings

My family goes through this granola so fast I barely get a chance to eat any! It's a definite favorite in my house because it's crunchy, coconutty and just slightly sweet.

WET INGREDIENTS

2 egg whites

⅓ cup (80 ml) pure maple syrup

1 Tbsp (15 ml) Sucanat or other unrefined sugar

½ tsp (2.5 ml) pure vanilla extract

Pinch sea salt

DRY INGREDIENTS

2 cups (480 ml) oats

¼ cup (60 ml) pecan pieces

¼ cup (60 ml) sliced raw almonds

¼ cup (60 ml) raw unsalted sunflower seed kernels

1 Tbsp (15 ml) flaxseed

1 Tbsp (15 ml) sesame seeds

2 Tbsp (30 ml) raw unsweetened coconut flakes

½ cup (120 ml) raisins

Preheat oven to 275°F (135°C).

In a large bowl, whisk together wet ingredients until thoroughly combined. Stir in dry ingredients until mixed well.

Spread mixture out on a baking sheet in a single layer and bake until dry and golden brown, about 60 to 70 minutes, stirring once.

Remove from oven, stir in coconut flakes and raisins, and set aside to cool completely. Store in an airtight container for up to two weeks – if it lasts that long!

TRY THIS!

This granola can be eaten alone as a snack, or it can be mixed with milk, milk substitute, low-fat yogurt or kefir to make a complete breakfast.

MAKE IT GLUTEN FREE!

Just make sure to choose uncontaminated oats.

NUTRITIONAL VALUE PER SERVING:
Calories: 173 | Calories from Fat: 65 | Protein: 5 g | Carbs: 23 g | Total Fat: 7 g | Saturated Fat: 0.6 g | Trans Fat: 0 g | Fiber: 3 g | Sodium: 17 mg | Cholesterol: 0 mg

Triple Berry Barley Crunch

PREP: 15 minutes | **COOK:** 50-60 minutes | **YIELD:** 8 x ¾-cup servings

At first, barley was an ingredient I used sporadically in the kitchen, but after trying this yummy recipe, I quickly changed my ways. This dish is extremely nutritious, and the sweet, tangy taste of berries is sure to balance out the crunch and brighten your day!

⅓ cup (80 ml) pure maple syrup

¼ cup (60 ml) plain or vanilla-flavored protein powder (as natural as possible, vegan if desired)

1 tsp (5 ml) pure vanilla extract (omit if using vanilla protein powder)

Pinch sea salt

2½ cups (600 ml) flaked barley

¼ cup (60 ml) oat bran

1 cup (240 ml) raw walnut halves and pieces

1 Tbsp (15 ml) chia seeds

1 Tbsp (15 ml) sesame seeds

½ cup (120 ml) unsweetened and unsulfured dried strawberries

½ cup (120 ml) unsweetened and unsulfured dried blueberries

¼ cup (60 ml) Ningxia goji berries (see tip at right)

Preheat oven to 275°F (120°C). In a large bowl, stir together maple syrup, protein powder, vanilla extract and sea salt until thoroughly combined. Stir in flaked barley, oat bran, walnuts, chia and sesame seeds until mixed well.

Spread out in a single layer on a baking sheet and bake, stirring halfway through, until golden brown and dry, 50 to 60 minutes. Remove from oven and stir in dried strawberries, blueberries and goji berries. Serve with low-fat milk, plain unsweetened soymilk or other milk substitute, plain low-fat kefir or soy yogurt. Can be stored in an airtight container for up to two weeks.

TOSCA'S TIP
Can't find Ningxia goji berries? Use regular goji berries, or if you can't find those, add ¼ cup dried cranberries or extra dried strawberries and blueberries instead!

NUTRITIONAL VALUE PER SERVING:
Calories: 439 | Calories from Fat: 106 | Protein: 12 g | Carbs: 74 g | Total Fat: 12 g | Saturated Fat: 1.3 g | Trans Fat: 0 g | Fiber: 13 g | Sodium: 28 mg | Cholesterol: 0 mg

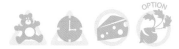

Blueberry and Citrus Breakfast Parfait

PREP: 15 minutes | **COOK:** 0 minutes | **YIELD:** 4 parfaits

Parfaits are a simple yet visually pleasing breakfast option. Best of all, you can pack them full of your favorite fruits. Here we've added tangy citrus and antioxidant-loaded blueberries to a crunchy walnut, flax and wheat germ mix. Top it with some yogurt and you will definitely be starting your day off right!

3 cups (710 ml) plain nonfat all-natural Greek
    yogurt or strained plain soy yogurt

1 Tbsp (15 ml) pure maple syrup

½ tsp (2.5 ml) pure vanilla extract

½ cup (120 ml) walnuts, chopped

2 Tbsp (30 ml) wheat germ

2 Tbsp (30 ml) cracked flaxseed

1 red grapefruit, peeled and cut into small slices

1 minneola, peeled and cut into small slices

1 cup (240 ml) fresh blueberries

Stir together the yogurt, maple syrup and vanilla.

In four parfait glasses, pour in some of the yogurt mixture. Then sprinkle in some of the walnuts, wheat germ and flaxseeds, and then add some of the grapefruit, minneola and blueberries.

Repeat the layering process until all of the ingredients are used.

ON THE GO

Assemble this in portable containers instead of parfait glasses and you can have a gourmet and good-for-you dish that goes anywhere!

NUTRITIONAL VALUE PER PARFAIT:
Calories: 305 | Calories from Fat: 110 | Protein: 20 g | Carbs: 33 g | Total Fat: 12 g |
Saturated Fat: 1 g | Trans Fat: 0 g | Fiber: 7 g | Sodium: 51 mg | Cholesterol: 0 mg

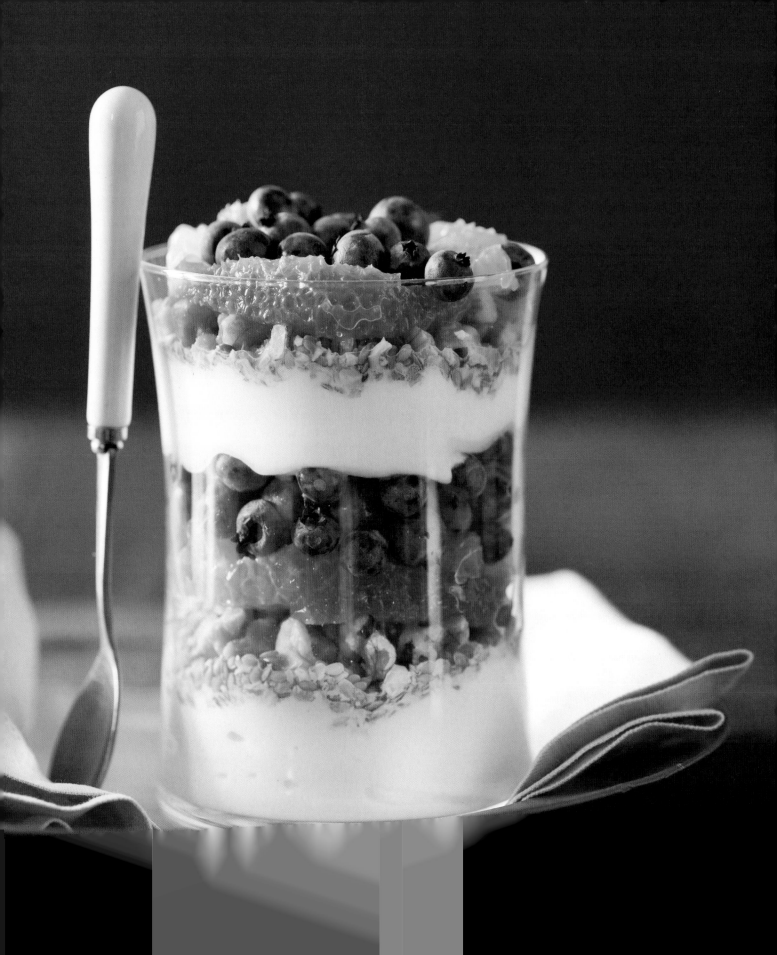

Suit Yourself!

Vegetarians have come a long way, baby. For the most part, they're no longer forced to order from the "sides" section of the menu, endure hemp-wearing-hippy assumptions or repeatedly assure pity-faced people that, no, they really don't miss meat. Also, as meatless becomes more and more mainstream (Martha and Oprah have devoted entire episodes to the pleasures of veganism), the available options, flavors and opportunities grow – and everyone wins!

Are you feeling the veggie love? Don't worry if you're not quite ready to relinquish all animal products. Choosing to follow a vegetarian or vegan lifestyle is a very personal decision and your reasons are all your own. It can also be a challenging decision to make, but don't feel like you've got to go all or nothing. Check out this list of the most popular vegetarian options to find one that works for you and includes everything you need to be healthy, happy and well fed. You will soon discover how easy it is to choose a lifestyle that fits, well, your life!

True Vegetarian Options

Vegan

This lifestyle eliminates all animal products including red meat, fish, poultry, eggs, dairy products, gelatins and even honey. Vegans often choose not to wear or use animal products such as leather, fur, wool, silk, bone china and beeswax.

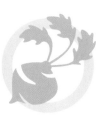

Lacto-Ovo Vegetarian

These vegetarians choose to keep dairy products and eggs in their diet (lacto means milk and ovo means eggs). Choosing to be a vegetarian of this nature gives you a lot of flexibility. You can enjoy yogurt, cheese, cottage cheese and more while also using eggs as a source of complete protein.

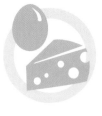

Ovo Vegetarian

These vegetarians are often called "eggetarians." Ovo vegetarians keep eggs in their diet, but unlike their lacto-ovo counterparts, they choose to keep all dairy products off the menu. The complete protein, vitamins, minerals and healthy fats present in the eggs is an easy and convenient way of helping them maintain a strong and healthy physique.

Lacto Vegetarian

What would a vegetarian diet be without variety? I'm sure you can figure out what lacto vegetarians keep in their diet: dairy products. You won't find any eggs, fish or chicken on their menus.

Semi-Vegetarian Options

Flexitarian

Also known as semi-vegetarianism, this is the most lax of the vegetarian diets. The flexitarian is mainly vegetarian, but chooses to eat meat, fish or poultry on occasion.

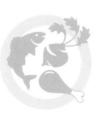

Pollotarian

Chicken, turkey and other poultry fit the bill as the meats of choice for pollotarians. They do not eat red meat, fish or other seafood. I have often heard this is one of the best types of semi-vegetarian to be. You can effortlessly get enough easily digestible protein without relying on meat products to be the center of every meal.

Pescatarian

Pescatarians choose to keep fish and seafood products in their diets. The rich flavors of tuna, salmon and sea bass keep them satisfied and well nourished with their abundant healthy fats and lean protein. Typically, pescatarians also choose to eat eggs and dairy products. Please see the profile of Jill Holland, *Eat-Clean Diet*® Ambassador and resident semi-vegetarian bodybuilder on p. 162 to learn more about this kind of diet.

Pollo-Pescatarian

Guess what? You can even be a pollo-pescatarian and keep both poultry and fish products in your diet!

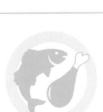

Meatless Done Right

When selecting the vegetarian diet that is right for you, remember to consider your health. I have highlighted some key things to consider in "Vegetarianism and Health" on p. 274. Please take a look at this information so you can make a well-informed decision.

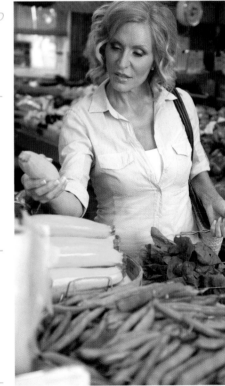

Snack
Break

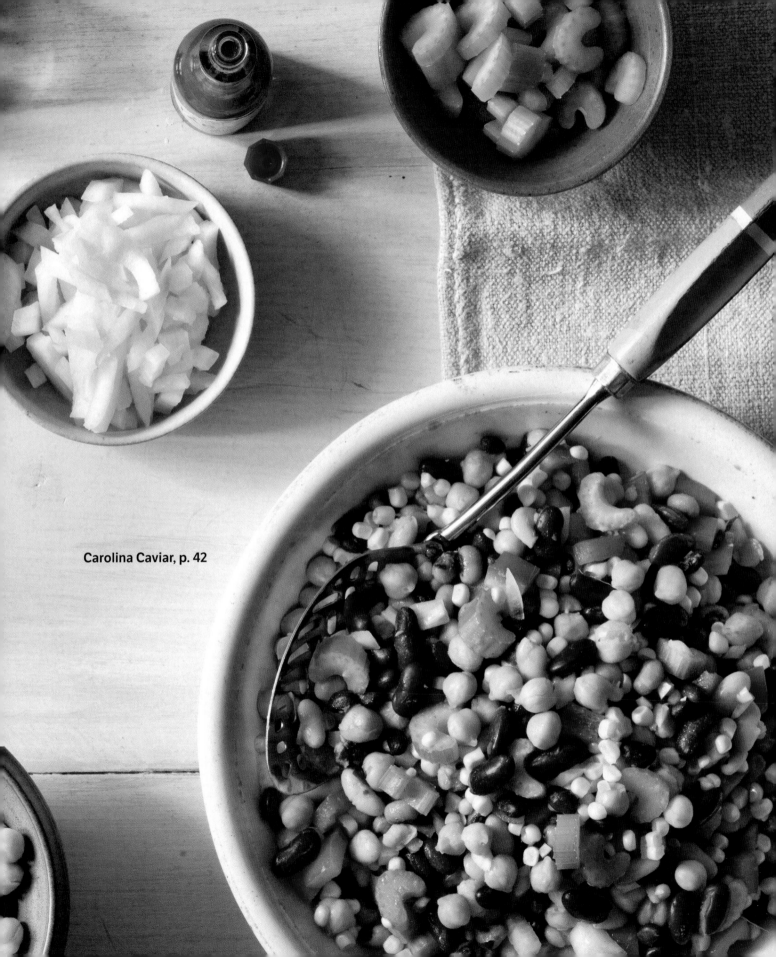

Carolina Caviar, p. 42

Carolina Caviar

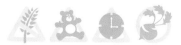

PREP: 20 minutes active, 1 hour inactive (optional) | **COOK:** 0 minutes | **YIELD:** 24 x ½-cup servings

This is the perfect potluck dish! Serve it as a dip alongside a batch of Bring the Heat Baked Blue Corn Chips (see p. 65). Yum!

2 cups (480 ml) frozen sweet yellow corn

2 cups cooked, drained and rinsed or 1 x 15-oz (440 ml) BPA-free can each no-salt-added red kidney beans, black-eyed peas, chickpeas, white kidney beans and black beans, drained and rinsed well

1 red bell pepper, seeded and diced into ½-inch pieces

3 ribs celery, diced into ½-inch pieces

½ white onion, diced into ¼-inch pieces

1 clove garlic

¾ tsp (3.75 ml) sea salt, divided

1 Tbsp (15 ml) extra virgin olive oil

3 Tbsp (45 ml) red wine vinegar

3 Tbsp (45 ml) aged sherry vinegar

1 Tbsp (15 ml) pure maple syrup

1 tsp (5 ml) hot sauce, such as Tabasco, or more to taste

½ tsp (2.5 ml) freshly ground black pepper

Place frozen corn in a bowl and cover with hot water to thaw. Drain and transfer to a large bowl. Add all of the beans, red bell pepper, celery and onion.

Mince garlic and then sprinkle it with ¼ tsp (1.25 ml) of sea salt. Using the side of a chef's knife, work salt into garlic and press it into a paste. Scrape garlic paste into a small bowl. Add remaining ½ tsp (2.5 ml) salt, olive oil, red wine vinegar, sherry vinegar, maple syrup, hot sauce and black pepper, and whisk to combine. Pour over beans and veggies and toss to coat. Refrigerate for about 1 hour to intensify flavors, if possible.

CHILL OUT
Will keep in the refrigerator for up to three days.

NUTRITIONAL VALUE PER SERVING:
Calories: 202 | Calories from Fat: 23 | Protein: 11 g | Carbs: 35 g | Total Fat: 3 g |
Saturated Fat: 0.3 g | Trans Fat: 0 g | Fiber: 10 g | Sodium: 41 mg | Cholesterol: 5 mg

Honey Nut Granola Bars

PREP: 15 minutes | **COOK:** 90 minutes | **YIELD:** 12 bars

Granola bars are the perfect portable option for on-the-go *Eat-Clean Diet*® followers. This hearty and delicious honey and nut version is perfect for tiding you over during a hike or while doing errands. Best of all, your kids will love them!

WET INGREDIENTS

¼ cup (60 ml) honey

¼ cup (60 ml) Sucanat or other unrefined sugar

2 Tbsp (30 ml) natural nut butter, such as
     almond, peanut or cashew

2 egg whites

½ tsp (2.5 ml) pure vanilla

½ tsp (2.5 ml) ground cinnamon

¼ tsp (1.25 ml) sea salt

DRY INGREDIENTS

2½ cups (600 ml) old-fashioned rolled oats

½ cup (120 ml) raw almonds, coarsely chopped

¼ cup (60 ml) shelled hemp seeds

Preheat oven to 275°F (135°C). Line a 9 x 9-inch baking pan with parchment paper, allowing a little extra to hang out two of the sides. This will make it easier to lift bars out of the pan.

In a large bowl, whisk together wet ingredients until combined. Stir in dry ingredients until mixed well. Scrape mixture into prepared baking pan and spread it out to the edges, pressing the top down very firmly to compact the mixture. Bake on middle oven rack for about 1 hour, then remove. Holding onto extra parchment, carefully lift partially cooked oat mixture out of pan and place on a cutting board. Using a large chef's knife, cut oat mixture into 12 bars. Mixture should be firm enough to hold its shape, but soft enough to cut.

Holding onto edges of parchment, carefully transfer bars to a baking sheet. Separate bars so heat can get in between each one, and place them back in oven to bake for another 30 to 45 minutes or until they're golden brown and firm (bars will continue to harden and get crunchier as they cool). Remove from oven and let cool to room temperature.

KEEP IT FRESH
Store in an airtight container for up to two weeks. These bars make great portable snacks!

MAKE IT GLUTEN FREE!
Just make sure to choose uncontaminated oats.

NUTRITIONAL VALUE PER BAR:
Calories: 154 | Calories from Fat: 55 | Protein: 6 g | Carbs: 19 g | Total Fat: 6 g | Saturated Fat: 0.5 g | Trans Fat: 0 g | Fiber: 3 g | Sodium: 23 mg | Cholesterol: 0 mg

Smoky Eggplant and Chickpea Spread

PREP TIME: 10 minutes | **COOK TIME:** 30-35 minutes | **YIELD:** 4½ cups (18 x ¼-cup servings)

Spreads can be used in any number of ways – on vegetables, crackers, sandwiches and more. When choosing your spread, be careful! Many are loaded with processed ingredients and harmful fats. Just say no to those guys and say yes to this delicious homemade spread, which is jam-packed with all the good stuff.

1 x 1½ to 2 lb (680 g to 908 g) eggplant

1 x 15-oz (440 ml) BPA-free can no-salt-added chickpeas, drained and rinsed

½ cup (120 ml) tahini, stirred well

¼ cup (60 ml) fresh lemon juice

2 Tbsp (30 ml) extra virgin olive oil

2 Tbsp (30 ml) water

1 clove garlic, chopped

1 tsp (5 ml) ground cumin

¼ tsp (1.25 ml) ground fresh chili paste, or more to taste

1 handful fresh parsley

¾ tsp (3.75 ml) sea salt

Pinch freshly ground black pepper

Preheat oven to 400°F (200°C). Heat a grill or grill pan to high.

Using a fork, poke eggplant five or six times so it won't explode when it cooks. Place eggplant on grill and cook, turning a few times, until skin is charred well, about 10 to 15 minutes. Transfer eggplant to a baking sheet to finish cooking in oven until very soft when pierced with a skewer, about 20 minutes. Remove eggplant and allow it to sit at room temperature until cool enough to handle. Peel away skin and discard.

Cut peeled eggplant into pieces so it will fit into a food processor or blender. Add chickpeas along with remaining ingredients and blend until smooth. If too thick, add water 1 Tbsp (15 ml) at a time, until mixture reaches desired consistency. Taste, and make any adjustments to seasoning with lemon juice, salt and pepper.

NUTRITIONAL VALUE PER SERVING:
Calories: 88 | Calories from Fat: 51 | Protein: 3 g | Carbs: 7 g | Total Fat: 6 g |
Saturated Fat: 1 g | Trans Fat: 0 g | Fiber: 3 g | Sodium: 8 mg | Cholesterol: 0 mg

THE EAT-CLEAN DIET VEGETARIAN COOKBOOK

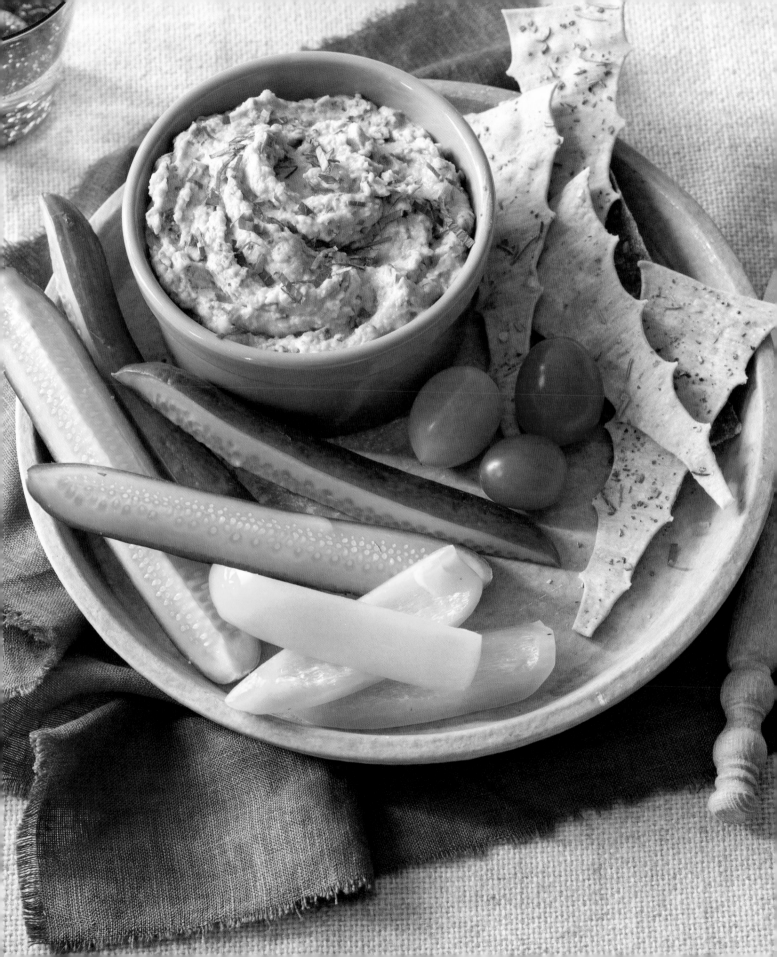

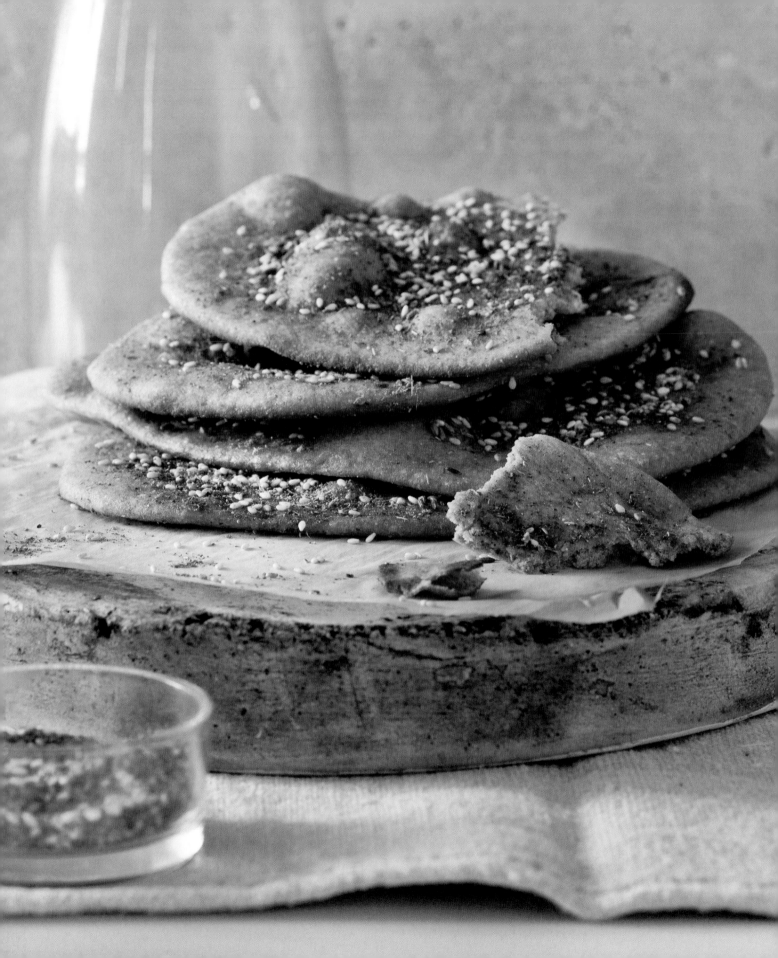

Flatbread with Za'atar and Sesame Seeds

PREP: 10 minutes | **COOK:** 11-14 minutes | **YIELD:** 4 x 6-inch flatbreads

When I discovered za'atar, I couldn't get enough of it! It is an absolutely incredible combination of spices that works perfectly as a pick-me-up for simple flatbread. Don't hesitate to try it in hummus, too. This might just be your next favorite spice!

1 lb (454 g) whole wheat pizza dough (store bought or see p. 277)

2 tsp (10 ml) extra virgin olive oil

4 tsp (20 ml) za'atar (see tip at right)

2 tsp (10 ml) sesame seeds

1 tsp (5 ml) cumin seeds, crushed in a mortar and pestle or spice grinder or 1 tsp (5 ml) ground cumin

Pinch each sea salt and freshly ground black pepper

Place rack in lower third of oven and preheat to 425°F (215°C).

Divide dough into four equal balls. Roll each ball out into a six-inch circle and place on a baking sheet. Brush each circle of dough with ½ tsp (2.5 ml) olive oil, and top with 1 tsp (5 ml) za'atar and ½ tsp (2.5 ml) sesame seeds. Sprinkle ¼ tsp (1.25 ml) crushed cumin seeds on top of each circle of dough and season with a small pinch of salt and pepper.

Bake until edges and bottom of flatbreads are golden brown, 11 to 14 minutes.

TOSCA'S TIP

Za'atar is a Middle Eastern spice blend usually containing sumac, ground dried thyme, sesame seeds and salt. It can also contain cumin, chilies and other ingredients, depending on the region it is from. If you aren't able to find za'atar, you can approximate the flavor by combining paprika, lemon pepper, dried ground thyme, ground dried sumac, sesame seeds and a pinch of sea salt.

NUTRITIONAL VALUE PER FLATBREAD:
Calories: 231 | Calories from Fat: 26 | Protein: 7 g | Carbs: 37 g | Total Fat: 2 g |
Saturated Fat: 0.4 g | Trans Fat: 0 g | Fiber: 2 g | Sodium: 256 mg | Cholesterol: 0 mg

Bruschetta with Tomato and Avocado

PREP: 15 minutes | **COOK:** 5-10 minutes | **YIELD:** 2½ cups tomato and avocado mixture

At my house, bruschetta is a definite family favorite. We love the contrasting textures of the juicy tomatoes and crispy bread. This recipe also includes some velvety avocado for a more well-rounded nutrient load.

1 whole grain French baguette, sliced into
　　½-inch diagonal slices
1 lb (454 g) tomatoes, cored and diced
1 tsp (5 ml) extra virgin olive oil
1 Tbsp (15 ml) fresh lemon juice
1 clove garlic, minced
¼ cup (60 ml) fresh basil leaves, thinly sliced
¼ tsp (1.25 ml) each sea salt and freshly ground
　　black pepper
1 avocado, pitted and diced
Lemon zest, to garnish

Heat oven to 350°F (175°C). Place baguette slices on a baking sheet and toast in oven until golden brown and slightly crisp, about 5 to 10 minutes. Remove and transfer to a platter.

Combine tomatoes and remaining ingredients, except avocado, and mix well. Add avocado and gently mix in. Top toasted baguette slices with tomato and avocado mixture. Garnish each with lemon zest and serve.

TOSCA'S TIP
The healthy fats in the avocado will satisfy your hunger and keep you from snacking on anything less than nutritious.

NUTRITIONAL VALUE PER SERVING (1 SLICE BAGUETTE + 2 TBSP TOMATO-AVOCADO MIXTURE):
Calories: 49 | Calories from Fat: 14 | Protein: 2 g | Carbs: 8 g | Total Fat: 2 g |
Saturated Fat: 0.2 g | Trans Fat: 0 g | Fiber: 1.3 g | Sodium: 76 mg | Cholesterol: 0 mg

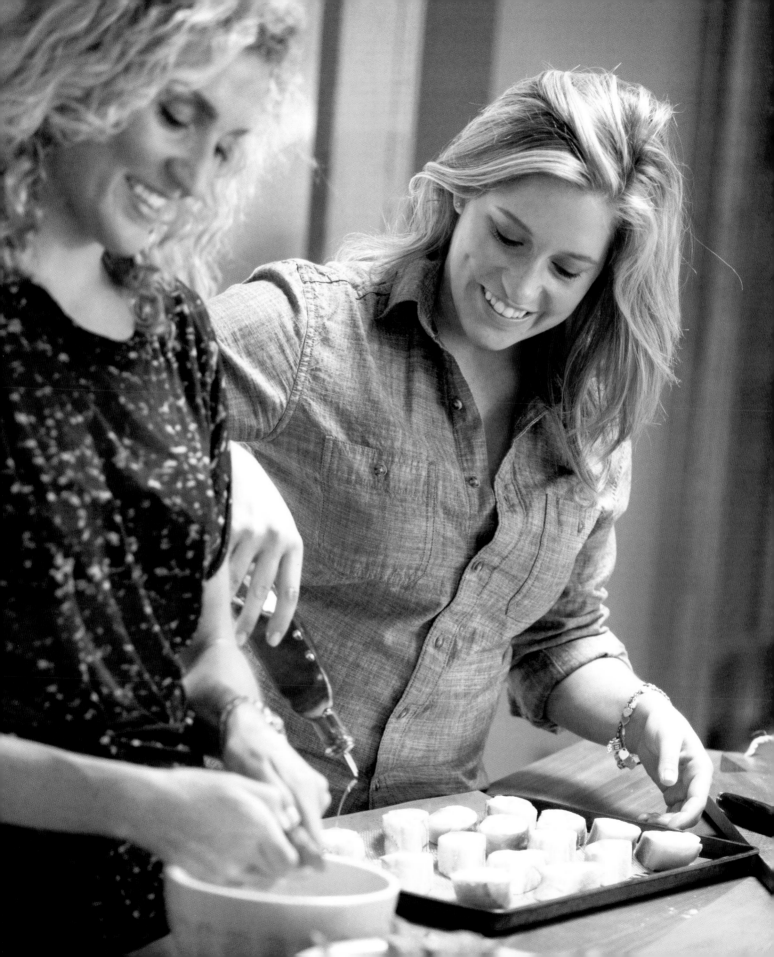

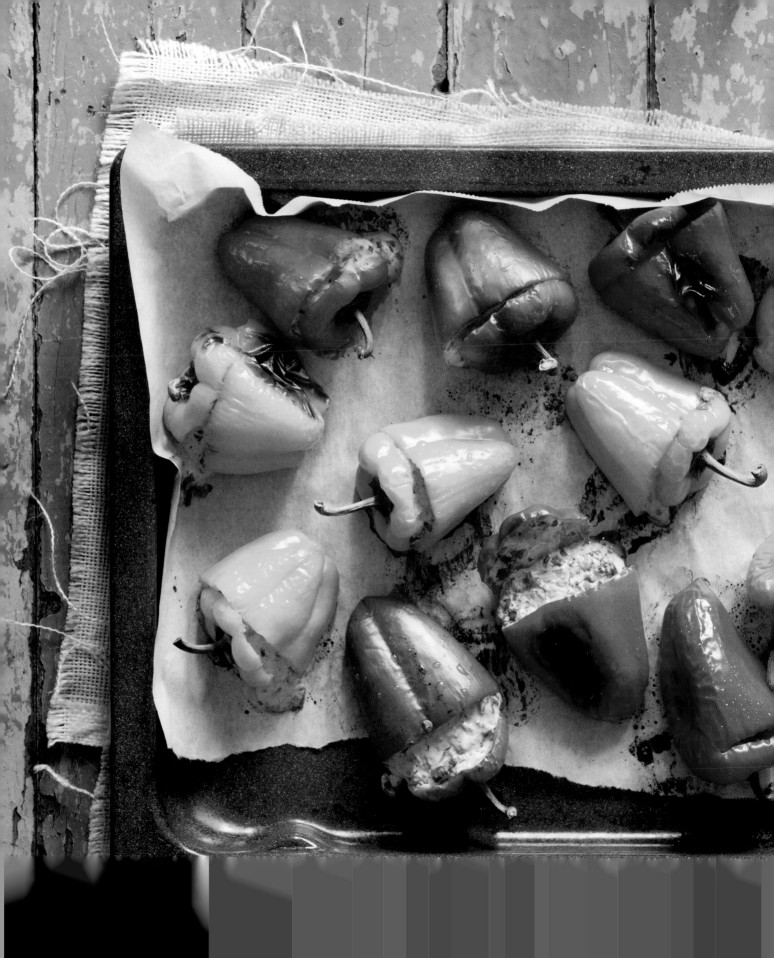

Baked Mini Pepper Poppers

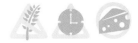

PREP: 20 minutes | **COOK:** 15 minutes | **YIELD:** About 30 stuffed peppers

This is my Eat-Clean version of jalapeño poppers, cleaned up by skipping the breading, using low-fat yogurt cheese and baking them instead of frying. They're a big hit at parties and no one misses the extra fat and calories!

2 cups (480 ml) Yogurt Cheese*, drained well (see p. 276)

1 large handful cilantro

2 chipotle peppers in adobo

2 tsp (10 ml) chopped shallots

Pinch sea salt and freshly ground black pepper

1½ lbs (680 g) sweet mini peppers (about 30 peppers)

Preheat oven to 400°F (200° C).

In a food processor, combine Yogurt Cheese, cilantro, chipotle peppers, shallots, salt and pepper. Whirl until blended and smooth. Pour into a food-grade squeeze bottle or pastry bag fitted with a tip. If you don't have either of these tools, see tip below.

Using a small sharp knife, make a slit crosswise at the top of pepper to create a "hinge," keeping stem intact. Open the top, or "lid," of pepper and remove any seeds. Fill pepper with yogurt cheese mixture and place on a baking sheet. Repeat until all peppers are filled. Place peppers close to one another on baking sheet and bake for about 15 minutes or until cheese is heated through and peppers are tender, but still slightly crisp. Serve warm.

> **NOTE**
> *Yogurt Cheese must be made ahead of time. For this recipe you will want it very thick.
>
> **EQUIPMENT TIP**
> If you don't have a pastry bag, just put the yogurt cheese mixture into a sealable plastic bag and fasten shut. With scissors, cut a hole in one corner so that you can squeeze the yogurt cheese into the peppers.

NUTRITIONAL VALUE PER SERVING (2 PEPPERS):
Calories: 46 | Calories from Fat: 4 | Protein: 4 g | Carbs: 6 g | Total Fat: 0.5 g |
Saturated Fat: 0.5 g | Trans Fat: 0 g | Fiber: 2 g | Sodium: 15 mg | Cholesterol: 2 mg

Cilantro and Pumpkin Seed Pesto

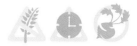

PREP: 10 minutes | **COOK:** 0 minutes | **YIELD:** 1 cup

This versatile sauce can be used in a variety of ways and can be made out of any number of ingredient combinations. I've branched out to combine cilantro (one of my favorite herbs) with pumpkin seeds (which are seriously wholesome!) for a taste that is zesty and refreshing.

1 bunch cilantro, including stems,
    washed and spun or patted dry
1 clove garlic
¼ cup (60 ml) raw shelled pumpkin seeds
    (pepitas)
1 lemon, zested and juiced
¼ tsp (1.25 ml) each sea salt and freshly
    ground black pepper
2 Tbsp (30 ml) extra virgin olive oil

Add all ingredients except olive oil to a food processor and pulse-blend until chopped. While processor is running, slowly stream in olive oil and let processor run until pesto comes together. Stop processor and scrape down sides. Let processor whirl for another minute until pesto is blended well. Pesto will be thick. If you prefer it thinner, you can add a little vegetable broth or more lemon juice until it reaches desired consistency.

TRY THIS!

This pesto tastes great tossed with whole grain pasta or steamed vegetables, but you can also use it instead of (or in addtion to!) tomato sauce when making your own pizza.

NUTRITIONAL VALUE PER 1-TBSP SERVING:
Calories: 26 | Calories from Fat: 17 | Protein: 1 g | Carbs: 1 g | Total Fat: 2 g |
Saturated Fat: 0.3 g | Trans Fat: 0 g | Fiber: 0.4 g | Sodium: 21 mg | Cholesterol: 0 mg

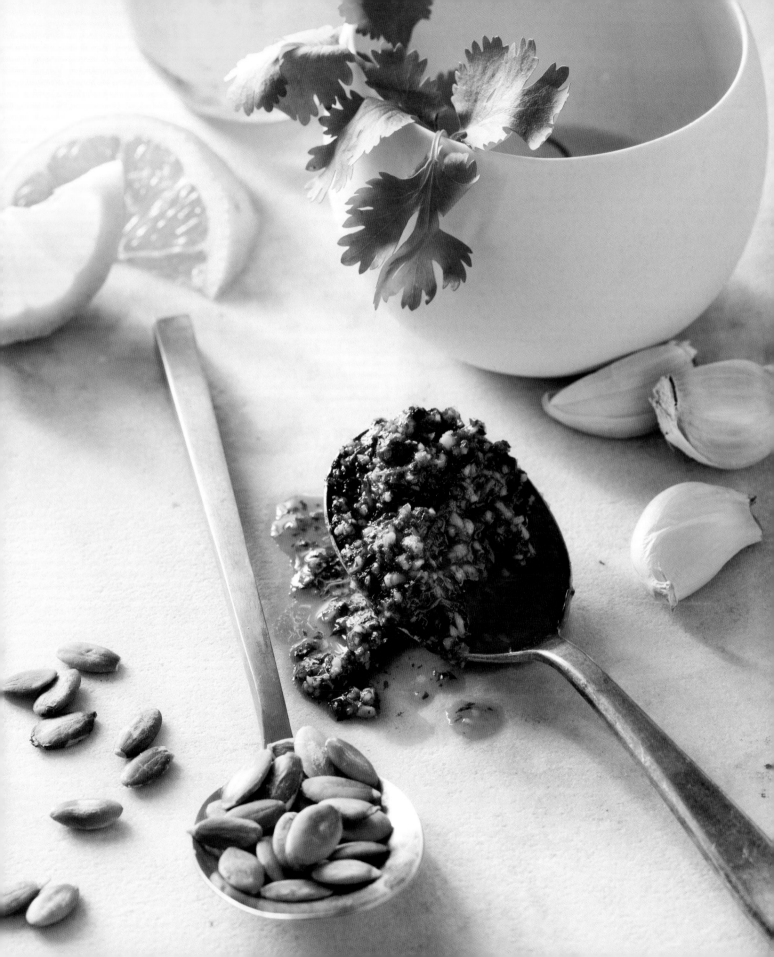

Artichoke and Roasted Red Pepper Tapenade

PREP: 10 minutes | **COOK:** 0 minutes | **YIELD:** 2 cups

It's a dip! It's a spread! It's also my daughter Rachel's favorite food. Whenever I serve it at family gatherings, she gobbles it right up. This recipe is her new favorite because it boasts artichoke hearts, which she loves. Now I really won't be able to keep it on the table!

1 x 14-oz (420 ml) BPA-free can artichoke hearts,
    drained and liquid pressed out

8 oz (225 g) roasted red bell peppers,
    about 1 cup (240 ml), drained and
    liquid pressed out

1 clove garlic

1 small or ½ large lemon, zested and juiced

1 Tbsp (15 ml) capers, drained and rinsed

Small handful fresh cilantro

Small handful fresh basil leaves

1 Tbsp (15 ml) extra virgin olive oil

¼ tsp (1.25 ml) each sea salt and freshly ground
    black pepper

Add all ingredients to a food processor and pulse-blend until chopped. Scrape down sides, and then let food processor whirl until the mix is well blended but still chunky. Scrape into a bowl and serve with raw cut vegetables, rice crackers or toasted whole wheat baguette slices, or use it as a tasty spread for sandwiches.

NUTRITIONAL VALUE PER 2-TBSP SERVINGS:
Calories: 12 | Calories from Fat: 4 | Protein: 0.1 g | Carbs: 1 g | Total Fat: 0.4 g |
Saturated Fat: 0.1 g | Trans Fat: 0 g | Fiber: 0.3 g | Sodium: 42 mg | Cholesterol: 0 mg

Sea Crunchie Snack Mix

PREP: 5 minutes | **COOK:** 25 minutes | **YIELD:** 8 x ½-cup servings

Sea palm is a variety of kelp also known as postelsia. It is found primarily on the western shores of North America. It is completely edible and serves as a delicious addition to spice up this snack mix.

1 cup (240 ml) raw almonds

2 tsp (10 ml) low-sodium tamari

Dash Worcestershire sauce, regular or vegan

Pinch Sucanat or other unrefined sugar

¾ oz (22 ml) dried raw sea palm, broken into 1- to 2-inch pieces, about 1 cup (240 ml)

½ cup (120 ml) dried unsulfured apricots, halved or quartered if large

½ cup (120 ml) prunes, halved or quartered if large

Preheat the oven to 250°F (120°C).

Place almonds on a baking sheet and add tamari, Worcestershire and Sucanat. Toss to coat, and then spread out in a single layer. Bake for about 25 minutes, stirring a few times. Transfer to a sealable container. Add sea palm, apricots and prunes and stir to combine.

KEEP IT FRESH
Snack mix will keep for up to two weeks in a sealed container.

NUTRITIONAL VALUE PER SERVING:
Calories: 145 | Calories from Fat: 63 | Protein: 4 g | Carbs: 17 g | Total Fat: 7 g | Saturated Fat: 0.5 g | Trans Fat: 0 g | Fiber: 3 g | Sodium: 152 mg | Cholesterol: 0 mg

Sun-Dried Tomato Olive Tapenade

PREP: 5 minutes | **COOK:** 0 minutes | **YIELD:** ¾ cup

I love the salty yet smooth bite of tapenade on a cracker. Delicious! In this version, we've raised the bar by adding sun-dried tomatoes and basil to the mix. It's refreshingly tasty and perfect for your next antipasto platter.

½ cup (120 ml) pitted kalamata olives

½ cup (120 ml) sun-dried tomatoes in extra virgin olive oil, drained

½ cup (120 ml) basil, lightly packed

1 clove garlic, chopped

½ tsp (2.5 ml) lemon juice

Pinch freshly ground black pepper

Add all ingredients to a food processor and pulse chop until blended but still chunky.

TRY THIS!
This tapenade is delicious on crackers, tossed with hot pasta, added to a salad or as a spread on sandwiches (try it on my Mediterranean Panini, see p. 207).

NUTRITIONAL VALUE PER 1-TBSP SERVING:
Calories: 22 | Calories from Fat: 13 | Protein: 0.5 g | Carbs: 1 g | Total Fat: 1 g | Saturated Fat: <0.1 g | Trans Fat: 0 g | Fiber: 0.1 g | Sodium: 60 mg | Cholesterol: 0 mg

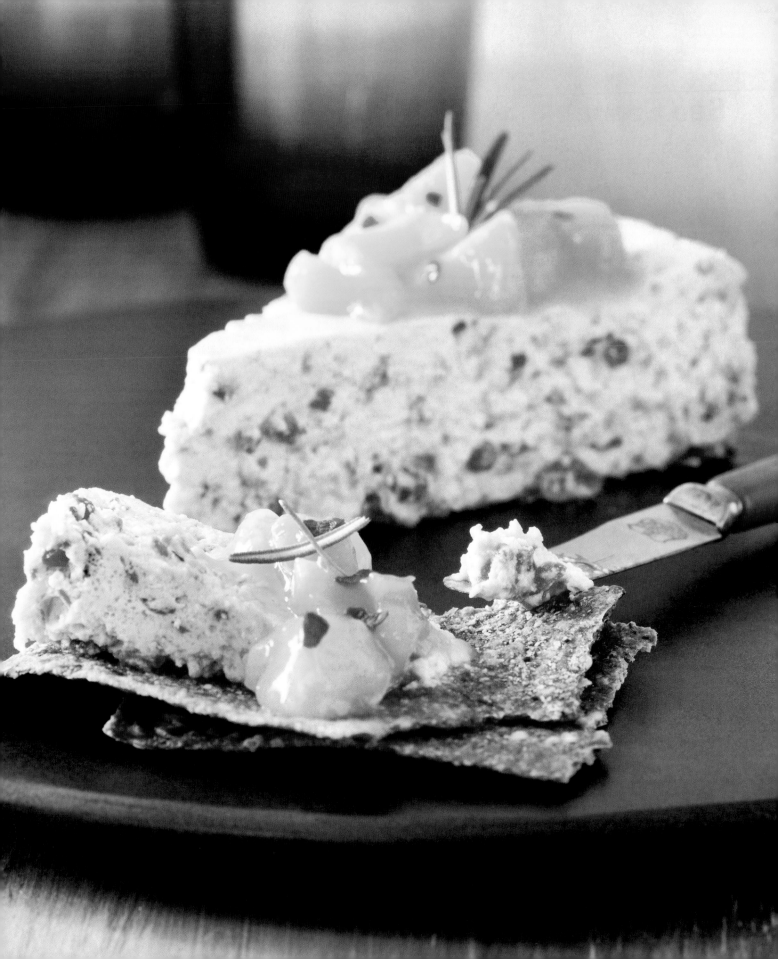

Red Pepper Cheesecake with Apricot Peach Compote

PREP: 15 minutes | **COOK:** 60 minutes | **YIELD:** 12 slices

Don't be confused by the word "cheesecake" – this savory dish actually makes a delicious appetizer or side dish! Made with yogurt, tofu and egg whites, it's high in protein, yet very low in fat. Bonus: It features a sweet and spicy topping that will send your taste buds on a roller-coaster ride.

2 cups (480 ml) low-fat Yogurt Cheese*
    (see p. 276)
2 x 12-oz (340 g) packages silken firm tofu,
    drained
2 egg whites
1 Tbsp (15 ml) lemon zest
Pinch sea salt
1 cup (240 ml) roasted red peppers, drained
    and liquid squeezed out, cut into thin strips
½ cup (120 ml) frozen peach slices,
    thawed slightly
½ cup (120 ml) dried apricots
½ cup (120 ml) orange juice
1 tsp (5 ml) orange zest
1 tsp (5 ml) arrowroot powder
1 tsp (5 ml) pure honey
Pinch red pepper flakes or ¼ tsp (1.25 ml)
    fresh chili paste

Preheat oven to 325°F (160°C).

In a food processor, blend Yogurt Cheese, tofu, egg whites, lemon zest and salt until smooth. Add red peppers and pulse-blend a few times until they are mixed in. Pour mixture into a 9-inch springform pan and bake on middle oven rack until edges are golden and center jiggles slightly when pan is shaken gently, about 60 minutes. Cake will firm up as it chills. Transfer cake to a wire rack to cool for about 1 hour.

While cheesecake cools, in a clean food processor, pulse-chop peaches and apricots into small chunks. Transfer to a small saucepan and stir in orange juice and zest, arrowroot powder, honey and red pepper flakes. Bring to a simmer and stir over low heat for about 2 minutes or until slightly thickened. Remove from heat and transfer to a small bowl. Can be served at room temperature or chilled.

To serve cheesecake, remove outer ring of springform pan, keep cake on bottom of pan, and transfer to a platter. Cut slices, top with a little Peach Apricot Compote and serve with baked whole grain pita chips or whole grain crackers.

NOTE
*Yogurt Cheese must be made ahead of time.

MAKE AHEAD
Cheesecake and Peach Apricot Compote can be made up to three days ahead of time and stored in the refrigerator until ready to serve.

NUTRITIONAL VALUE PER SLICE (¹⁄₁₂ OF CHEESECAKE):
Calories: 81 | Calories from Fat: 12 | Protein: 7 g | Carbs: 10 g | Total Fat: 2 g |
Saturated Fat: 1 g | Trans Fat: 0 g | Fiber: 0.4 g | Sodium: 97 mg | Cholesterol: 2 mg

Dried Fruit and Nut Bars

PREP: 20 minutes | **COOK:** 30 minutes | **YIELD:** 16 x 2-inch squares

This bar recipe is very flexible, as long as you keep the proportions the same. Feel free to make it your own by changing up the dried fruits and nuts to suit your tastes.

½ cup (120 ml) whole oat flour

2 Tbsp (30 ml) oat bran

2 Tbsp (30 ml) Sucanat or other unrefined sugar

¼ tsp (1.25 ml) baking soda

¼ tsp (1.25 ml) baking powder

¼ tsp (1.25 ml) ground cinnamon

Pinch freshly grated nutmeg

¼ tsp (1.25 ml) sea salt

2 Tbsp (30 ml) flaxseed

¼ cup (60 ml) hulled hemp seeds

1½ cups (360 ml) combination almonds, walnuts and pecans, coarsely chopped

½ cup (120 ml) dried cranberries

½ cup (120 ml) dried blueberries

½ cup (120 ml) dried cherries

½ cup (120 ml) dried dates or prunes, coarsely chopped

½ cup (120 ml) dried apricots, coarsely chopped

½ cup (120 ml) dried pears or apples, coarsely chopped

1 whole egg + 2 egg whites

½ tsp (2.5 ml) vanilla extract

Preheat the oven to 325ºF (160ºC). Line an 8 x 8-inch square baking pan with parchment paper, allowing a little extra to hang out the two opposite sides.

In a large bowl, whisk together flour, oat bran, Sucanat, baking soda, baking powder, cinnamon, nutmeg and salt. Stir in flaxseed, hemp seeds, almonds, walnuts, pecans and dried fruit, and mix well.

In a separate bowl, beat whole egg, egg whites and vanilla extract until thick and foamy. Add to fruit and nut mixture and mix thoroughly.

Scrape into prepared pan, pressing mixture into edges. Bake on center rack of oven for about 30 minutes. Remove and let cool slightly. Lift bars out of pan by holding onto edges of parchment paper. Let finish cooling on a wire rack. Use a sharp chef's knife to cut into 16 bars.

CHILL OUT
These bars will keep at room temperature for one week or individually wrapped in the freezer for up to three months.

NUTRITIONAL VALUE PER SERVING:
Calories: 193 | Calories from Fat: 79 | Protein: 5 g | Carbs: 28 g | Total Fat: 9 g | Saturated Fat: 1 g | Trans Fat: 0 g | Fiber: 3 g | Sodium: 32 mg | Cholesterol: 0 mg

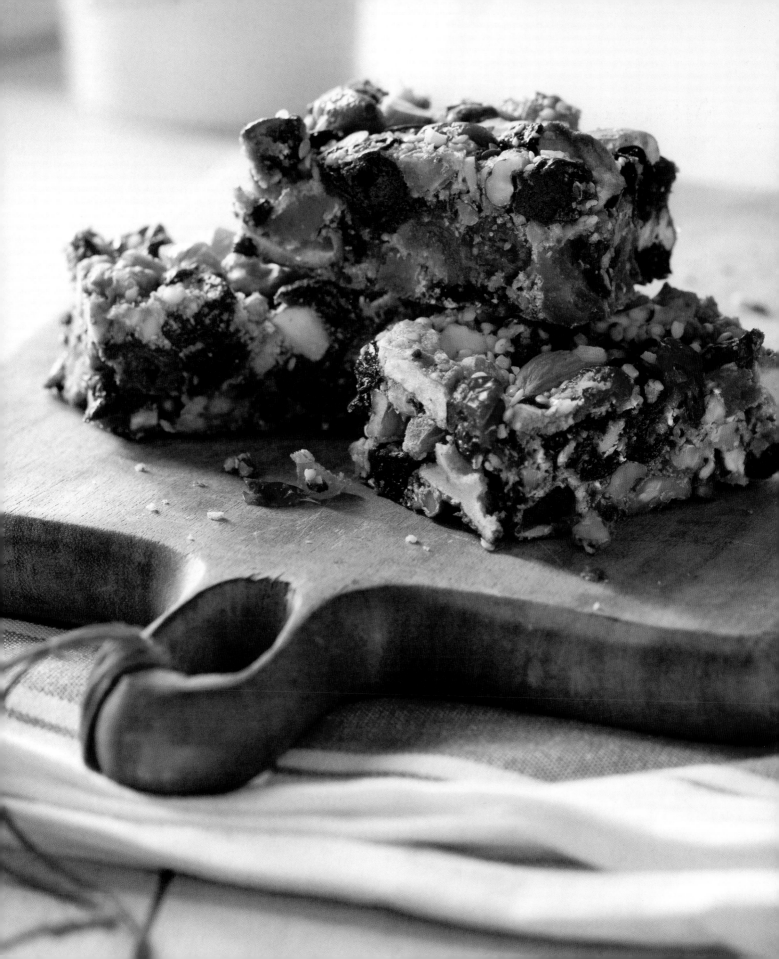

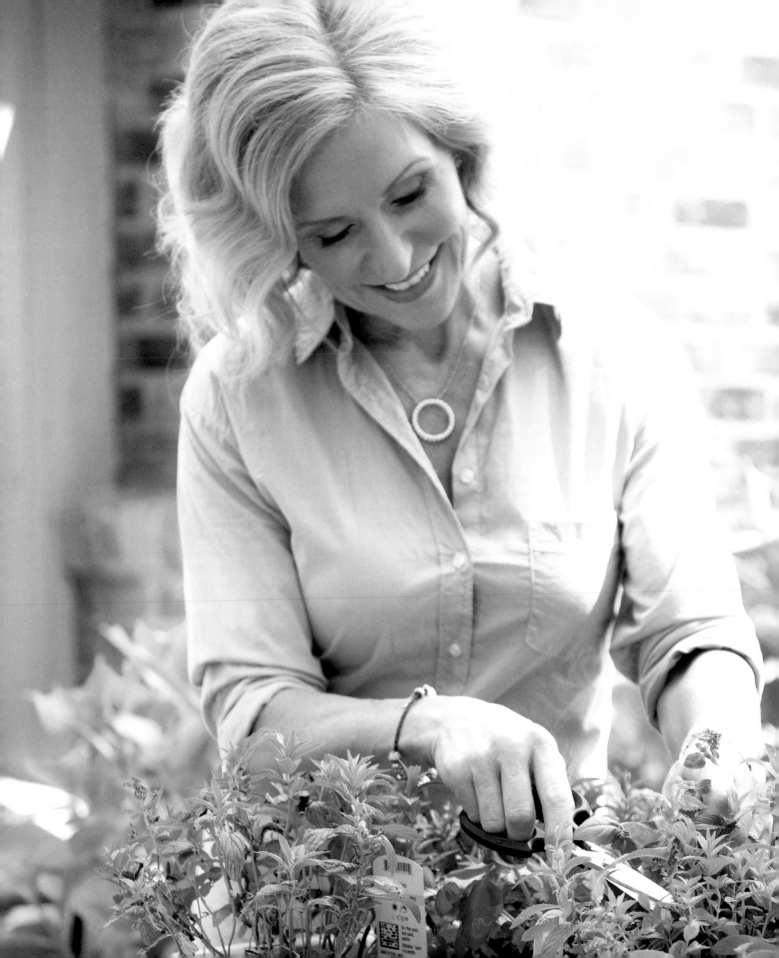

Moroccan Chickpea Spread

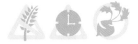

PREP: 15 minutes | **COOK:** 0 minutes | **YIELD:** 2½ cups

Like hummus, this spread is based on chickpeas – a hearty legume high in protein and starch. Throw in some truly Moroccan ingredients, like cumin and turmeric, and you've got yourself a tasty spread that's sure to disappear in as little time as it took to make it!

2 cups cooked, rinsed and drained or 1 x 15-
oz (440 ml) BPA-free can no-salt-added
chickpeas

1 carrot, peeled, trimmed and chopped

1 large clove garlic

½ cup (120 ml) sun-dried tomatoes, not in oil,
rehydrated, drained and liquid reserved

1 tsp (5 ml) ground cumin

½ tsp (2.5 ml) turmeric powder

½ tsp (2.5 ml) smoked paprika

¼ tsp (1.25 ml) ground cinnamon

Pinch cayenne, or to taste

2 Tbsp (30 ml) tahini (sesame seed paste)

1 Tbsp (15 ml) extra virgin olive oil

¼ cup (60 ml) fresh lemon juice

½ tsp (2.5 ml) sea salt

¼ tsp (1.25 ml) freshly ground black pepper

¼ cup (60 ml) cilantro

2 Tbsp (30 ml) fresh mint

Add all ingredients except cilantro and mint to a food processor, and pulse-blend until finely chopped. Mixture will be thick. Add reserved sun-dried tomato water, 1 Tbsp (15 ml) at a time, until spread comes together. You may need up to ½ cup (120 ml) of tomato water. If you run out of tomato water, you can use low-sodium vegetable broth or plain water.

Once desired consistency is achieved, add cilantro and mint, and let processor whirl for about 1 minute or until herbs are blended into the spread.

TRY THIS!
You can serve this spread with vegetable crudités, baked whole-grain tortilla chips or Bring the Heat Baked Blue Corn Chips (see p. 65). It is also adds a healthy zip to sandwiches and wraps.

NUTRITIONAL VALUE PER ¼-CUP SERVING:
Calories: 84 | Calories from Fat: 34 | Protein: 3 g | Carbs: 8 g | Total Fat: 4 g |
Saturated Fat: 0.5 g | Trans Fat: 0 g | Fiber: 2 g | Sodium: 21 mg | Cholesterol: 0 mg

Brown Rice Squares with Coconut Cashew Dipping Sauce

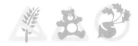

PREP: 15 minutes | **COOK:** 45-50 minutes | **YIELD:** 20 squares

This flavorful and unique appetizer is likely to become the life of your next party. Plus, it's perfect for gluten-free guests!

COCONUT CASHEW DIPPING SAUCE

½ cup (120 ml) reduced-fat coconut milk

1 Tbsp (15 ml) lime juice

1 tsp (5 ml) low-sodium tamari

½ tsp (2.5 ml) ground fresh chili paste (sambal oelek)

1 tsp (5 ml) honey, brown rice syrup or yacon syrup

1 tsp (5 ml) natural unflavored rice vinegar

¼ tsp (1.25 ml) sea salt

2 Tbsp (30 ml) creamy unsalted cashew butter

BROWN RICE SQUARES

2 cups (480 ml) medium grain brown rice

In a medium bowl, combine all sauce ingredients except cashew butter and whisk. Slowly start to incorporate cashew butter and then mix more vigorously until sauce is smooth. Refrigerate until ready to serve.

In a medium-sized heavy-bottomed saucepan, rinse and drain rice well. Add 4 cups (960 ml) water and bring to a boil on high heat. Cover and reduce heat to simmer for 45 to 50 minutes or until water is absorbed and rice is cooked through. Remove from heat. Scoop out 1 cup (240 ml) of rice and place in a food processor. Blend until as smooth as possible. Stir blended rice back into cooked rice until mixed well.

Line two 9 x 5-inch loaf pans with plastic wrap. Divide rice mixture evenly between the two pans. Using a rubber spatula, smooth out rice and press it down firmly. Holding onto edges of plastic wrap, lift rice out of pans and place on a cutting board. Dip a chef's knife in warm water and cut each "loaf" of rice into 10 squares, dipping knife in warm water in between each cut to prevent it from sticking to rice. Transfer rice squares to a platter and serve with Coconut Cashew Dipping Sauce .

TIME SAVER
Don't have time to make the brown rice squares, but still want to enjoy the bright and exotic flavors of this dish? Cook the rice, scoop it into a bowl and pour the sauce on top.

NUTRITIONAL VALUE PER SQUARE + ¹⁄₂₀ OF DIPPING SAUCE:
Calories: 36 | Calories from Fat: 12 | Protein: 1 g | Carbs: 5 g | Total Fat: 1 g |
Saturated Fat: 0.5 g | Trans Fat: 0 g | Fiber: 0.4 g | Sodium: 18 mg | Cholesterol: 0 mg

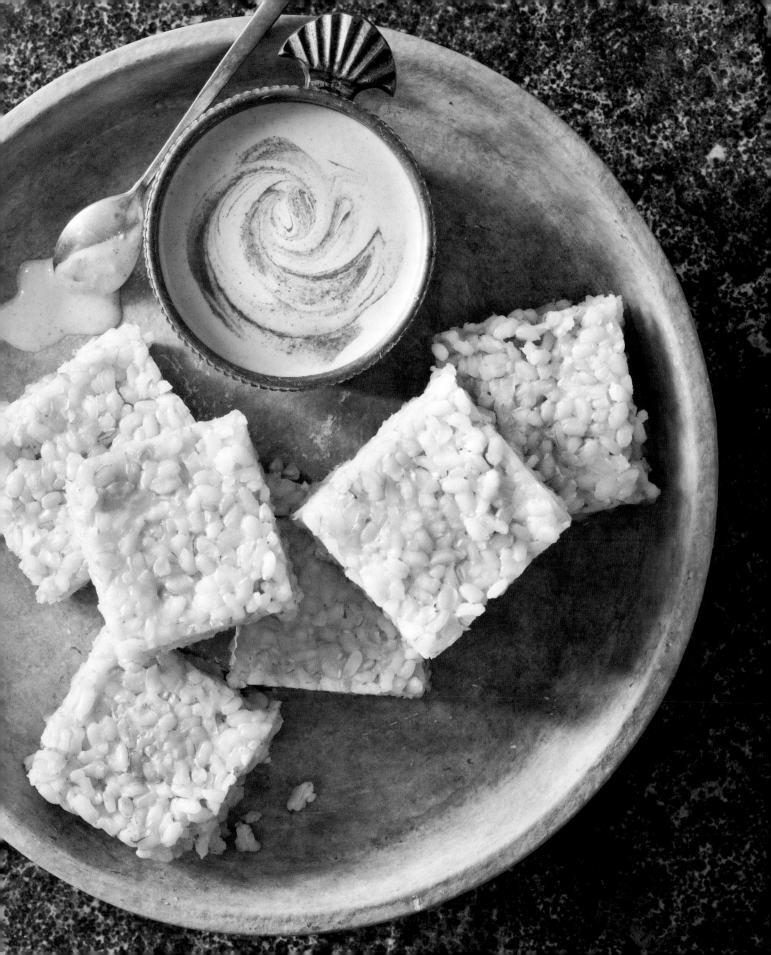

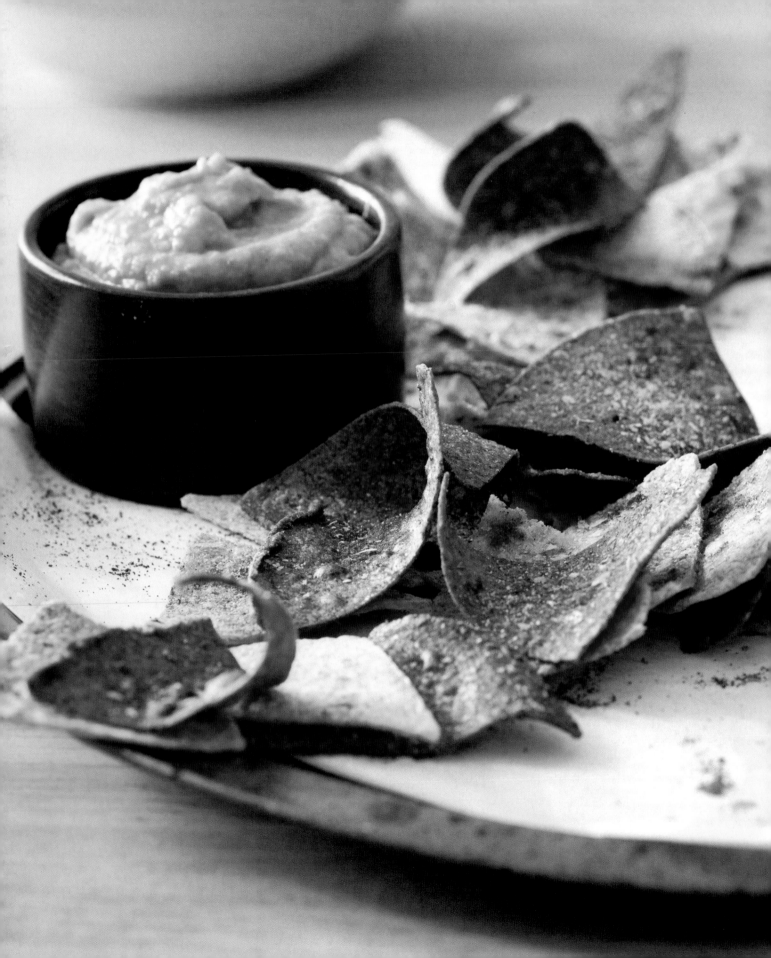

Bring the Heat Baked Blue Corn Chips

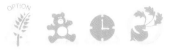

PREP: 10 minutes | **COOK:** 10-12 minutes | **YIELD:** 48 chips

Clean corn chips? Enough said! This perfectly tasty snack packs a sassy kick that will keep your guests grabbing for "just one more handful!"

8 whole grain blue corn tortillas (6 inches in diameter)
Eat-Clean Cooking Spray (see p. 277)

SPICE COATING

½ tsp (2.5 ml) nutritional yeast
¼ tsp (1.25 ml) smoked paprika
¼ tsp (1.25 ml) sweet paprika
¼ tsp (1.25 ml) Mexican chili powder
Pinch onion powder
Pinch cayenne (or to taste)
Pinch sea salt

Heat oven to 350°F (175°C). Cut each tortilla into six wedges and spread wedges out in a single layer on a baking sheet. It's okay if they overlap a little.

Mix Spice Coating ingredients together. If nutritional yeast is "large flake," grind it with a mortar and pestle or use a spoon to press it into a fine powder. Spray tortilla wedges with Eat-Clean Cooking Spray and sprinkle them with Spice Coating mixture. Bake 10 to 12 minutes or until crisp and lightly browned on edges. These chips are delicious eaten by themselves or dipped into hummus or Clean guacamole.

KEEP IT FRESH
Store uneaten chips in an airtight container or seal in a plastic bag.

MAKE IT GLUTEN FREE!
Choose gluten-free nutritional yeast.

NUTRITIONAL VALUE PER 6-CHIP SERVING:
Calories: 91 | Calories from Fat: 38 | Protein: 1 g | Carbs: 12 g | Total Fat: 4 g |
Saturated Fat: 0.3 g | Trans Fat: 0 g | Fiber: 2 g | Sodium: 108 mg | Cholesterol: 0 mg

The Lowdown on Legumes

Legumes! Although the word may stump some of our meat-eating friends, most vegetarians know this superfood intimately. For the uninitiated among us, though, let's get up close and personal with these nutrient-packed little gems that have been unfortunately burdened with a sometimes-smelly reputation (see sidebar for tips on dealing with this issue).

Lentils, chickpeas, kidney beans, snap peas, black beans and soybeans are some of the more popular members of the legume crowd. Basically, the term "legume" is used to describe a vegetable plant whose seeds are enclosed in two-sided pods. In some cases, you can eat the whole pod (think snow peas), otherwise you just eat the seed inside (think sweet green peas).

Pod Power

There's quite a bit of truth in that childish chant – beans really are good for your heart (and the rest of your body for that matter). They are cholesterol free, low in fat, and the fiber they contain helps lower LDL ("bad") cholesterol levels. This fiber also slows the absorption of carbohydrates, which stabilizes blood sugar levels and can help prevent diabetes. Legumes are also high in folate (and other B vitamins), iron and magnesium, and they contain healthy fats as well as disease-fighting antioxidants. Who knew so much could be packed into these little wonders?

You Complete Me

Legumes can be used to add variation to a diet that may otherwise depend entirely on meat, or as a substitute for meat. For vegetarians, the most important thing about legumes is that they are extremely high in protein, making them an excellent staple. Vegetarians (and omnivores, too) need to be aware that legumes are not a source of complete protein. This means they are missing one or two key amino acids necessary for maintaining the human body. For this reason, grains are often paired with legumes; grains have what legumes lack and vice versa. One key amino acid is lysine, which grains contain and legumes don't. They make a cute couple for this reason! Think of pairing rice and beans in Mexican cooking or lentils and rice in Indian cooking.

How to Cook Dried Legumes

In order to be fully enjoyed, legumes need to be cooked at low temperatures and with the right additions. A common rule of thumb is to use three cups of water for every cup of dried legumes. Then toss in your favorite herbs and spices. (Don't add salt yet, though, as it will toughen the beans!) Bring water and legumes to a boil and then simmer by removing the lid, reducing the heat and stirring every so often until legumes are tender. Cooking time will vary based on the type of legume, so refer to your package directions and keep checking after 45 minutes. You should be able to mash the legumes between two fingers once they're cooked. Salt and any acidic ingredients can be added near the end of the cooking time, when the beans are just tender.

Common Legumes

Alfalfa
Chickpeas
Clover
Peas
String beans
Dried beans (adzuki, anasazi, black, black-eyed peas, red kidney, fava, lima)
Lentils
Lupins
Mesquite
Carob
Soy
Peanuts

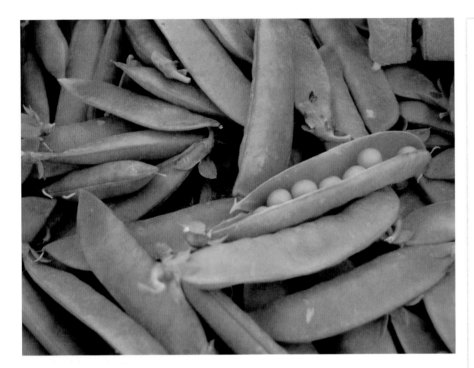

> "Legumes are easy to prepare, tasty and they nourish you from the inside out. There are tons of different ways to enjoy legumes – hot or cold, whole or pureed."

Back in the Day

Legume consumption began more than 20,000 years ago. Our earlier ancestors served legumes as a supplement to the diet when meat was in scarce supply. The Ancient Greeks and Romans deemed legumes a "poor man's food," causing them to go out of style. But with the dawn of the Middle Ages came the resurgence of legume usage. They have maintained their popularity as a staple in the diets of many cultures since then.

Nowadays, experts recommend that we eat at least three cups of legumes per week – and why not? Legumes are easy to prepare, tasty and they nourish you from the inside out. There are tons of different ways to enjoy legumes – hot or cold, whole or pureed. Keep an eye out for these little powerhouses in many of the recipes used in *The Eat-Clean Diet Vegetarian Cookbook*, including Carolina Caviar (see p. 42), Moroccan Chickpea Spread (see p. 61) and Cuban Black Beans (see p. 190), to name just a few!

Beat the Bloat!

On a typical day, the average adult releases enough gas to fill a party balloon – and likely more if they've been eating beans! Despite the multiple health benefits of legumes, many people are deterred by this pungent fact of life. Don't give up on these musical fruits just yet! Here are some tips to help reduce the gas factor:

Drink plenty of water. I know, I know, I sound like a broken record, but believe me, it helps!

Chew, chew, chew your food! The more you pre-digest your food, the less gas you'll have after you eat.

Move your body and your bowels will follow. Physical activity helps strengthen and stimulate the intestinal muscles, which keeps things running smoothly.

Experiment! Various beans affect people differently. Find your digestive system's faves!

Soak 'em. To rehydrate dried beans, add 1 pound of beans to 10 cups of water and boil for 2 to 3 minutes. Cover and set aside overnight. By the next day, most of the indigestible, gas-inducing sugars will have dissolved into the water. If you can change the water several times during soaking, even better.

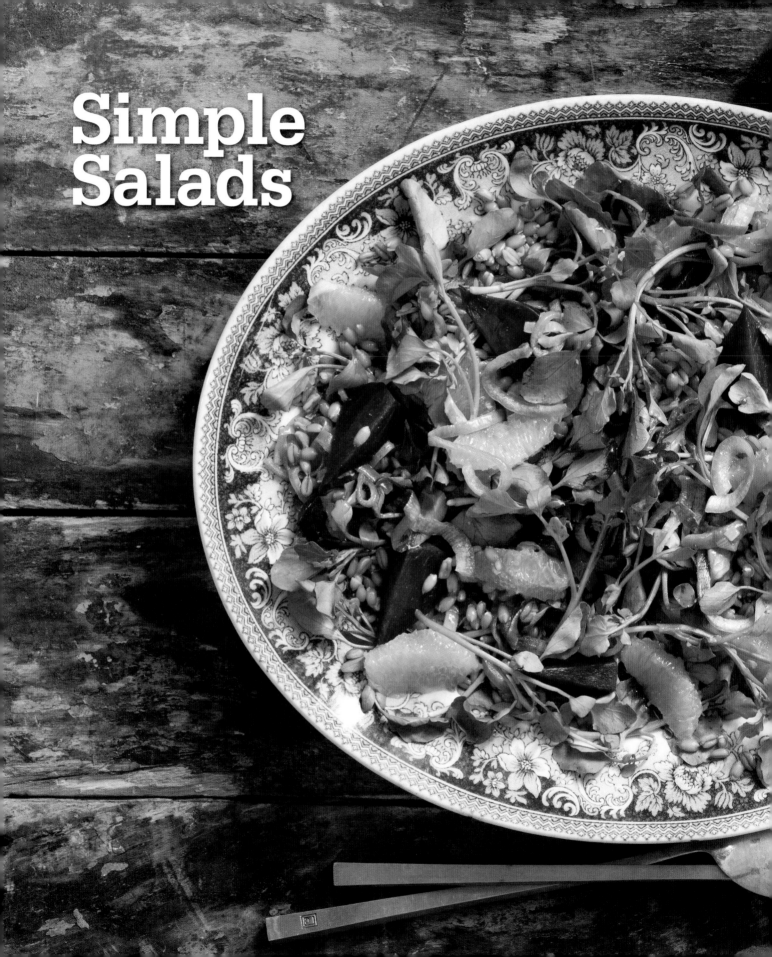

Simple
Salads

Farro Salad with Watercress,
Beets and Caramelized Onions p. 70

Farro Salad with Watercress, Beets and Caramelized Red Onions

PREP: 15 minutes | **COOK:** 1 hour | **YIELD:** 5 x 1-cup servings

Farro, a type of wheat, is crunchy and hearty and provides tons of fiber to keep your digestive system running smoothly. Don't take my word for it, though! Try this recipe and I'm sure that you too will soon be adding farro to your weekly grocery list.

1 medium beet, scrubbed

½ cup (120 ml) farro

1 red onion, thinly sliced

1 tsp (5 ml) extra virgin olive oil

Pinch each sea salt and freshly ground
    black pepper

1 bunch watercress, root ball removed and
    discarded, cress washed well

1 red grapefruit, peeled and the segments cut
    from the membrane (save the membrane
    for the vinaigrette)

1 Tbsp (15 ml) grapefruit juice, squeezed from
    the leftover membrane

1 Tbsp (15 ml) aged sherry vinegar

1 Tbsp (15 ml) extra virgin olive oil

Pinch each sea salt and freshly ground
    black pepper

Preheat oven to 400°F (200°C). Place beet in a loaf pan and add enough water to come a quarter of the way up the side of the beet. Cover tightly with aluminum foil and cook in the oven for about 1 hour, or until tender when pierced with a skewer.

In the meantime, combine farro and 2½ cups (600 ml) water in a heavy-bottomed saucepan on high heat. Bring to a boil, stir and reduce heat to simmer, covered, for about 50 minutes or until tender but firm to the bite (al dente). Drain and set aside.

While farro and beet are cooking, place red onion on a baking sheet and toss with 1 tsp olive oil, salt and pepper. Spread out in a single layer and roast in oven for 15 to 20 minutes or until caramelized, stirring once.

Remove beet from oven when done. Uncover and let cool until comfortable to handle. The skin should slip right off, but you can use a paring knife to assist the process. Chop beet into bite-sized pieces.

To a large bowl, add cooked farro, chopped beet, half of caramelized onions, watercress and grapefruit segments. In a small bowl, whisk together grapefruit juice, sherry vinegar, 1 Tbsp olive oil and salt and pepper. Pour mixture over salad and toss to combine. Divide among plates and top with remaining caramelized onions. Serve immediately.

NUTRITIONAL VALUE PER SERVING:
Calories: 96 | Calories from Fat: 34 | Protein: 2 g | Carbs: 16 g | Total Fat: 4 g |
Saturated Fat: 0.5 g | Trans Fat: 0 g | Fiber: 3 g | Sodium: 17 mg | Cholesterol: 0 mg

Bulgur with Black Kabuli Chickpeas

PREP: 1 hour | **COOK:** 30 minutes | **YIELD:** 8 x 1-cup servings

Bulgur, a staple of Middle Eastern cuisine, is absolutely packed full of fiber. Pair it with black chickpeas and you've got a meal that's pleasing to both the eye and the digestive system!

1 cup (240 ml) dried black kabuli chickpeas (use regular chickpeas if you can't find black kabuli)

1 cup (240 ml) bulgur

4 green onions or scallions, thinly sliced

½ cup (120 ml) drained and diced roasted red bell peppers

½ cup (120 ml) finely chopped fresh mint

2 cups (480 ml) chopped parsley

¼ cup (60 ml) pitted and chopped kalamata olives

Juice of 1½ lemons

2 Tbsp (30 ml) extra virgin olive oil

1½ tsp (7.5 ml) ground cumin

2 heaping tsp (10 or 11 ml) harissa or fresh chili paste

¾ tsp (3.75 ml) sea salt

½ tsp (2.5 ml) freshly ground black pepper

Add chickpeas to a heavy-bottomed saucepan and cover with just over two inches of water. Place on stove and bring to a boil on high heat. Cover, remove from heat and let stand for about 1 hour. Alternatively, you can soak garbanzo beans overnight in plenty of water in the refrigerator. Once beans are done soaking, drain, rinse and cover with two times their volume in cold water. Place on stove and simmer until beans are tender but still hold their shape, about 30 minutes. Drain.

In the meantime, cook bulgur according to package directions.

To a large bowl, add chickpeas, bulgur, green onions, roasted red peppers, mint, parsley and kalamata olives. In a separate small bowl, whisk together lemon juice, olive oil, cumin, harissa, salt and pepper. Pour into the large bowl with chickpeas and toss well to combine. Taste, and make any adjustments to seasoning with more lemon juice and/or harissa.

Can be served hot, at room temperature or chilled.

NUTRITIONAL VALUE PER SERVING:
Calories: 210 | Calories from Fat: 53 | Protein: 10 g | Carbs: 31 g | Total Fat: 6 g | Saturated Fat: 0.5 g | Trans Fat: 0 g | Fiber: 11 g | Sodium: 330 mg | Cholesterol: 0 mg

Delightful Strawberry, Spinach and Broccoli Salad with Macadamia Nuts

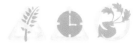

PREP: 15 minutes | **COOK:** 0 minutes | **YIELD:** 8 x 1-cup servings

Aren't the salads in this book unique? It's amazing how inspiring a few new ingredients can be. For this dish, I took my favorite nuts and paired them with my favorite berries to add some interest to spinach and broccoli. It's almost too pretty to eat!

4 cups (950 ml) baby spinach, lightly packed

2 cups (480 ml) raw broccoli florets, cut into small bite-sized pieces

2 cups (480 ml) sliced fresh strawberries

½ avocado, diced

¼ cup (60 ml) unsalted macadamia nuts, coarsely chopped

DRESSING

1 Tbsp (15 ml) low-sodium soy sauce or tamari

2 tsp (10 ml) rice vinegar

2 tsp (10 ml) sesame oil

1 tsp (5 ml) honey, brown rice syrup or yacon syrup

½ tsp (2.5 ml) Dijon mustard

1 Tbsp (15 ml) chia seeds

To a salad bowl, add spinach, broccoli florets, sliced strawberries, avocado and macadamia nuts.

In a small bowl, whisk together soy sauce, rice vinegar, sesame oil, honey, Dijon mustard and chia seeds. Pour mixture over salad and toss gently to combine. Serve immediately.

NUTRITIONAL VALUE PER SERVING:
Calories: 86 | Calories from Fat: 55 | Protein: 2 g | Carbs: 7 g | Total Fat: 6 g | Saturated Fat: 1 g | Trans Fat: 0 g | Fiber: 2 g | Sodium: 98 mg | Cholesterol: 0 mg

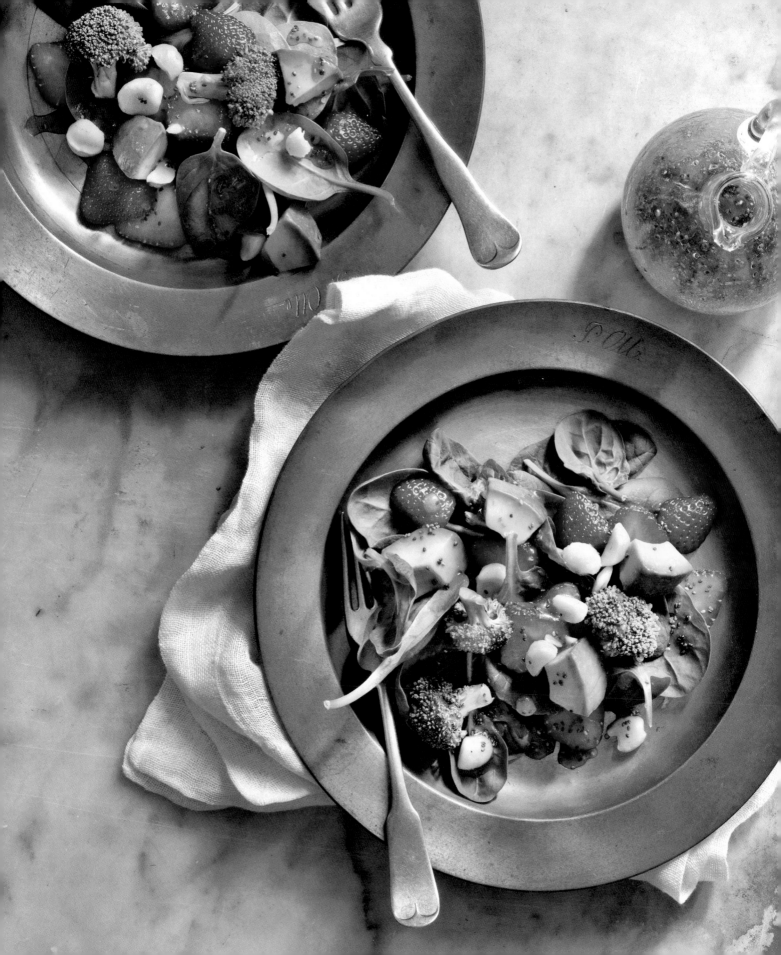

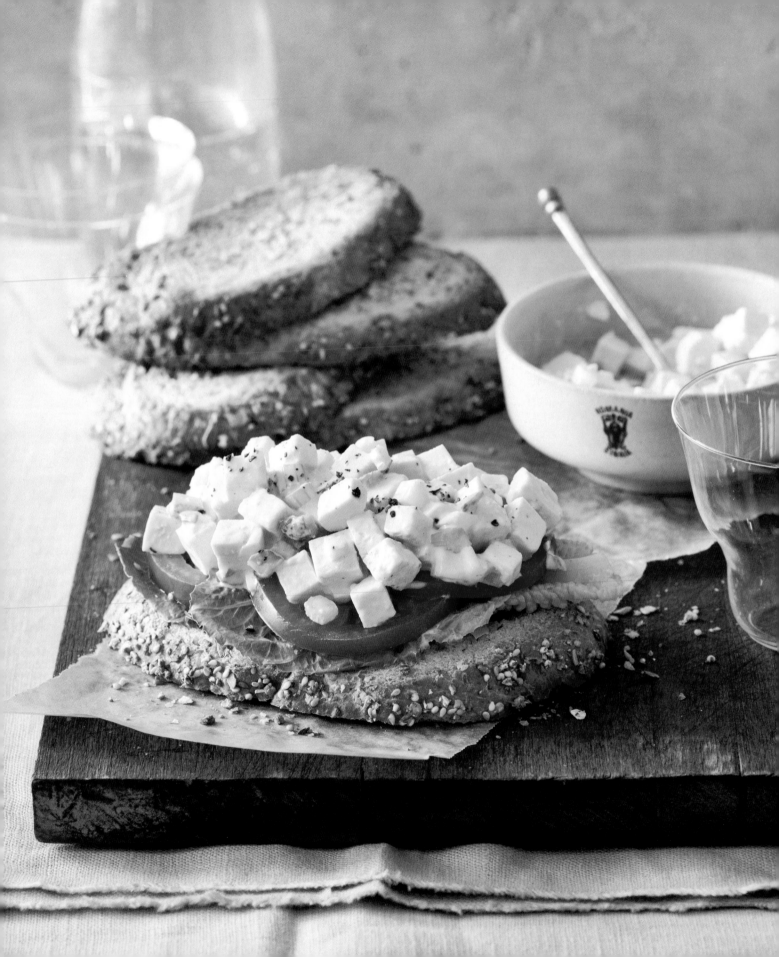

Eggless Egg Salad

PREP: 15 minutes | **COOK:** 0 minutes | **YIELD:** 4 x ¾-cup servings

I love this tofu-based egg salad because it's easy, cholesterol free and it tastes just like the real thing. (Psst, the secret is the black salt.)

2 Tbsp (30 ml) all-natural vegan mayonnaise
(Try: Vegenaise or Nayonaise)

1 tsp (5 ml) prepared mustard

1 tsp (5 ml) white wine vinegar

¼ tsp (1.25 ml) black salt (see Prep Tip at right)

¼ tsp (1.25 ml) freshly ground black pepper

¼ cup (60 ml) finely diced celery

2 Tbsp (30 ml) finely diced dill pickle
or cornichon

1 Tbsp (15 ml) minced white or yellow onion

1 lb (454 g) extra-firm tofu, drained and diced
into ½-inch pieces

In a medium bowl, thoroughly mix together mayonnaise, mustard, vinegar, black salt and pepper. Stir in celery, pickle, onion and tofu until mixed well. Refrigerate until ready to use.

PREP TIP
Black salt, also known as Kala Namak or Sanchal, is often used in vegan cooking to help mimic the taste of eggs. If you can't find any in your neighborhood, it is definitely worth seeking out from a reputable online source. If you're in a pinch, though, you can use sea salt instead.

TRY THIS!
Why not try an Eggless Egg Salad sandwich on toasted whole grain bread with lettuce and tomato?

NUTRITIONAL VALUE PER SERVING (WITHOUT BREAD):
Calories: 112 | Calories from Fat: 60 | Protein: 8 g | Carbs: 3 g | Total Fat: 7 g |
Saturated Fat: 0.3 g | Trans Fat: 0 g | Fiber: 0.3 g | Sodium: 197 mg | Cholesterol: 0 mg

Spelt, Asparagus and Pea Salad

PREP: 15 minutes | **COOK:** 45 minutes | **YIELD:** 10 x 1-cup servings

It's time to toss your salad prejudices out the window! That's right, I'm here to remind you that this dish doesn't always need to be based on a bed of leafy greens. In this salad, spelt, an ancient grain that is also a good source of vitamin B2, manganese and fiber, acts as the perfect nutty and nutritious base.

1 cup (240 ml) spelt

1 cup (240 ml) frozen peas

1 bunch asparagus, stalk ends trimmed, cut into 1-inch pieces on the diagonal

1 cup (240 ml) sun-dried tomatoes, not in oil, rehydrated with hot water, drained and coarsely chopped

½ cup (120 ml) finely chopped fresh basil

¼ cup (60 ml) finely chopped fresh mint

¼ cup (60 ml) finely chopped fresh parsley

½ cup (120 ml) toasted walnuts, coarsely chopped

Zest and juice of 1 large lemon

1 small or ½ large clove garlic, finely minced

1 Tbsp (15 ml) extra virgin olive oil

½ tsp (2.5 ml) each sea salt and freshly ground black pepper

Pinch red pepper flakes

In a medium pot, combine spelt and 4 cups (950 ml) water and bring to a boil over high heat. Reduce heat to simmer, partially cover and cook for about 45 minutes, until tender but still chewy. Drain in a small-holed colander.

Meanwhile, steam peas and set aside.

While spelt cooks, prepare a large bowl of ice water. Bring a large pot of water to boil over high heat and add asparagus. Boil asparagus for no more than about 10 seconds, and then immediately drain and add to ice bath to cool down, then drain again.

To a large bowl, add cooked spelt, steamed peas, blanched asparagus, sun-dried tomatoes, basil, mint, parsley and walnuts. In a small bowl, whisk together lemon zest and juice, garlic, olive oil, salt, pepper and red pepper flakes. Pour over spelt salad ingredients and toss to combine.

CHILL OUT
This salad can be served hot, at room temperature or chilled. Will keep in the refrigerator for up to three days.

NUTRITIONAL VALUE PER SERVING:
Calories: 157 | Calories from Fat: 53 | Protein: 6 g | Carbs: 21 g | Total Fat: 6 g | Saturated Fat: 1 g | Trans Fat: 0 g | Fiber: 5 g | Sodium: 75 mg | Cholesterol: 0 mg

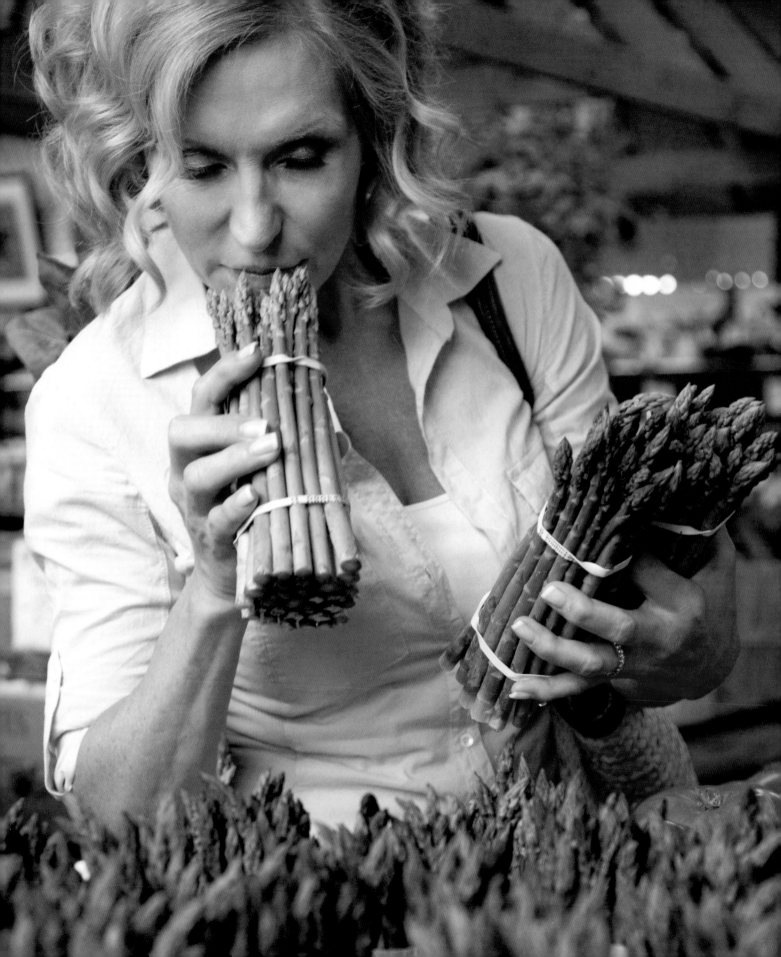

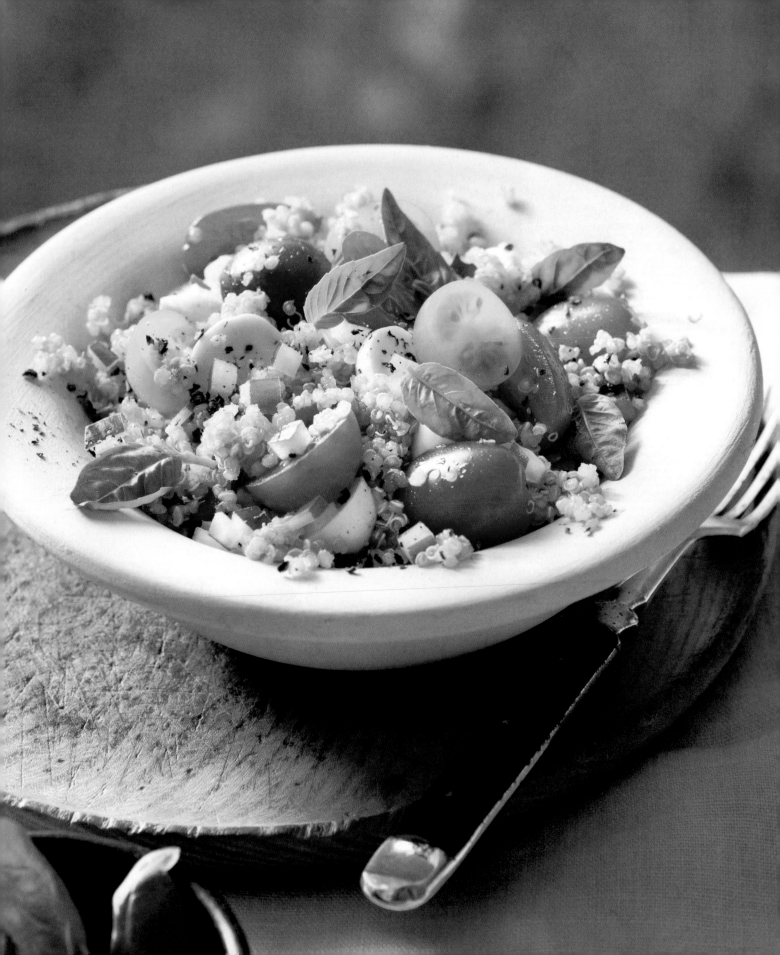

Caprese Quinoa Salad

PREP: 10 minutes | **COOK:** 10-15 minutes | **YIELD:** 5 x 1-cup servings

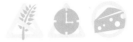

Wouldn't it be nice to be basking on the Isle of Capri enjoying a delicious, Clean meal? This salad will help you feel like you're right there. Fashioned in the style of Capri, the tomatoes, quinoa and cheese blend together to create a light and tasty meal that will leave you with the same glow you'd get from a Mediterranean sojourn.

½ cup (120 ml) uncooked quinoa

1½ cups (360 ml) mixed cherry and mini pear tomatoes, halved

½ cup (120 ml) thinly sliced basil

1 cup (240 ml) fresh mozzarella balls, halved (see prep tip)

2 Tbsp (30 ml) minced red onion or shallot

2 Tbsp (30 ml) balsamic vinegar

1 Tbsp (15 ml) extra virgin olive oil

¼ tsp (1.25 ml) sea salt

Pinch freshly ground black pepper

Cook quinoa according to package directions. Scrape into a mixing bowl. Add tomatoes, basil and mozzarella. In a separate small bowl, whisk together minced red onion, balsamic vinegar, olive oil, salt and pepper. Pour over quinoa and toss to coat. Best served at room temperature.

PREP TIP

For this recipe, I recommend fresh ciliegine mozzarella, which is shaped into cherry-sized balls. If you can't find it, golf-ball-sized bocconcini cut into quarters will do the trick.

NUTRITIONAL VALUE PER SERVING:
Calories: 177 | Calories from Fat: 76 | Protein: 10 g | Carbs: 15 g | Total Fat: 8 g | Saturated Fat: 3 g | Trans Fat: 0 g | Fiber: 2 g | Sodium: 56 mg | Cholesterol: 14 mg

Seven Citrus Salad with Mint

PREP: 20 minutes active, 15 minutes inactive | **COOK:** 0 minutes | **YIELD:** 4 x 1-cup servings

When you combine seven exotic citrus fruits with the snap of mint you wind up with one of the freshest salads around. The crisp colors, tangy flavors and juicy texture make winter feel like summer. Ahhh!

1 Cara Cara orange

1 pink or red grapefruit

1 blood orange

2 mandarin oranges

1 cocktail citrus (omit if you can't find)

1 ugli fruit (Jamaican tangelo)

4 kumquats, peels washed well, halved
   lengthwise and thinly sliced, removing
   any seeds

2 Tbsp (30 ml) finely chopped fresh mint leaves

Using a knife, or by hand, remove peels from Cara Cara orange, grapefruit, blood orange and mandarins. Pull apart sections, cut into bite-sized pieces and add to a bowl. Using a knife, cut away peel of cocktail citrus and ugli fruit. Then, using a paring knife, cut between membranes to remove fruit segments. Place segments in bowl. Add kumquats and mint. Toss to combine and refrigerate for about 15 minutes before serving.

NUTRITIONAL VALUE PER SERVING:
Calories: 148 | Calories from Fat: 2 | Protein: 2 g | Carbs: 36 g | Total Fat: 0.2 g | Saturated Fat: <0.1 g | Trans Fat: 0 g | Fiber: 5 g | Sodium: 9 mg | Cholesterol: 0 mg

Chilled Asparagus Salad

PREP: 10 minutes active, 1 to 2 hours inactive | **COOK:** 1 minute | **YIELD:** 5 x 1-cup servings

Asparagus is one of my absolute favorite veggies. It's crisp, satisfying and pairs well with just about anything. In this case, we've spiced it up with wasabi paste and red pepper flakes, dressed it with sesame seeds and balanced it all out with a dash of sweetness. Perfect? You'd better believe it!

2 lbs (908 g) asparagus, cut into 2- to 3-inch
   pieces, stalk ends trimmed

½ tsp (2.5 ml) prepared wasabi paste

½ tsp (2.5 ml) Dijon mustard, or to taste

1 Tbsp (15 ml) rice vinegar

½ tsp (2.5 ml) honey, brown rice syrup
   or yacon syrup

2 tsp (10 ml) sesame oil

Pinch sea salt

Pinch red pepper flakes

1 tsp (5 ml) sesame seeds

Prepare a large bowl of ice water.

Steam asparagus until tender-crisp, about 1 minute. Transfer asparagus to bowl of ice water to stop cooking. Drain.

In a large bowl, whisk together wasabi paste, Dijon mustard, rice vinegar, honey or syrup, sesame oil, sea salt and red pepper flakes. Add asparagus and sesame seeds and toss to coat. Refrigerate until chilled, about 1 to 2 hours. Can be made a day ahead.

NUTRITIONAL VALUE PER SERVING:
Calories: 60 | Calories from Fat: 21 | Protein: 4 g | Carbs: 8 g | Total Fat: 2 g | Saturated Fat: 0.5 g | Trans Fat: 0 g | Fiber: 4 g | Sodium: 40 mg | Cholesterol: 0 mg

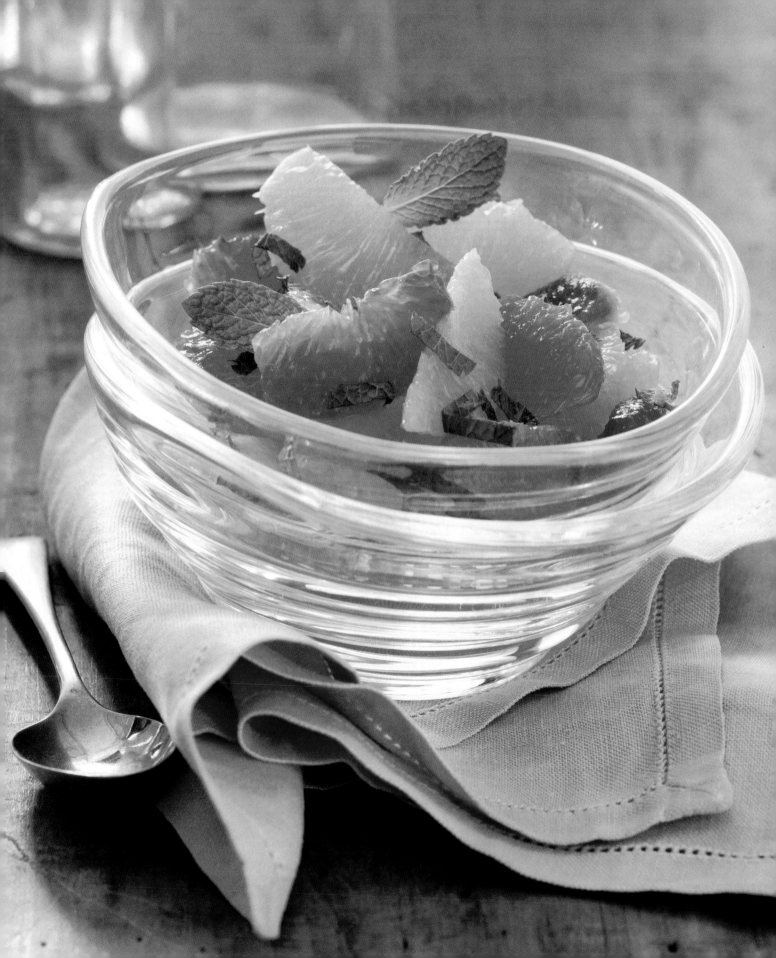

Ethiopian-Style Bread Salad

PREP: 10 minutes active + 10 minutes inactive | **COOK:** 0 minutes | **YIELD:** 12 x 1-cup servings

Bread salad is a favorite of mine. It has a unique texture and quality that makes it hearty and fresh all at the same time. You won't have to worry about the bread getting soggy because with all the mouthwatering flavors in this dish, it will be gone before you know it!

About 10 cups (2.4 L) lightly packed chopped green leaf lettuce

2 medium tomatoes, chopped

2 jalapeños, quartered lengthwise, seeds and ribs removed, finely chopped (or leave intact for a spicier salad)

4 cups (950 ml) whole wheat sourdough bread or levain, cut into ½-inch cubes (can be day old)

Juice of 1 large lemon

2 Tbsp (30 ml) extra virgin olive oil

½ tsp (2.5 ml) sea salt

¼ tsp (1.25 ml) freshly ground black pepper

To a large bowl add lettuce, tomatoes, jalapeños and bread cubes. In a separate small bowl, whisk together lemon juice, olive oil, salt and pepper. Pour the dressing over the salad and toss well to combine. Let sit, refrigerated, for about 10 minutes so the bread can soak up the lemon dressing and soften.

MAKE-AHEAD TIP
This salad will last in the fridge for one day dressed, so it can be made ahead on the same day it will be served.

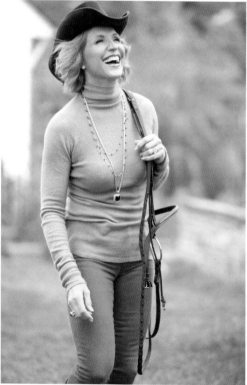

NUTRITIONAL VALUE PER SERVING:
Calories: 58 | Calories from Fat: 21 | Protein: 1 g | Carbs: 8 g | Total Fat: 2 g | Saturated Fat: 0.3 g | Trans Fat: 0 g | Fiber: 1 g | Sodium: 64 mg | Cholesterol: 0 mg

Stone Fruit and Beet Salad

PREP: 5 minutes | **COOK:** 1 to 1½ hours | **YIELD:** 8 servings

Remember Rule #8 from my book *Just the Rules*? "Color up! The more color on your plate, the healthier you will be!" The deep yellows of the nectarines and corn, the lush red beets and the vibrant mixed greens mean that this salad is packed with nutrients – and it's pretty as a picture!

¾ lb (340 g) beets (about 1 large or 2 small)

1 ear corn, husked

1 lb (454 g) ripe nectarines (about 2 medium), pitted and cut into bite-sized pieces

¾ lb (340 g), ripe red plums (about 2 medium), pitted and cut into bite-sized pieces

½ tsp (2.5 ml) Dijon mustard

½ tsp (2.5 ml) pure maple syrup

1 tsp (5 ml) lemon juice

1 Tbsp (15 ml) white balsamic vinegar

1 Tbsp (15 ml) extra virgin olive oil

Pinch each sea salt and freshly ground black pepper

8 cups (1.9 L) mixed greens

2 Tbsp (30 ml) finely chopped basil leaves

Heat oven to 400°F (200°C). Place the beet(s) in a dish or pan with one inch of water and cover. Bake in oven until tender when pierced, about 1 hour for medium-sized beets and about 1½ hours for large. Remove and let cool until comfortable to handle. Slide off skin and dice into bite-sized pieces.

Meanwhile, steam ear of corn for a few minutes and set aside to cool. Cut kernels from cob.

Whisk together Dijon mustard, maple syrup, lemon juice, balsamic vinegar, olive oil and salt and pepper. Pour half of vinaigrette over greens and toss to coat. Place greens on plates, and add diced beets, nectarines, plums and corn. Drizzle with remaining vinaigrette and sprinkle with chopped basil.

TIME SAVER
Want to make assembling this salad a snap? Cook the beet a day ahead, and it will take only minutes to put this salad together.

NUTRITIONAL VALUE PER SERVING:
Calories: 134 | Calories from Fat: 27 | Protein: 3 g | Carbs: 28 g | Total Fat: 3 g |
Saturated Fat: 0.3 g | Trans Fat: 0 g | Fiber: 4 g | Sodium: 28 mg | Cholesterol: 0 mg

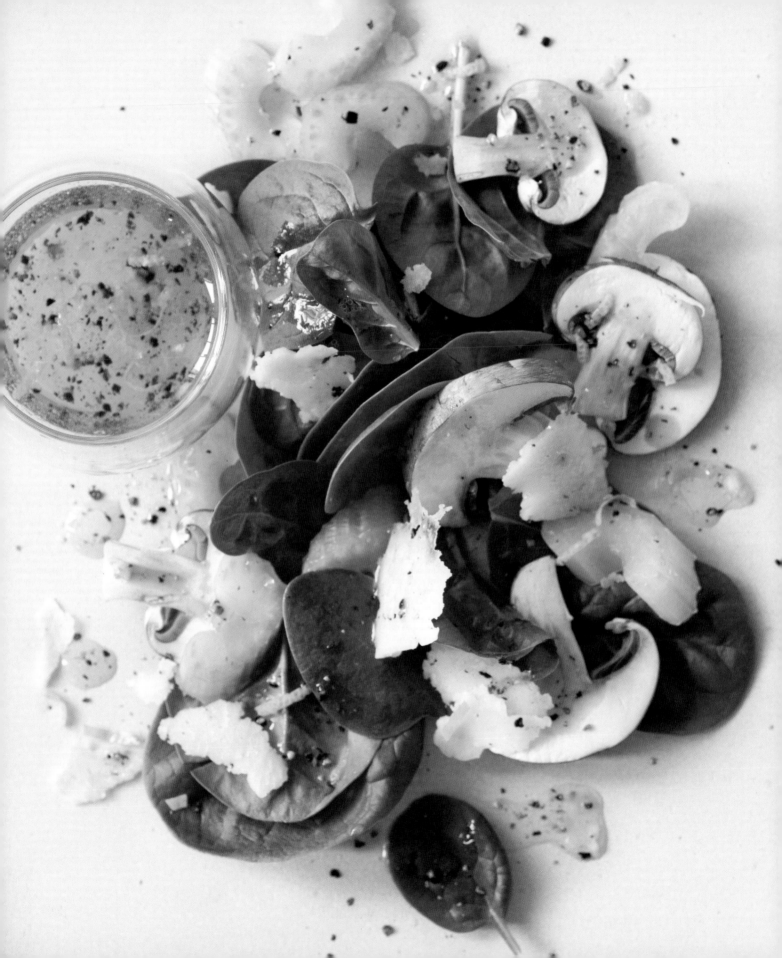

Meyer Lemon, Mushroom, Celery and Spinach Salad

PREP: 15 minutes | **COOK:** 0 minutes | **YIELD:** 8 x 1-cup servings

Meyer lemons are thought to be a cross between a regular lemon and a mandarin orange, so you can imagine how unique they taste. In fact, the flavor is so distinctive it offers the perfect base for this salad full of vegetables. One bite and you'll be a lifelong meyer lemon fan.

½ lb (225 g) white button mushrooms, thinly sliced

2 large ribs celery, thinly sliced crosswise

4 cups (950 ml) baby spinach, lightly packed

1 Meyer lemon, zested and juiced

1 Tbsp (15 ml) extra virgin olive oil

¼ tsp (1.25 ml) each sea salt and freshly ground black pepper

1 Tbsp (15 ml) Pecorino Romano or Asiago, freshly grated

To a large bowl, add mushrooms, celery and spinach. In a small bowl, whisk together Meyer lemon zest and juice, olive oil and salt and pepper. Pour over salad, add Pecorino Romano or Asiago and toss to combine.

MAKE IT VEGAN!
Simply leave out the cheese or replace it with nutritional yeast.

NUTRITIONAL VALUE PER SERVING:
Calories: 35 | Calories from Fat: 19 | Protein: 2 g | Carbs: 3 g | Total Fat: 2 g |
Saturated Fat: 0.4 g | Trans Fat: 0 g | Fiber: 1 g | Sodium: 48 mg | Cholesterol: 0.5 mg

Spring Fling Pasta Salad

PREP: 15 minutes | **COOK:** 10 minutes | **YIELD:** 8 x 1-cup servings

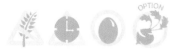

A pasta dish packed full of vegetables is one of the best kinds to enjoy. It will make you feel light, satisfied and well nourished. Bon appétit!

12 oz (340 g) whole grain or gluten-free fusilli

1½ cups (360 ml) frozen petite or baby peas

1 yellow pepper, seeded and thinly sliced
   into 2-inch strips

2 scallions, thinly sliced crosswise

1 Tbsp (15 ml) capers, drained

Zest of 1 large lemon

Juice of ½ lemon

1 Tbsp (15 ml) extra virgin olive oil

2 Tbsp (30 ml) thinly sliced fresh basil leaves

1 Tbsp (15 ml) finely chopped fresh
   tarragon leaves

1 Tbsp (15 ml) finely chopped fresh mint leaves

¼ tsp (1.25 ml) each sea salt and freshly
   ground black pepper

Bring a large pot of water to boil on high heat. Add pasta and cook according to package directions for al dente. When pasta has 1 to 2 minutes left to cook, add peas. When pasta has finished cooking, drain pasta and peas into a colander. Do not rinse.

Transfer peas and pasta to a large bowl and add yellow pepper, scallions and capers.

In a small bowl, whisk together lemon zest, juice and olive oil. Pour mixture over pasta and add basil, tarragon, mint and salt and pepper. Toss to combine. Can be served hot, at room temperature or cold.

ON THE GO
This salad travels well! Toss it into a sealable container and take it to work, a garden party or a picnic.

MAKE IT VEGAN!
Be sure to use an egg-free pasta.

NUTRITIONAL VALUE PER SERVING:
Calories: 196 | Calories from Fat: 27 | Protein: 7 g | Carbs: 37 g | Total Fat: 3 g |
Saturated Fat: 0.2 g | Trans Fat: 0 g | Fiber: 6 g | Sodium: 124 mg | Cholesterol: 0 mg

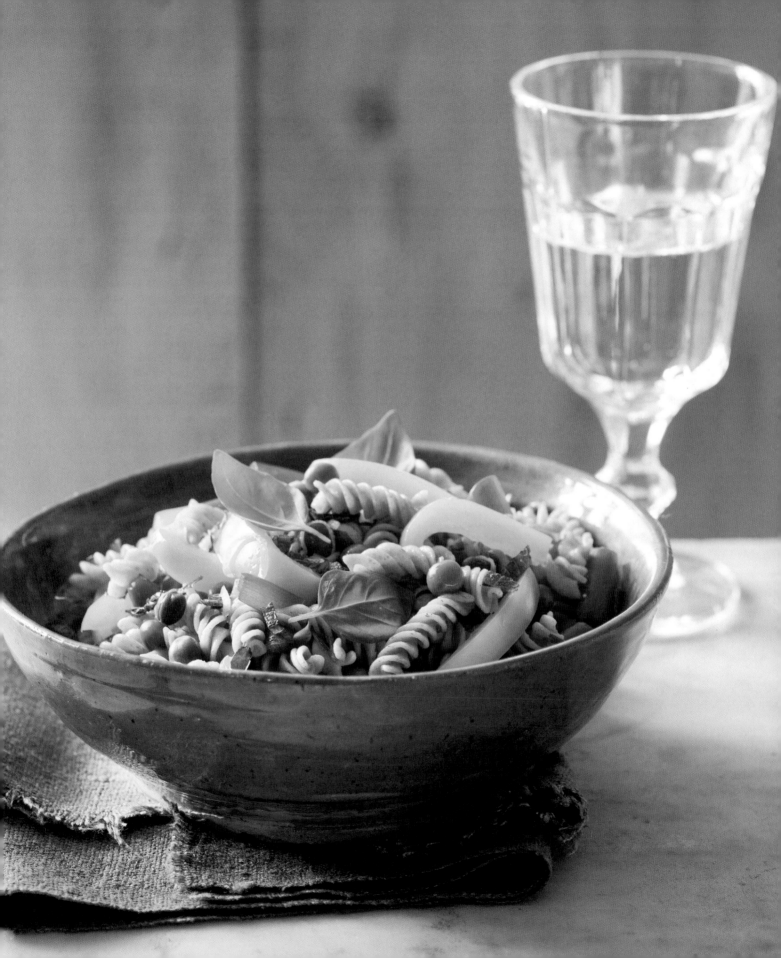

Sweet Potato Picnic Salad

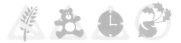

PREP: 20 minutes | **COOK:** 7 minutes | **YIELD:** 10 x 1-cup servings

It's too bad potato salad has a reputation for being laden with sodium, saturated fats, chemicals and preservatives. Rest assured, though, this version of the perfect summer side dish is as good for you as it is easy to make. I recommend serving up a big batch at your next picnic or BBQ!

2 lbs (908 g) sweet potatoes (about 4 medium), peeled and cut into 1-inch pieces

2 medium apples, diced into 1-inch pieces

2 ribs celery, diced into ½-inch pieces

4 scallions, thinly sliced crosswise

⅓ cup (80 ml) golden raisins

¼ cup (60 ml) finely chopped flat leaf parsley

3 Tbsp (45 ml) cider vinegar

1 Tbsp (15 ml) extra virgin olive oil

½ tsp (2.5 ml) Dijon mustard

Pinch curry powder

Pinch smoked paprika

½ tsp (2.5 ml) sea salt

¼ tsp (1.25 ml) freshly ground black pepper

Place sweet potatoes in a large pot or Dutch oven and cover with cold water. Put on stove and bring to a boil on high heat. Reduce heat to simmer and cook potatoes until just tender, about 7 minutes. Drain, transfer to a large bowl and let cool slightly.

Add apples, celery, scallions, raisins and parsley.

In a separate small bowl, whisk together vinegar, olive oil, Dijon mustard, curry powder, smoked paprika, salt and pepper. Pour over sweet potato salad and toss gently to coat.

CHILL OUT
This salad can be served immediately or refrigerated for up to three days.

NUTRITIONAL VALUE PER SERVING:
Calories: 128 | Calories from Fat: 14 | Protein: 2 g | Carbs: 27 g | Total Fat: 1.5 g |
Saturated Fat: 0.2 g | Trans Fat: 0 g | Fiber: 4 g | Sodium: 81 mg | Cholesterol: 0 mg

Warm Farro and Arugula Salad with Roasted Fennel, Delicata Squash and Red Onion

PREP: 30 minutes | **COOK:** 50 minutes | **YIELD:** 6 x 1-cup servings

Warm salads are perfect for fall and winter enjoyment. Their ingredients are typically wholesome and hearty, but they won't leave you feeling weighed down and in need of a post-meal nap. The lightness of farro paired with the digestive encouragement of fennel make this a warming salad that benefits you from the inside out.

½ cup (120 ml) uncooked farro, rinsed

1 large bulb fennel, cut lengthwise into 8 wedges

½ large delicata squash, rind washed well and left on, quartered lengthwise and cut crosswise into ½-inch slices

1 medium red onion, peeled and root end trimmed but left intact, halved through each axis, and each half cut into 6 wedges (12 wedges total)

Eat-Clean Cooking Spray (see p. 277)

4 cups (950 ml) baby arugula

1 large pink grapefruit, segmented, membrane reserved

1 tsp (5 ml) Dijon mustard

1 Tbsp (15 ml) extra virgin olive oil

Pinch each sea salt and freshly ground black pepper

Cook farro according to package directions, or bring 3 cups (710 ml) of water to boil on high heat and add farro. Reduce heat to simmer, stirring occasionally, for 25 to 50 minutes (cooking time will vary depending on the brand), until tender but still chewy. Drain in a fine mesh sieve, rinse under cold water, drain again and set aside.

In the meantime, heat oven to 450°F (230°C). Spread prepared fennel, squash and onion in a single layer on one or two baking sheets. Spray vegetables with Eat-Clean Cooking Spray and season with salt and pepper. Roast in oven for about 20 minutes or until golden brown at the edges and cooked through, stirring once. If vegetables look like they're getting dry while cooking, mist with a little more Eat-Clean Cooking Spray. Once done, remove and set aside to cool slightly.

To a large bowl, add arugula and grapefruit segments. Add roasted fennel, squash, red onions and cooked farro.

Squeeze juice from reserved grapefruit membrane into a small bowl. Discard membrane. Add mustard, olive oil and salt and pepper. Whisk together and pour over salad. Toss gently to combine.

PREP TIP
When baking the fennel, squash and onion, make sure they are spread out in a single layer and not crowded in any way, otherwise they won't cook evenly.

NUTRITIONAL VALUE PER SERVING:
Calories: 127 | Calories from Fat: 27 | Protein: 4 g | Carbs: 23 g | Total Fat: 3 g | Saturated Fat: 0.3 g | Trans Fat: 0 g | Fiber: 4 g | Sodium: 57 mg | Cholesterol: 0 mg

Macronutrients: the BIG Picture

When you adopt a vegetarian lifestyle, you will have to pay close attention to getting enough nutrients. Finding balance will take your health and wellness to the next level. The big picture items are the macronutrients we rely on every day to maintain our steadily burning metabolism. These include protein, fat, and carbohydrates – they give us what we need to burn baby burn all day long!

All Eyes on Protein

Protein is our friend. It builds us, maintains us, helps us communicate both inside and out, and much more. But how do we get enough of it? Getting adequate protein can be hard when eating a vegetarian diet. Vegetarians who have excluded all or most animal proteins normally choose sources that are not easy for the body to extract and use. I've written an entire information page on protein (p. 144) for help on choosing the best sources.

Get a variety of protein sources throughout the day. And don't just stop there. Keep a close eye on the way you are feeling – are you tired, fatigued, overly sore, or not recovering well from your workouts? While these symptoms may result from many other causes, too little protein is a common culprit, especially among vegetarians. So don't let those beautiful muscles you are sculpting wilt away. Get your protein, eat it, and be able to use it too!

Fat Is Good!

When we hear the word "fat" we have been conditioned to instantly think of a wobbly, wiggly mass of flesh hobbling down the street. But this is far from being its only form. Fat is a primeval food. When there were no grocery stores, primitive peoples ate animal protein, plants growing in the ground and in the sea, and they ate fat too, in abundance. Understand something very simple – fat is survival food. Without it we lose our ability to think, to make hormones, to function or to have a decent quality of health and life. Certain vitamins (think A, D, E and K) are fat soluble, and you will not be able to use them without fat in your diet. If you want moist skin, you need fat. If you want your metabolism to operate efficiently, you need fat. If you want to stay warm, you need fat. If you want to have sex, you need fat. If you want your food to taste good, you need fat. If you want to have cushioning and protection for your organs, you need fat. Your brain loves fat – it is made up mostly of fat, and so are your nerves.

Fat is not the evil it is purported to be, unless it comes from concentrated feedlot animals, deep-fried foods, rancid oils and nuts, hydrogenated or trans sources. You should avoid these sources like the plague. Bacteria do. Try this test for yourself: Put a dish of butter on the counter and leave it there for a week or two. You will see organisms growing on the butter because there are nutrients in the butter they love. Smart! Now do the same with a dish of margarine. It will sit for a century collecting dust and melting into a puddle, but nothing will eat it. Smart little bacteria. Why would you want to eat something even single-celled creatures wouldn't touch?

Mono and polyunsaturated fats (from olive oil, pumpkinseed oil, grapeseed oil, seeds, nuts and nut butters, in addition to fish and fish oils) are excellent forms of healthy fat, which can be consumed on a daily basis in moderate amounts. Saturated fats (from coconut oil and avocados, in addition to meats) are also important, but should be consumed in much smaller amounts.

So when do you eat which kind of fat? Stick to mainly unsaturated fats. I use about one tablespoon of olive oil on my salads to ensure I am getting all of the vitamins out of the veggies, two tablespoons of flaxseed on my oatmeal in the morning for

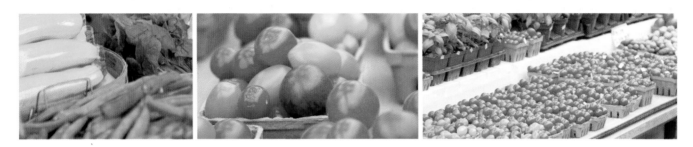

healthy heart and colon function, one tablespoon of nut butter or a handful of nuts and seeds as a snack most days of the week, and one tablespoon of coconut oil when cooking dinner. I also have fish once or twice each week, and fish oil supplements daily.

So you see you don't need to eat loads of fat, but you do need to eat the right kinds of fat in moderation on a daily basis for optimal health.

The Right Kinds of Carbohydrates

When you choose to follow a vegetarian diet it's important to ensure your diet is as balanced as possible. One thing to watch carefully is your intake of starchy carbohydrates from whole grains. Many people follow what they call a "vegetarian" diet that is actually extremely low in vegetables. They fill their plates with pasta, bread and rice, often with high-saturated-fat cheese piled on top. Without careful monitoring of starch intake, vegetarians run the risk of seriously damaging their health. First of all they can become deficient in any number of the important elements mentioned on p. 240. They also bring themselves closer to developing type II diabetes. I remember my daughter telling me the story of her classmate, who considered herself to be very healthy as a vegetarian until she was diagnosed with Type II Diabetes. Her doctor chalked it up to a vegetarian diet too high in carbohydrates from whole grains and too low in lean protein, fruit and, most importantly, veggies!

If you are choosing to follow a vegetarian diet, it is important that you manage your starchy carbohydrate intake. Your plate should be full of veggies, balanced with legumes and other protein sources, along with small amounts of starches such as sweet potatoes or brown rice. After all, the word isn't "vege"tarian for nothing!

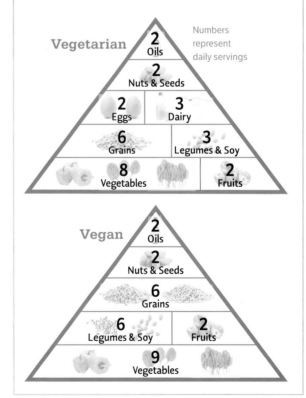

Portion Sizes

Oils – 2 Tbsp
Nuts & Seeds – 1 handful
Dairy – ½ to 1 cup low fat
Eggs – 2-3 eggs
Legumes & Soy – 1 handful
Fruit – 1 handful
Vegetables – 2 handfuls
Grains – 1 handful

Vegetarian — Numbers represent daily servings

2 Oils
2 Nuts & Seeds
2 Eggs | 3 Dairy
6 Grains | 3 Legumes & Soy
8 Vegetables | 2 Fruits

Vegan

2 Oils
2 Nuts & Seeds
6 Grains
6 Legumes & Soy | 2 Fruits
9 Vegetables

Savory Soups &
One Pot Meals

Hawaiian Curry with Sweet
Potatoes and Bananas p. 94

Hawaiian Curry with Sweet Potatoes and Bananas

PREP: 20 minutes | **COOK:** 18-23 minutes | **YIELD:** 6 servings

Aloha! Get ready to enjoy a curry so delicious you might just have to book a trip to Hawaii to test its authenticity! And this dish has more than just a pretty taste – it is full of vegetables, hearty whole grains and beans, making it one of the healthiest curries around.

1 Tbsp (15 ml) raw unrefined coconut oil

1 sweet onion, chopped

1 rib celery, chopped

1 carrot, chopped

1 clove garlic, finely chopped

1 Tbsp (15 ml) fresh ginger, peeled and grated

1 Tbsp (15 ml) curry powder

½ tsp (2.5 ml) cayenne

¾ tsp (3.75 ml) sea salt

¼ tsp (1.25 ml) black pepper

2 cups cooked, drained and rinsed or 1 x 15-oz (440 ml) BPA-free can kidney beans, drained and rinsed

12 oz (340 g) extra firm tofu, drained and diced into 1-inch cubes

1 large garnet red sweet potato, peeled and diced into ½-inch pieces

1 x 13.5-oz (405 ml) BPA-free can light unsweetened coconut milk

½ cup (120 ml) golden raisins

½ cup (120 ml) chopped walnuts

½ cup (120 ml) flaked unsweetened coconut

2 bananas, sliced into ¼-inch rounds

3 cups (710 ml) steamed brown jasmine rice

Heat coconut oil in a large, heavy-bottomed pot on medium. Add onion, celery, carrot, garlic, ginger, curry powder, cayenne, salt and pepper, and allow rice to sweat until onion is soft and translucent, about 3 minutes.

Add kidney beans, tofu, sweet potato, coconut milk and raisins, and stir to combine. Cover and simmer for 15 to 20 minutes or until sweet potato is tender.

In the meantime, toast walnuts and flaked coconut in a preheated 350°F (175°C) oven until golden brown, about 3 minutes.

To serve, spoon ½ cup (120 ml) rice into each bowl and ladle Hawaiian Curry over top. Top with banana slices and sprinkle with chopped walnuts and flaked coconut.

NUTRITIONAL VALUE PER SERVING (1 CUP CURRY + ½ CUP RICE):
Calories: 571 | Calories from Fat: 169 | Protein: 20 g | Carbs: 79 g | Total Fat: 19 g | Saturated Fat: 7 g | Trans Fat: 0 g | Fiber: 15 g | Sodium: 222 mg | Cholesterol: 0 mg

Avocado Gazpacho

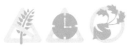

PREP: 20 minutes | **COOK:** 0 minutes | **YIELD:** 6 x ⅔-cup servings

This no-cook soup is full of zing and packed with goodies! It's also served cold, which makes it perfect for enjoying on hot summer days. Plus, it's a great way to clear your fridge of any leftover veggies. Practical and delicious… what could be better?

1 avocado, pitted and diced

¾ lb (340 g) ripe tomatoes (about 3 medium), diced

1 green bell pepper, seeded and diced

½ English cucumber, diced

¼ red onion, finely diced

1 clove garlic, passed through a garlic press or very finely minced

1 x 5.5-oz (165 ml) BPA-free can low-sodium tomato juice

3 Tbsp (45 ml) red wine vinegar

1 Tbsp (15 ml) aged sherry vinegar

2 Tbsp (30 ml) fresh lemon juice

¼ tsp (1.25 ml) sea salt

½ tsp (2.5 ml) freshly ground black pepper

Dash hot sauce, or to taste

Place all ingredients in a food processor or blender and pulse-chop until blended but still chunky. Taste, and make any adjustments to seasoning with more vinegar, lemon juice and/or hot sauce. Refrigerate for three hours and then serve chilled.

CHILL OUT
This soup will last in the fridge up to three days – the flavors will meld and improve as it sits.

NUTRITIONAL VALUE PER SERVING:
Calories: 69 | Calories from Fat: 34 | Protein: 2 g | Carbs: 8 g | Total Fat: 4 g |
Saturated Fat: 0.4 g | Trans Fat: 0 g | Fiber: 2 g | Sodium: 105 mg | Cholesterol: 0 mg

Broccoli "Cheddar" Soup

PREP: 10 minutes | **COOK:** 38 minutes | **YIELD:** 4 x 1-cup servings

Any meal that encourages the consumption of broccoli is fine by me. In fact, the more the better! But to make this classic soup as vegetarian-friendly as possible, we've removed the cheddar cheese and replaced it with nutritional yeast. After trying this, I think you'll agree that sometimes even the classics can be improved upon.

2 Tbsp (30 ml) extra virgin olive oil

1 medium yellow onion, chopped

1 clove garlic, chopped

2 Tbsp (30 ml) whole wheat flour

1½ cups (360 ml) low-fat milk, plain
    unsweetened soy milk, almond milk
    or other milk substitute

1½ cups (360 ml) low-sodium vegetable broth

2 bay leaves

¼ tsp (1.25 ml) fresh grated nutmeg

½ tsp (2.5 ml) sea salt

½ tsp (2.5 ml) pepper

1 large carrot, peeled and chopped

½ lb (225 g) broccoli, chopped

¼ cup (60 ml) nutritional yeast

Heat olive oil in a Dutch oven or soup pot on medium. Add onion and garlic, and cook until onion is translucent but not brown, about 3 minutes. Stir in flour. Whisk in milk and vegetable broth until thoroughly combined and no lumps remain.

Add bay leaves, nutmeg, salt and pepper. Increase heat to bring broth to a boil, then cover, reduce heat to simmer, and cook for about 20 minutes, stirring occasionally to make sure the bottom isn't burning. Remove bay leaves and discard. Add carrot and broccoli, and stir.

Cover and simmer about 15 minutes longer, or until veggies are tender. Uncover, add nutritional yeast, and blend using a handheld immersion blender or a stand blender, working in batches, if necessary. Ladle into bowls and serve hot.

NUTRITIONAL VALUE PER SERVING:
Calories: 202 | Calories from Fat: 77 | Protein: 10 g | Carbs: 24 g | Total Fat: 9 g |
Saturated Fat: 2 g | Trans Fat: 0 g | Fiber: 6 g | Sodium: 378 mg | Cholesterol: 6 mg

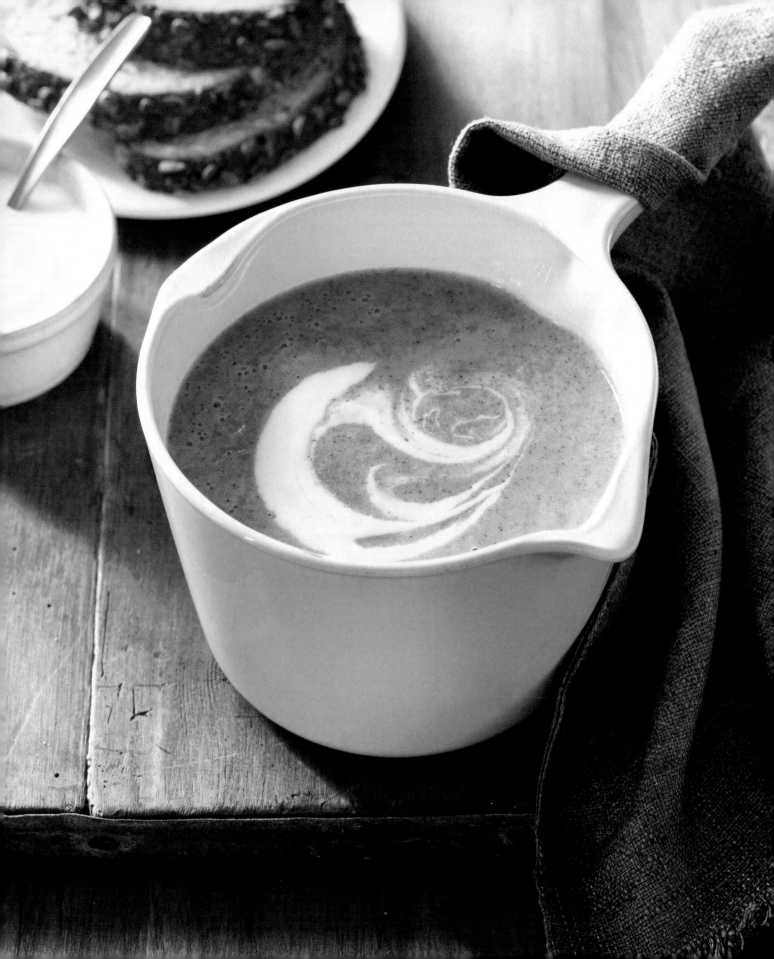

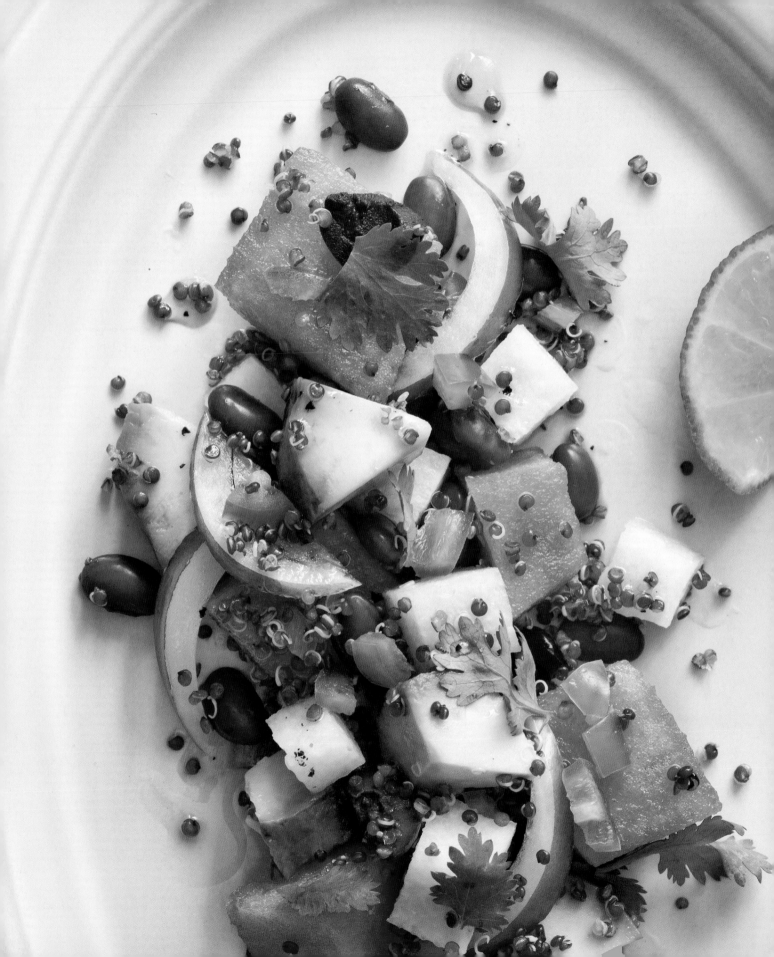

Mexican Fiesta Bowl

PREP: 20 minutes | **COOK:** 20 minutes | **YIELD:** 5 x 2-cup servings

This dish has everything to make a complete meal. And there are so many fresh flavors and textures that each bite is like a fiesta in your mouth. Arriba!

½ cup (120 ml) red quinoa

1 cup (240 ml) diced jicama

¼ cup (60 ml) diced red onion

½ cup (120 ml) coarsely chopped black olives

½ cup (120 ml) chopped cilantro

2 cups cooked, drained and rinsed or 1 x 15-oz (440 ml) BPA-free can black beans, drained and rinsed

1 avocado, diced

3 cups (710 ml) diced watermelon

1 jalapeño, seeds and ribs removed, finely diced

Juice of 1 lime

2 tsp (10 ml) avocado oil or extra virgin olive oil

2 tsp (10 ml) white balsamic vinegar

2 tsp (10 ml) honey, brown rice syrup or yacon syrup

½ tsp (2.5 ml) ground cumin

¼ tsp (1.25 ml) each sea salt and freshly ground black pepper

In a small saucepan, combine quinoa and 1 cup (240 ml) water and simmer, covered, until plumped up and all water is absorbed, about 15 minutes. Remove from heat and let sit for about 5 minutes. To a large bowl, add jicama and the rest of the ingredients up to and including jalapeño. Fluff quinoa with a fork and add to bowl.

In a small bowl, whisk together lime juice, avocado or olive oil, vinegar, honey or syrup, cumin, salt and pepper. Pour over the ingredients in the large bowl and toss to combine. Serve immediately.

NUTRITIONAL VALUE PER SERVING:
Calories: 296 | Calories from Fat: 99 | Protein: 9 g | Carbs: 42 g | Total Fat: 11 g |
Saturated Fat: 1.5 g | Trans Fat: 0 g | Fiber: 11 g | Sodium: 167 mg | Cholesterol: 0 mg

Butternut and Bean Soup

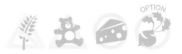

PREP: 10 minutes | **COOK:** 40 minutes | **YIELD:** 8 x 1-cup servings

This soup is thick and creamy thanks to the beans, which also lend a healthy dose of protein and fiber. It is also a great make-ahead dish: If you blend it ahead of time, all you have to do is heat and eat when hunger strikes. See below for an additional time-saving trick.

1 butternut squash, about 3 lbs (1.36 kg), halved
    lengthwise and seeds scooped out
Eat-Clean Cooking Spray (see p. 277)
1 tsp (5 ml) extra virgin olive oil
1 onion, halved and thinly sliced
1 tsp (5 ml) herbes de Provence
1 clove garlic, minced
2 cups cooked, drained and rinsed or 1 x 15-oz
    (440 ml) can cannellini beans or white
    kidney beans
1½ cups (360 ml) low-fat milk, plain
    unsweetened soy milk, almond milk or
    other milk substitute
½ tsp (2.5 ml) ground cinnamon
¼ tsp (1.25 ml) ground cumin
Pinch freshly grated nutmeg
Pinch cayenne
½ tsp (2.5 ml) sea salt
¼ tsp (1.25 ml) pepper
¼ tsp (1.25 ml) pure vanilla extract

Preheat oven to 400°F (200°C). Spray the flesh of the squash with Eat-Clean Cooking Spray and place on a baking sheet, flesh side down. Bake until tender when pierced with a skewer, about 40 minutes. Remove and let cool until comfortable to handle.

While the squash cools, heat olive oil in a large skillet on medium high. Add onion and herbes de Provence, and cook, stirring occasionally, until starting to brown, about 3 minutes. Reduce heat to medium and continue to cook until very soft and well browned, 5 to 10 minutes more. Stir in garlic and cook for 2 or 3 minutes or until fragrant. Transfer to a blender.

Scoop squash out of skin and transfer to blender. Add beans, milk, spices, salt, pepper and vanilla extract. Blend until very smooth. Transfer the soup to a pot and bring to a gentle simmer to heat through. The soup is ready to serve.

TIME SAVER
Want to cut down on the cooking time for this soup? Substitute 4 cups (950 ml) puréed pumpkin (not the pie mix) or sweet potato purée. You can have the soup ready to eat in less than 20 minutes.

NUTRITIONAL VALUE PER SERVING:
Calories: 156 | Calories from Fat: 18 | Protein: 2 g | Carbs: 25 g | Total Fat: 2 g |
Saturated Fat: 0.5 g | Trans Fat: 0 g | Fiber: 1 g | Sodium: 274 mg | Cholesterol: 2 mg

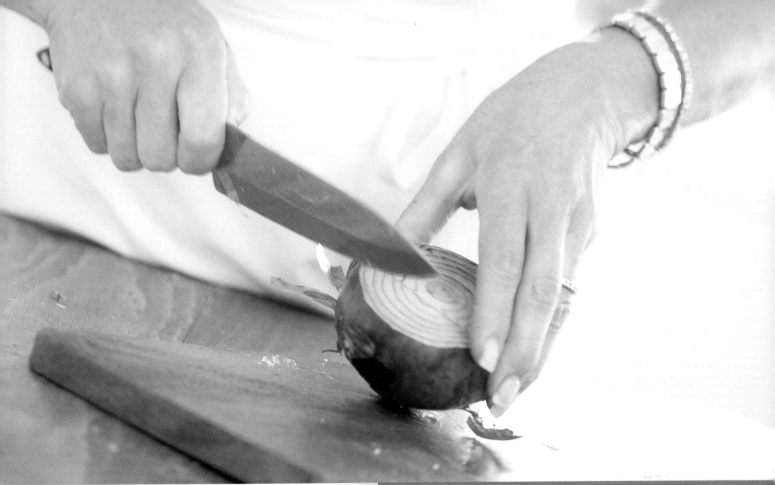

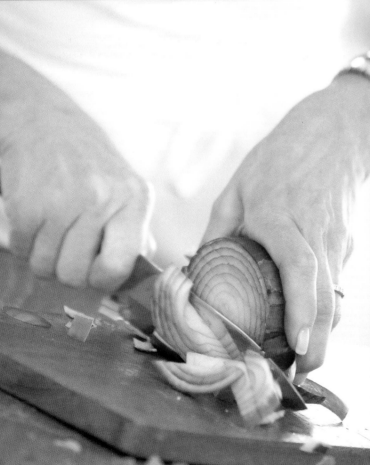

"Your best weapon against the waterworks that come with chopping onions? A very sharp chef's knife because it causes less damage to cell walls, which means fewer tear-inducing enzymes are released."

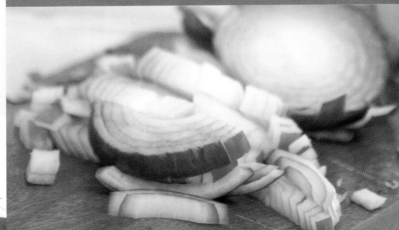

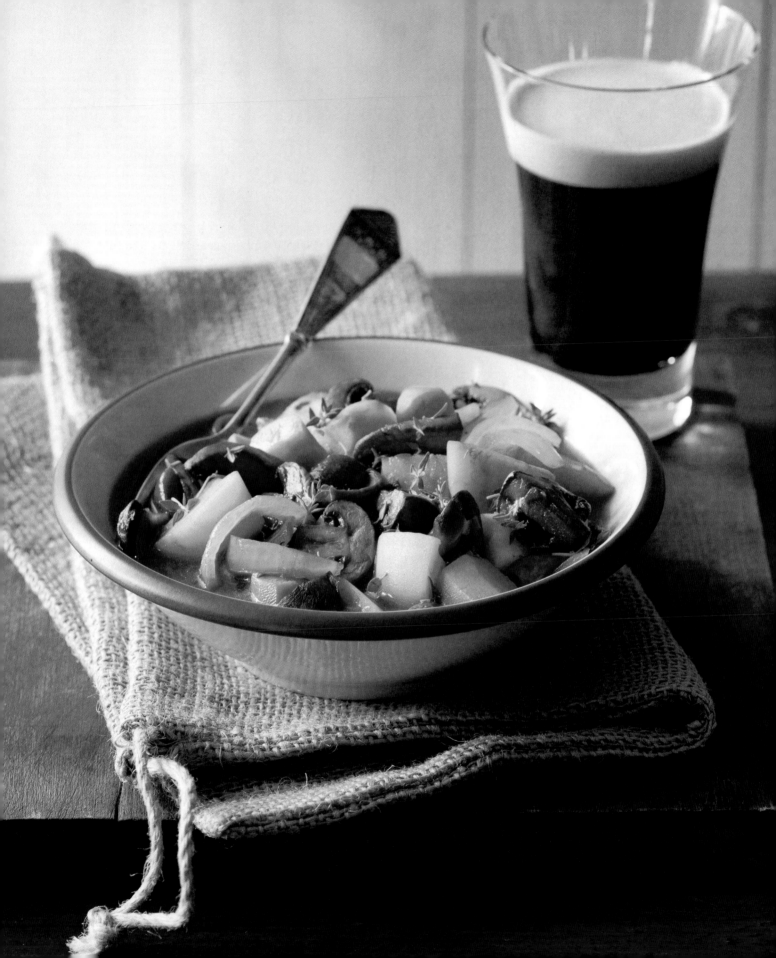

St. Patrick's Day Celebration Stew

PREP: 30 minutes | **COOK:** 40 minutes | **YIELD:** 8 x 1½-cup servings

Of course you aren't limited to enjoying this stew only on St. Patty's Day, but that celebration does beg for it. After all, who wouldn't want a little Irish beer in their meal? What a treat!

2 Tbsp (30 ml) extra virgin olive oil, divided

2 large Portobello mushrooms, stems removed, gills scraped out, cut into 1-inch pieces

½ lb (225 g) cremini mushrooms, quartered

6 cloves garlic, minced

½ cup (120 ml) dry red wine

1 cup (240 ml) dark Irish beer, such as Guinness

6 cups (1.44 L) low-sodium mushroom broth

2 Tbsp (30 ml) chopped fresh thyme

1 Tbsp (15 ml) Bragg's Liquid Aminos

2 Tbsp (30 ml) vegan Worcestershire sauce

2 Tbsp (30 ml) tomato paste

2 bay leaves

1 large onion, quartered and sliced

2 large carrots, peeled and cut into ½-inch pieces

2 large parsnips, peeled and cut into ½-inch pieces

2 russet potatoes, peeled and diced into ¾-inch pieces

GARNISH

Freshly ground black pepper

Finely chopped Italian flat leaf parsley

In a large soup pot or Dutch oven, work in batches heating ½ to 1 Tbsp (7.5 to 15 ml) olive oil on medium and adding a single layer of mushrooms to cook until brown, about 3 minutes. Transfer to a bowl and repeat with more olive oil and mushrooms until they're all cooked. Return all the mushrooms to pot and stir in garlic. Cook until fragrant, about 1 minute. Add wine and beer, and scrape up any crusty bits that might have formed on bottom of pot.

Add broth and remaining ingredients, stirring to combine. Increase heat and bring stew to a boil, then reduce heat and simmer partially covered. Cook for about 30 minutes or until vegetables are tender, stirring occasionally. Remove bay leaves and discard. Ladle stew into bowls and garnish with pepper and parsley.

CHILL OUT
Leftovers will be even better the next day, and will keep up to three days in the fridge.

NUTRITIONAL VALUE PER SERVING:
Calories: 169 | Calories from Fat: 42 | Protein: 4 g | Carbs: 26 g | Total Fat: 5 g | Saturated Fat: 0.5 g | Trans Fat: 0 g | Fiber: 5 g | Sodium: 328 mg | Cholesterol: 0 mg

Elegant Mushroom and Winter Vegetable Stew

PREP: 30 minutes | **COOK:** 45 minutes | **YIELD:** 12 x 1-cup servings

Love mushrooms? Then this is the recipe for you! This warm and hearty stew is packed full of our little fungi friends (and a few of my favorite winter root vegetables for good measure). This is a true immune-boosting stew that's perfect for cold winter days.

½ cup (120 ml) dried morel mushrooms

½ cup (120 ml) dried porcini mushrooms

2 cups (480 ml) boiling water

2½ Tbsp (37.5 ml) extra virgin olive oil, divided

1 lb (454 g) cremini mushrooms, quartered or halved if small

1 lb (454 g) portobello mushrooms, stemmed, gills scraped out and cut into 1-inch pieces

½ lb (225 g) shiitake mushrooms, stemmed and quartered, or halved if small

1 leek, white and light green parts only, washed well, thinly sliced crosswise

2 carrots, peeled and cut into ½-inch pieces

6 cloves garlic, minced

3 Tbsp (45 ml) Cognac (optional)

4 cups (950 ml) low-sodium mushroom broth, gluten free if necessary

1 Tbsp (15 ml) Dijon mustard

1 Tbsp (15 ml) vegan Worcestershire sauce

1½ Tbsp (22.5 ml) Bragg's Liquid Aminos

1 tsp (5 ml) tomato paste

2 bay leaves

1 cup (240 ml) each parsnip, rutabaga and celery root, cut into ½-inch pieces

2 tsp (10 ml) each finely chopped fresh savory, sage and marjoram

½ tsp (2.5 ml) finely chopped fresh rosemary

¾ tsp (3.75 ml) freshly ground black pepper

2 cups (480 ml) frozen pearl onions

1 tsp (5 ml) aged sherry vinegar

Optional: Truffle-infused extra virgin olive oil, to garnish

In a small bowl, place morel and porcini mushrooms and cover with boiling water. Set aside to rehydrate.

In a Dutch oven or large heavy-bottomed soup pot, heat 1 Tbsp (15 ml) olive oil on medium. Add half of cremini, Portobello and shiitake mushrooms. Cook, stirring rarely, until browned, about 5 minutes. Transfer to a bowl. Repeat with an additional 1 Tbsp (15 ml) olive oil and remaining fresh mushrooms. Transfer to the same bowl.

Heat remaining ½ Tbsp (7.5 ml) olive oil. Add leek and carrots, and cook, stirring rarely, until lightly browned and starting to soften, about 5 minutes. Stir in garlic and cook about 1 minute longer. Add Cognac, if using, and use a wooden spoon to scrape up any crusty bits that have formed on bottom of pot. Add mushroom broth and remaining ingredients up to and including black pepper. Strain mushroom-rehydrating liquid through a chinoise or China cap (if you don't have one, see Equipment Tip below). Add mushrooms and strained liquid to the stew.

Increase heat and bring stew to a boil. Cover, reduce heat to simmer and cook for about 25 minutes or until vegetables are tender. Stir in pearl onions, cover and cook about 5 minutes longer. Remove bay leaves and stir in sherry vinegar.

Ladle into bowls and sprinkle with a few drops of truffle oil if desired. Serve warm.

EQUIPMENT TIP
A chinoise and China cap are both cone-shaped strainers made with extremely fine mesh and small perforated holes, respectively. If you don't have either, just line a fine mesh strainer with four layers of cheesecloth and you'll be good to go!

CHILL OUT
This soup will keep in the refrigerator for up to five days.

NUTRITIONAL VALUE PER SERVING:
Calories: 168 | Calories from Fat: 34 | Protein: 7 g | Carbs: 22 g | Total Fat: 4 g | Saturated Fat: 0.6 g | Trans Fat: 0 g | Fiber: 5 g | Sodium: 253 mg | Cholesterol: 0 mg

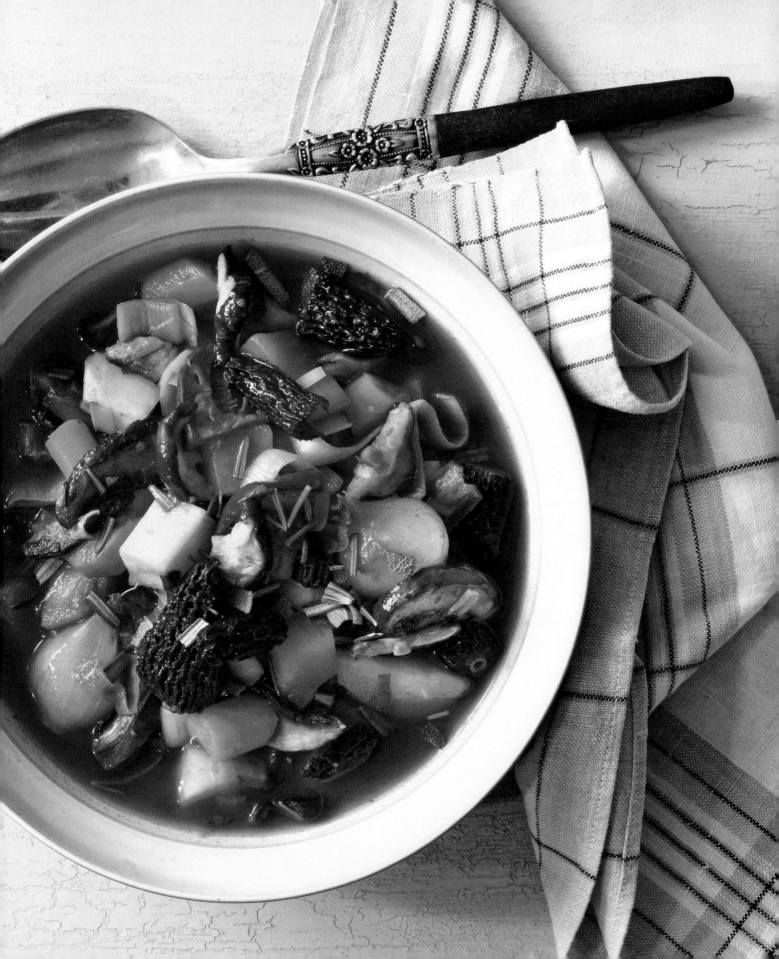

Catalan Lentil and Vegetable Soup

PREP: 25 minutes | **COOK:** 35-45 minutes | **YIELD:** 8 x 1½-cup servings

Catalan lentils are a brown variety of the pulse family. They are tasty and pair well with the crunchy sweetness of the onion, celery, carrots and bell pepper found in this soup. Perfect for a casual lunch on a cold day or even entertaining, this bowl of goodness will leave your guests satisfied and nourished from the inside out!

2 Tbsp (30 ml) extra virgin olive oil

1 large onion, finely chopped

2 cups finely chopped celery, including leaves

2 cups peeled, finely chopped carrots

1 red bell pepper, seeded and finely chopped

½ tsp (2.5 ml) each sea salt and freshly ground black pepper

4 cloves garlic, minced

1 lb (454 g) brown lentils, rinsed and picked through

1 tsp (5 ml) smoked paprika

¼ tsp (1.25 ml) cayenne

2 bay leaves

4 cups (950 ml) low-sodium vegetable broth, gluten free if necessary

1 Tbsp (15 ml) tomato paste

1 Tbsp (15 ml) Bragg's Liquid Aminos

2 Tbsp (30 ml) aged sherry vinegar

Finely chopped flat leaf parsley, to garnish

Heat olive oil in a very large heavy-bottomed soup pot or Dutch oven on medium high. Add onion, celery, carrots, red bell pepper, salt and pepper. Cook, stirring occasionally, until soft and decreased in volume but not brown, about 10 minutes.

Stir in garlic and cook for 1 or 2 minutes longer. Add lentils, paprika, cayenne, bay leaves, vegetable broth, 5 cups (1.2 L) water and tomato paste. Bring soup to a gentle boil, then cover, tilting the lid to allow steam to escape. Reduce heat to simmer, stirring occasionally until lentils are tender, 25 to 30 minutes.

Occasionally skim foam that appears on the surface and discard it. When lentils are cooked through, turn off heat and stir in Bragg's Liquid Aminos and sherry vinegar. The soup will be thick. If you desire more liquid, stir in more vegetable broth or water ½ cup (120 ml) at a time until desired consistency is achieved.

Taste soup and make any adjustments to seasoning with salt, pepper and/or sherry vinegar. Ladle into bowls and serve with a sprinkle of finely chopped flat leaf parsley.

CHILL OUT
This soup will keep in the refrigerator for up to five days, or in the freezer for three months.

NUTRITIONAL VALUE PER SERVING:
Calories: 144 | Calories from Fat: 35 | Protein: 6 g | Carbs: 19 g | Total Fat: 4 g |
Saturated Fat: 0.6 g | Trans Fat: 0 g | Fiber: 7 g | Sodium: 354 mg | Cholesterol: 0 mg

Roman "Little Rag" Soup with Spinach

PREP: 10 minutes | **COOK:** 5 minutes | **YIELD:** 4 x 1¼-cup servings

This is an Italian egg drop soup called "stracciatella," which means "little rags," for the shapes the eggs form in the broth. It's super quick and easy to make, and is full of protein from the egg whites and spinach. When you need a meal in a hurry, this one is ready pronto!

4 cups (960 ml) low-sodium vegetable
    broth, divided
4 cups (950 ml) baby spinach, roughly chopped
5 egg whites
2 Tbsp (30 ml) semolina or farina
2 Tbsp (30 ml) freshly grated Parmesan cheese
1 Tbsp (15 ml) each chopped basil and
    flat leaf parsley
Pinch freshly grated nutmeg
Pinch sea salt and freshly ground black pepper

Heat 3½ cups (840 ml) of vegetable broth in a medium-sized, heavy-bottomed soup pot. Add spinach. In a bowl, whisk together reserved ½ cup (120 ml) vegetable broth, egg whites, semolina, Parmesan, basil, parsley, nutmeg, salt and pepper. Bring vegetable broth to a boil, and slowly pour in egg mixture. Remove pot from heat and slowly stir back and forth with a fork until "rags" appear. Ladle into bowls and serve.

NUTRITIONAL VALUE PER SERVING:
Calories: 60 | Calories from Fat: 7 | Protein: 7 g | Carbs: 7 g | Total Fat: 1 g |
Saturated Fat: 0.4 g | Trans Fat: 0 g | Fiber: 1.4 g | Sodium: 170 mg | Cholesterol: 2 mg

Split Pea Soup

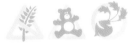

PREP: 15 minutes | **COOK:** 1½ hours | **YIELD:** 8 x 1-cup servings

This thick and comforting soup is full of warmth and flavor. Every spoonful boasts healthful ingredients to nourish you on the coldest of winter days.

1 Tbsp (15 ml) extra virgin olive oil
1 large onion, chopped
2 large carrots, peeled and chopped
2 ribs celery, chopped
2 cloves garlic, chopped
1½ cups (360 ml) green split peas,
    picked through and rinsed
5 cups (1.2 L) water
Pinch ground cloves
1 bay leaf
¾ tsp (3.75 ml) sea salt
½ tsp (2.5 ml) freshly ground black pepper
2 to 3 drops all-natural mesquite seasoning
    (liquid smoke)

In a heavy-bottomed soup pot, heat olive oil on medium. Add onion, carrots, celery and garlic, and cook for about 5 minutes, stirring. Add peas and remaining ingredients, and stir to combine. Increase heat and bring to a boil, then cover pot and reduce heat to simmer for about 1½ hours, or until peas are very tender. Stir pot occasionally to make sure nothing is sticking to bottom. Remove bay leaf and discard. Purée soup with a handheld immersion blender, or in batches in a blender until peas are smooth, but there are still little chunks of vegetables. Ladle into bowls and serve.

NUTRITIONAL VALUE PER SERVING:
Calories: 117 | Calories from Fat: 17 | Protein: 9 g | Carbs: 24 g | Total Fat: 2 g |
Saturated Fat: 0.3 g | Trans Fat: 0 g | Fiber: 9 g | Sodium: 131 mg | Cholesterol: 0 mg

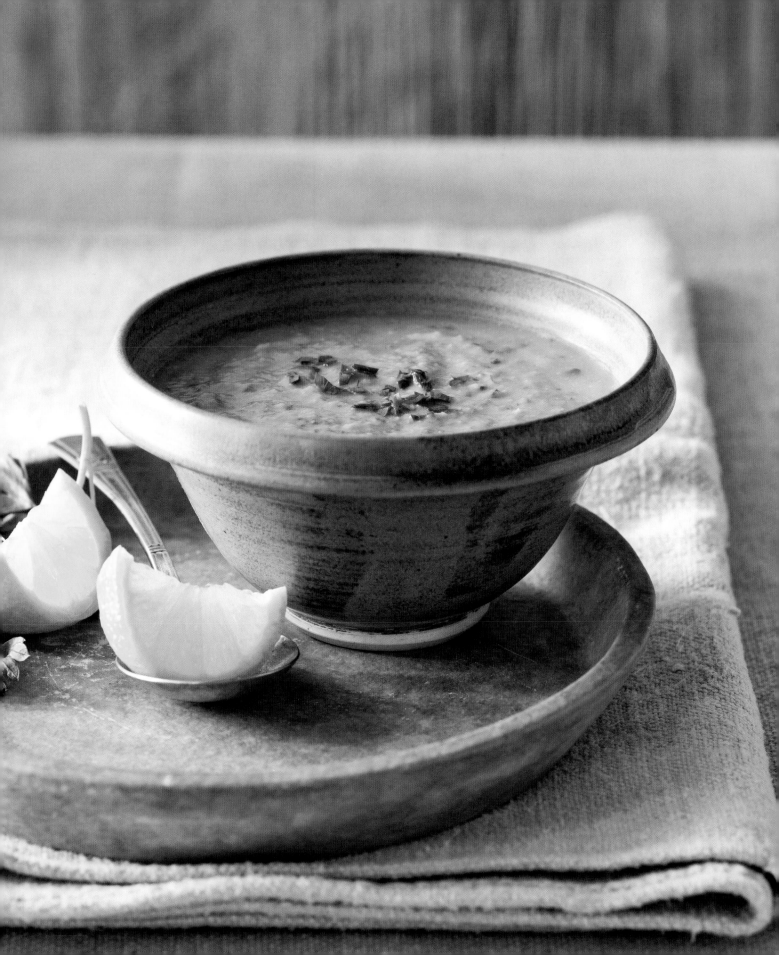

The Soup-er Cleanse

PREP: 15 minutes | **COOK:** 13-18 minutes | **YIELD:** 6 x 1-cup servings

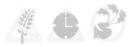

Need we say more? Full of nutrition and effective at cleansing out your digestive tract, this is a "soup-er" star recipe full of your favorite flavors.

1 Tbsp (15 ml) extra virgin olive oil

½ medium yellow onion, chopped

3 ribs celery, finely chopped

3 cloves garlic, chopped, divided

1 small zucchini, chopped

2 cups cooked or 1 x 15-oz (440 ml) BPA-free
    can no-salt chickpeas, drained and rinsed

1½ tsp (7.5 ml) ground cumin

Pinch cayenne

¾ tsp (3.75 ml) sea salt

½ tsp (2.5 ml) freshly ground black pepper

½ cup (120 ml) chopped raw walnuts

1 cup (240 ml) parsley, including stems,
    roughly chopped

Juice of 2 lemons

Heat olive oil in a heavy-bottomed soup pot on medium. Add onion, celery and two cloves of chopped garlic. Sweat for about 3 minutes or until onion is translucent. Add 3 cups (710 ml) water, zucchini, chickpeas, cumin, cayenne, salt and pepper, and bring to a simmer.

Cover and cook on low heat until vegetables are tender, 10 to 15 minutes.

Pour into a blender and add reserved clove of chopped garlic, walnuts, parsley and lemon juice. Blend until smooth, working in batches if necessary. Can be eaten hot or cold.

NUTRITIONAL VALUE PER SERVING:
Calories: 200 | Calories from Fat: 91 | Protein: 6 g | Carbs: 23 g | Total Fat: 10 g |
Saturated Fat: 1 g | Trans Fat: 0 g | Fiber: 5 g | Sodium: 364 mg | Cholesterol: 0 mg

Roasted Red Pepper Minestrone Soup

PREP: 30 minutes | **COOK:** 40 minutes | **YIELD:** 10 x 1½-cup servings

If there is one soup my family would reach for more than any other, this would be it! My kids, who are all in their 20s, still love the pasta shapes that make an appearance, but they also appreciate the variety of veggies a little more now.

1 Tbsp (15 ml) extra virgin olive oil

1 white or yellow onion, finely chopped

1 carrot, peeled, trimmed and finely chopped

½ tsp (2.5 ml) each sea salt and freshly ground black pepper

4 cloves garlic, minced

¼ cup (60 ml) dry red wine (optional)

4 cups (950 ml) low-sodium vegetable broth

2 cups (480 ml) water

1 tsp (5 ml) dried Italian herbs

1 x 8-oz (240 ml) jar roasted bell peppers, drained and finely chopped

2 cups cooked or 1 x 15-oz (440 ml) BPA-free can no-salt-added diced tomatoes plus juice

2 cups cooked or 1 x 15-oz (440 ml) BPA-free can no-salt-added kidney beans, drained and rinsed

2 cups cooked or 1 x 15-oz (445 ml) BPA-free can no-salt-added great northern white beans, white kidney beans, or cannellini beans, drained and rinsed

1 medium zucchini, ends trimmed and diced

1 cup (240 ml) trimmed fresh or frozen green beans, cut into 2-inch pieces

2 bay leaves

2 Tbsp (30 ml) finely chopped fresh parsley

2 cups (480 ml) small-size whole grain pasta such as shells, elbow macaroni or petite penne, cooked al dente

4 cups (950 ml) baby spinach, lightly packed

Heat olive oil in a large soup pot or Dutch oven on medium. Add onion, carrot, salt and pepper, and cook until soft but not brown, about 5 minutes. Stir in garlic and cook about 1 minute longer. Add red wine and scrape up any crusty bits that might have formed on bottom of pot.

Add remaining ingredients up to, but not including, pasta. Increase heat to bring soup to a boil, then partially cover and reduce heat to simmer for about 30 minutes or until vegetables are tender. Uncover, remove bay leaves and stir in spinach. Ladle into bowls and sprinkle with cooked pasta.

PREP TIP
If you are serving all of the soup at once, you can stir the cooked pasta into the pot. If you are planning for leftovers, keep the pasta separate and stir it into each batch as you heat it up. This will prevent the pasta from getting mushy.

NUTRITIONAL VALUE PER SERVING:
Calories: 264 | Calories from Fat: 21 | Protein: 12 g | Carbs: 46 g | Total Fat: 2 g | Saturated Fat: 0.3 g | Trans Fat: 0 g | Fiber: 10 g | Sodium: 362 mg | Cholesterol: 0 mg

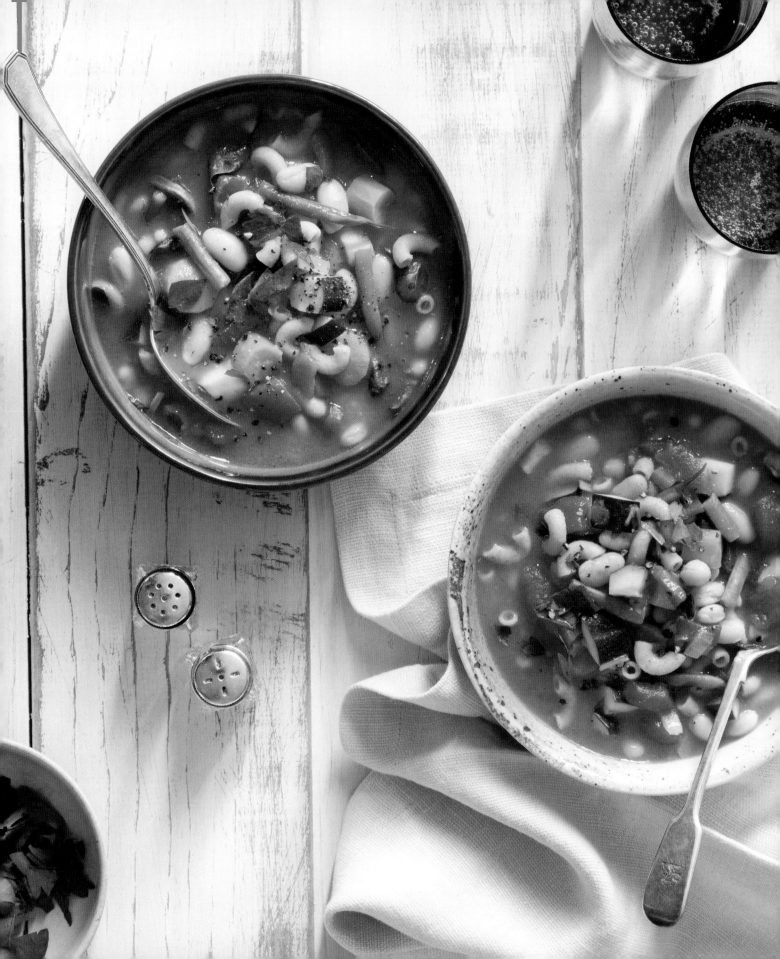

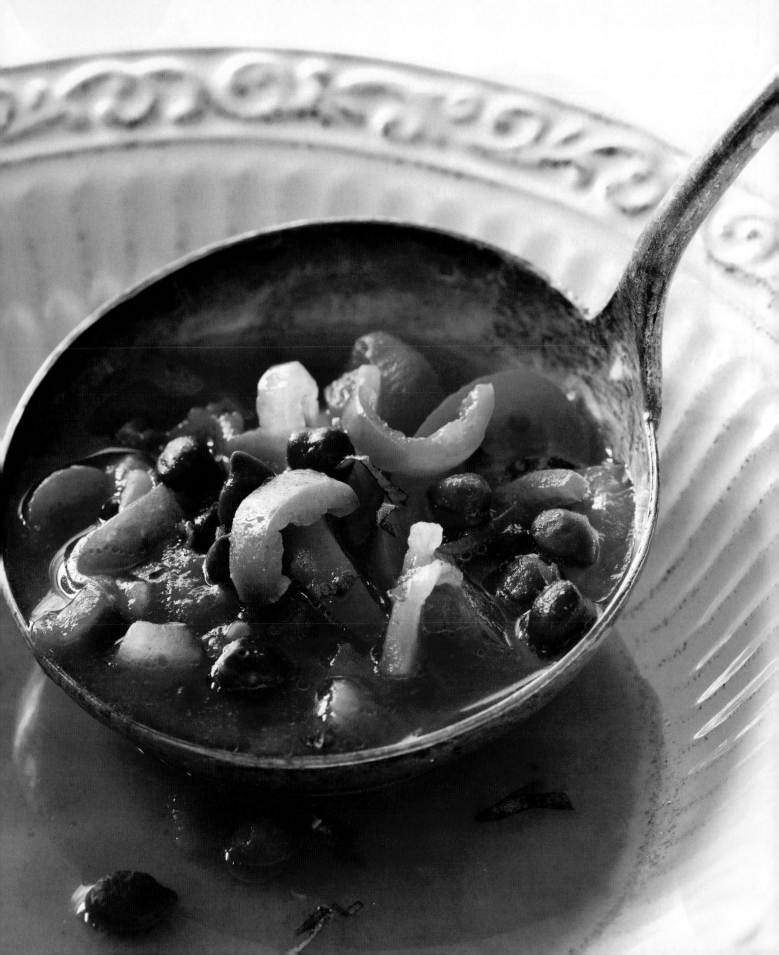

Mexican Pepper and Black Chickpea "Stoup"

PREP: 15 minutes + overnight soaking of chickpeas | **COOK:** 26 minutes | **YIELD:** 6 x 1½-cup servings

Are you wondering what a "stoup" is? It's a combination of a soup and stew – and that's just what this spicy Mexican dish is. Heartier than a soup, but not as thick as a stew, it's the perfect dish to warm up your body and wake up your taste buds.

1 cup (240 ml) black kabuli chickpeas, soaked overnight in plenty of water, drained and rinsed (use regular chickpeas if you cannot find black kabuli)

1 Tbsp (15 ml) extra virgin olive oil

1 onion, halved and thinly sliced

1 jalapeño, halved lengthwise and thinly sliced

½ red bell pepper, thinly sliced into 2-inch strips

¾ tsp (3.75 ml) sea salt

½ tsp (2.5 ml) black pepper

2 cloves garlic, chopped

2 tsp (10 ml) ground cumin

1 tsp (5 ml) chili powder

¼ tsp (1.25 ml) dried Mexican oregano

1 x 7-oz (210 ml) BPA-free can whole green chilis, drained and thinly sliced

1 x 28-oz (840 ml) BPA-free can no-salt-added diced tomatoes, including their juice

2 cups (480 ml) low-sodium vegetable broth, gluten free if necessary

1 bay leaf

ACCOMPANIMENTS (optional)

Lime wedges

Hot sauce

Plain low-fat yogurt

Drain soaked chickpeas, place them in a medium pot and cover with plenty of water. Simmer for 20 to 30 minutes or until just tender but still firm to the bite. Drain.

Heat olive oil in a large soup pot or Dutch oven on medium. Add onion, jalapeño, red bell pepper, salt and pepper, and cook about 5 minutes or until soft. Add garlic, cumin, chili powder and oregano, and cook for about 1 minute longer. Add chickpeas, green chilies, chopped tomatoes plus juice, vegetable broth and bay leaf. Simmer for about 20 minutes to let flavors combine. Ladle into bowls and serve with a wedge of lime, hot sauce and a dollop of yogurt, if desired.

NUTRITIONAL VALUE PER SERVING:
Calories: 134 | Calories from Fat: 28 | Protein: 4 g | Carbs: 22 g | Total Fat: 3 g | Saturated Fat: 0.4 g | Trans Fat: 0 g | Fiber: 4 g | Sodium: 324 mg | Cholesterol: 0 mg

Thriving Vegetarian Cultures

Vegetarianism isn't some new fancy craze. In fact, many cultures have been thriving on a vegetarian diet for centuries. The term vegetarian is itself English-based, but many cultures adopted vegetarian ways of eating without calling it vegetarianism.

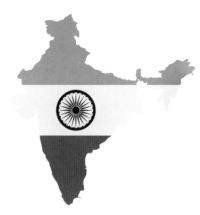

India most people have no issue with meat dishes, as long as the cow remains sacred. Indian culture has survived for years; in fact, India is currently one of the fastest-developing nations, and nearly a quarter of its population follows a vegetarian diet.

India

Centuries ago in India, Brahmins, also known as the priestly caste, swore to observe a meat-free lifestyle by the virtue of Ahimsa or non-violence. In Gujarat followers of the Jain faith employ the same principles of non-violence, non-absolutism and non-possession. They choose to eat meat-free, fish-free, egg-free diets and seldom use dairy products. Instead they feast on curries, Dhokra, Dal Bhajia and other dishes heavy in lentils and Ayurvedic spices to increase digestibility and bioavailability. Hindus in Rajasthan, Punjab, Haryana, and Uttar Pradesh also maintain a vegetarian lifestyle due to their faith. In other parts of

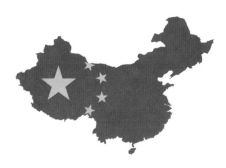

China

Buddhists thrive on the principles of mercy, respect and compassion for all living beings. They choose to follow a vegetarian diet for this reason. In China, where Buddhist culture maintains a stronghold today, you can find a host of vegetarian ingredients, including soy – miso, tempeh, soy milk, tofu, soy flour and soy cheese. While the issue is controversial, the high consumption of soy products in Buddhist, Chinese and Japanese diets

SPICE UP YOUR VEGETARIAN DIET

France – Bouquet garni – parsley, thyme and bay leaf

India – Garam masala – cumin, coriander seeds, cardamom, cloves, mace, cinnamon, bay leaf and black pepper

China – 5-spice powder – star anise, Sichuan pepper, cassia or cinnamon, fennel seeds and cloves

has appeared to reduce the discomfort of menopause while also reducing the incidence of breast cancer and coronary heart disease. According to Buddhist scripture, "All Buddhust disciples should abstain from killing, practice vegetarianism, and cultivate a spirit of great mercy. They should look upon all living beings in equality." They also believe in reincarnation, meaning injuring the soul of an animal could therefore harm the soul of a human inhabiting an animal. With a count of 312 million Buddhists worldwide, clearly they are surviving quite well on a vegetarian diet.

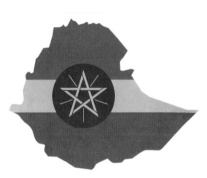

Ethiopia

Many Ethiopians incorporate vegetarianism into their lifestyle in a limited fashion. Orthodox Christians, making up 50 percent of the population, maintain a meat-free diet for 208 days of each year including Lent, one month of summer, and Wednesdays and Fridays of every week. Ethiopians receive much of their nutrition from t'ef (an Ethiopian ancient grain), wheat, barley, corn, sorghum and millet. T'ef is used to make the popular Injera bread – a staple of Ethiopian cuisine. T'ef itself is high in protein and minerals such as calcium. Ethiopians also rely on quite a few legumes as their principle source of protein. Of course, tons of vegetables make up the remainder of the colorful Ethiopian diet, including cabbage, carrots and greens that you scoop up with your hands and savor!

Health and prosperity can be maintained while living a vegetarian lifestyle, as demon-strated by the cultures listed above. If you're not ready to completely convert to vegetarianism, try to incorporate more legumes, vegetables and grains in your diet, including the occasional meat-free dish. Spice it up and you will no doubt be well on your way to a veggie-friendly lifestyle.

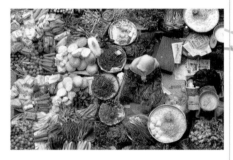

Other Parts of Southern Asia

Vegetarian cultures seem to thrive throughout Southern Asia. Large numbers of those living in Pakistan, Bangladesh and Malaysia follow a vegetarian lifestyle. Malaysia's unique combination of Chinese, Indian and European inhabitants fosters its vegetarian roots. These traditions are easily maintained because of the wealth of vegetables, fruits, seeds, pulses (lentils and other legumes), spices and sweeteners available in these parts. Like Malaysia, other areas of the world have seen their vegetarian populations soar because of a mix of cultures and availability of a variety of foods. This can certainly be said of the United States and Canada.

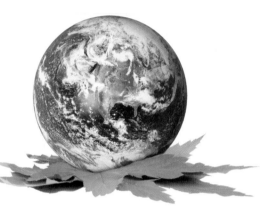

VEGETARIAN EATING WHEN TRAVELING

Traveling can throw a wrench into anyone's healthy diet, but it can be even more difficult when you are vegetarian. This is especially true in regions with strong cultural holds in meat eating. According to expatify.com, here are the top ten countries to visit that will fully support your vegetarian lifestyle:

Canada	Taiwan
Israel	Thailand
China	United Kingdom
India	United States
Malaysia	Vietnam

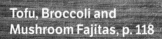
Tofu, Broccoli and
Mushroom Fajitas, p. 118

The Main
Course

Tofu, Broccoli and Mushroom Fajitas

PREP: 30 minutes | **COOK:** 30 minutes | **YIELD:** 8 fajitas

As you're probably well aware, tofu has the habit of taking on the flavors of whatever it is cooked with. In this quick and easy dish, the spices give the tofu a fajita-worthy kick that will definitely keep you coming back for more!

SEASONING

1 tsp (5 ml) ground cumin

1 tsp (5 ml) chili powder

½ tsp (2.5 ml) smoked paprika

½ tsp (2.5 ml) garlic powder

½ tsp (2.5 ml) each sea salt and freshly ground black pepper

1 green pepper, seeded and thinly sliced

2 poblano peppers, seeded and thinly sliced

1 orange or red pepper, seeded and thinly sliced

2 jalapeño peppers, seeded and thinly sliced (optional)

½ onion, thinly sliced

½ lb (225 g) cremini mushrooms, sliced, about 4 cups (950 ml)

4 cups (950 ml) broccoli florets, cut into large bite-sized pieces

2 lbs (908 g) extra-firm tofu, drained, pressed dry with paper towels, and cut into 1-inch cubes

2 Tbsp (30 ml) Bragg's Liquid Aminos

Eat-Clean Cooking Spray (see p. 277)

8 sprouted-grain tortillas, such as Ezekiel, warmed in the oven

Combine seasoning ingredients in a small bowl. You will use half of the seasoning for the vegetables (peppers, mushrooms and broccoli), and half for the tofu.

Heat a very large cast-iron skillet thoroughly on medium and spray with Eat-Clean Cooking Spray. Working in batches, add peppers to skillet in a single layer and sprinkle with a little of the seasoning. Cook for 3 to 5 minutes until lightly browned and tender-crisp, stirring occasionally. Transfer to a bowl, spray skillet with a little more Eat-Clean Cooking Spray, and repeat until all peppers are cooked. Now repeat this process with mushrooms, and then broccoli.

Wipe out skillet with a paper towel and return to heat. Spray with Eat-Clean Cooking Spray and add tofu. Sprinkle with remaining half batch of the seasoning. Cook, stirring occasionally, until heated through and lightly browned, about 3 minutes. Remove from heat and stir in Bragg's Liquid Aminos.

To build your fajitas, lay out tortillas and divide veggies among them, about 1 cup (240 ml) per tortilla, and top each with tofu. If desired, add some Mexican hot sauce and plain low-fat yogurt. Fold up and enjoy!

NUTRITIONAL VALUE PER SERVING (1 FAJITA WITH 4 OZ TOFU + 1 CUP VEGGIES):
Calories: 296 | Calories from Fat: 55 | Protein: 23 g | Carbs: 36 g | Total Fat: 6 g |
Saturated Fat: 0.7 g | Trans Fat: 0 g | Fiber: 9 g | Sodium: 512 mg | Cholesterol: 0 mg

Italian Marinara Beanball Subs

PREP: 20 minutes | **COOK:** 35-40 minutes | **YIELD:** 5 servings

My daughter, Rachel, loves the classic Italian meatball sub, but she doesn't like to splurge too often. This vegetarian version ups the nutritional quality without sacrificing adequate protein or taste. It's become Rachel's new favorite sandwich.

BEANBALL INGREDIENTS

½ yellow or white onion, cut into large chunks

2 cloves garlic, peeled

½ cup (120 ml) basil leaves, packed

½ cup (120 ml) flat leaf parsley, packed

2 cups cooked, rinsed and drained or 1 x 15-oz (440 ml) BPA-free can organic great northern, white kidney or cannellini beans, drained and rinsed

1 cup (240 ml) cooked red quinoa

2 Tbsp (30 ml) Bragg's Liquid Aminos

2 Tbsp (30 ml) nutritional yeast, plus more to garnish

Pinch red pepper flakes

¼ cup (60 ml) whole wheat dry bread crumbs

¼ cup + 2 Tbsp (60 ml + 30 ml) wheat germ

2 Tbsp (30 ml) extra virgin olive oil

¼ tsp (1.25 ml) each sea salt and black pepper

1½ cups (360 ml) Clean Marinara Sauce (see p. 276) or any jarred Clean spaghetti sauce

5 x 6-inch sections whole-grain baguette, sliced in half lengthwise, keeping enough of the bread intact to create a hinge

Preheat the oven to 350°F (175°C).

To a food processor, add onion, garlic, basil and parsley. Pulse chop until smooth. Scrape into a large bowl. Add beans to processor and pulse chop until chunky. Scrape out into bowl. Add remaining beanball ingredients to bowl and stir to combine thoroughly.

Roll one beanball to check the consistency. If mixture is too moist to easily hold its shape, add 2 Tbsp (30 ml) more bread crumbs and 1 Tbsp (15 ml) more wheat germ, and stir to combine.

Once the mixture has the right consistency, roll into golf-ball-sized balls and place on a baking sheet lined with parchment. Bake 35 to 40 minutes, until firm to the touch and lightly browned.

To assemble subs, pour ½ cup (120 ml) of marinara inside each section of baguette, add four beanballs and top with a sprinkle of nutritional yeast, if desired. Serve hot.

NUTRITIONAL VALUE PER SERVING (EACH SERVING: 6-INCH SECTION OF BAGUETTE, 4 BEANBALLS, ½ CUP MARINARA):
Calories: 456 | Calories from Fat: 94 | Protein: 19 g | Carbs: 77 g | Total Fat: 11 g |
Saturated Fat: 1 g | Trans Fat: 0 g | Fiber: 9 g | Sodium: 871 mg | Cholesterol: 0 mg

Beluga Lentils with Porcini Mushrooms, Asparagus and a Sunny Egg

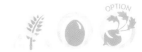

PREP: 15 minutes | **COOK:** 25 minutes | **YIELD:** 4 servings

Don't be afraid of the unique ingredients used in this recipe! You can use beluga lentils and porcini mushrooms in so many other recipes that I'm sure any extras won't go to waste. Or you could make seconds and thirds of this recipe – it's sure to be a hit!

1 cup (240 ml) black beluga lentils, rinsed

1 clove garlic, peeled and slightly smashed

1 bay leaf

½ cup (120 ml) dried porcini mushrooms

1 cup (240 ml) boiling water

1 tsp (5 ml) extra virgin olive oil

1 clove garlic, minced

½ tsp (2.5 ml) chopped fresh thyme

Optional: 1 tsp (5 ml) truffle-infused extra virgin olive oil

¼ tsp (1.25 ml) each sea salt and freshly ground black pepper

1 small bunch baby asparagus, stalk ends trimmed

Eat-Clean Cooking Spray (see p. 277)

4 eggs

Combine lentils, garlic, bay leaf and 2½ cups (600 ml) water in a pot and bring to a simmer. Partially cover and simmer until lentils are tender but still holding their shape, 15 to 20 minutes. Drain and discard garlic and bay leaf.

While lentils cook, place mushrooms in a small bowl and cover with boiling water. Allow to rehydrate, about 5 minutes, and then drain thoroughly. Heat olive oil in a skillet on medium. Add mushrooms and cook until lightly browned, about 3 minutes. Stir in garlic and thyme and cook for about 1 minute more. Transfer mushrooms to lentils and add truffle oil (if using), salt and pepper. Stir to combine.

Steam asparagus 1 or 2 minutes until tender-crisp.

Turn on broiler. Heat a large, ovenproof nonstick skillet on medium and spray with Eat-Clean Cooking Spray. Crack eggs carefully into skillet, taking care to keep yolks intact. Cook until whites are mostly set, 3 to 4 minutes. Put skillet under broiler for about 15 seconds to finish cooking whites. Remove and season with a pinch of salt and pepper.

To serve, mound lentils on plates, lay 6 to 7 asparagus spears over lentils, and place egg on top. Serve immediately.

MAKE IT VEGAN!
Simply omit the eggs.

NUTRITIONAL VALUE PER SERVING (EACH CONTAINING ¾ CUP LENTILS, 6 TO 7 SPEARS ASPARAGUS AND 1 EGG):
Calories: 345 | Calories from Fat: 95 | Protein: 25 g | Carbs: 38 g | Total Fat: 11 g |
Saturated Fat: 2 g | Trans Fat: 0 g | Fiber: 14 g | Sodium: 172 mg | Cholesterol: 210 mg

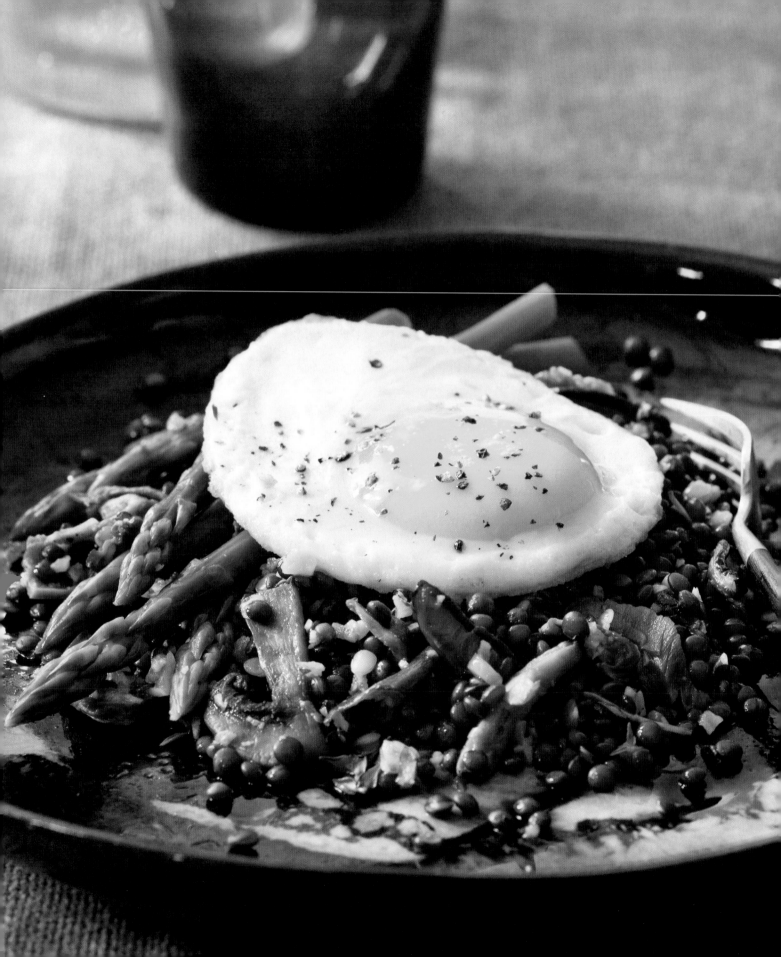

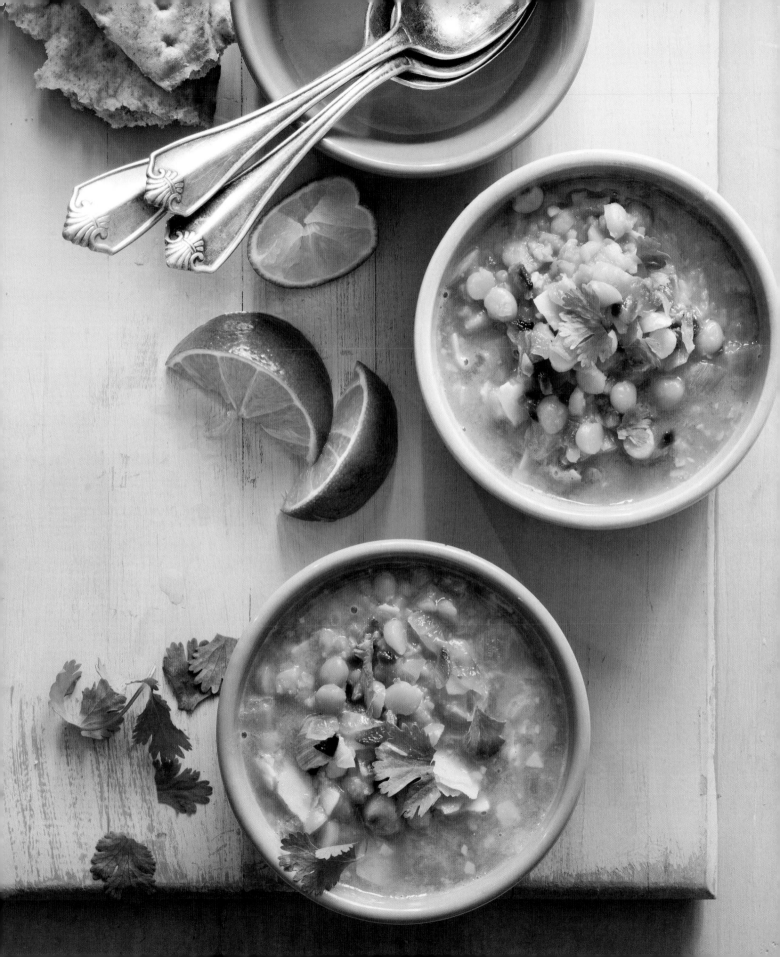

Chana Dal with Caramelized Onions and Coconut

PREP: 10 minutes | **COOK:** 60 minutes | **YIELD:** 5 x 1-cup servings

Chana dal and the chickpea are very similar legumes, but the chana is smaller, sweeter and has a much lower glycemic index. If you're in a pinch, you can substitute chickpeas for the chana dal in this recipe.

2 cups (480 ml) chana dal (split desi chickpeas), picked through and rinsed

1 Tbsp (15 ml) finely grated fresh ginger

1 tsp (5 ml) garam masala

½ tsp (2.5 ml) ground turmeric

½ tsp (2.5 ml) ground coriander

¼ tsp (1.25 ml) cayenne

½ tsp (2.5 ml) sea salt

¼ tsp (1.25 ml) freshly ground black pepper

1 Tbsp (15 ml) coconut oil

1 large onion, finely chopped

2 Tbsp (30 ml) unsweetened flaked coconut

2 Tbsp (30 ml) fresh lime juice

¼ cup (60 ml) chopped fresh cilantro, to garnish

In a large pot or Dutch oven, combine chana dal, 6 cups (1.44 L) water, ginger, garam masala, turmeric, coriander, cayenne, salt and pepper. Bring to a boil, stir, then cover and reduce heat to simmer for about 60 minutes, stirring occasionally.

While chana dal cooks, heat coconut oil in a large skillet on medium high. Add onions and cook until they start to brown, about 3 minutes. Reduce heat to medium low and continue to cook until onions are well browned, 8 to 10 minutes more. Stir in flaked coconut and cook for about 1 minute. Remove from heat.

Blend chana dal with a handheld immersion blender or stand blender until slightly smooth with some of the chickpeas still intact. Stir in lime juice, half of browned onions and coconut.

Ladle into bowls, top with remaining browned onions and coconut, and sprinkle with chopped cilantro.

NUTRITIONAL VALUE PER SERVING:
Calories: 163 | Calories from Fat: 49 | Protein: 7 g | Carbs: 23 g | Total Fat: 6 g |
Saturated Fat: 3.5 g | Trans Fat: 0 g | Fiber: 6 g | Sodium: 101 mg | Cholesterol: 0 mg

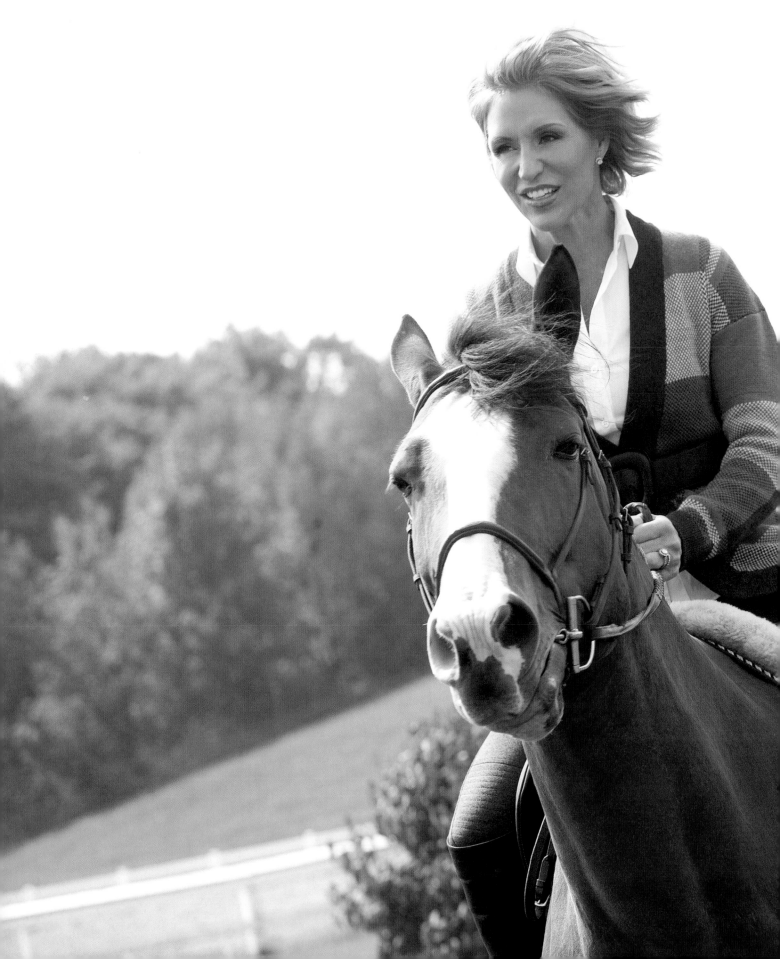

"Taking a day of active rest is a great way to help keep your workout routine fresh and fun. Any low-impact activity, such as horseback riding, hiking or skating with the kids, will do wonders for your mind, body and muscles."

Stuffed Shells

PREP: 25 minutes | **COOK:** 45 minutes | **YIELD:** 8 servings; about 3 stuffed shells per serving

Hearty, comforting and Clean – this is the stuff your Italian dreams are made of!

10 oz (284 g) jumbo shell pasta

8 oz (225 g) tempeh

1 Tbsp (15 ml) extra virgin olive oil

½ yellow onion, finely chopped

½ tsp (2.5 ml) herbes de Provence

½ tsp (2.5 ml) sweet paprika

½ tsp (2.5 ml) garlic powder

Pinch freshly grated nutmeg

Sea salt and freshly ground black pepper,
    to taste

15 oz (425 g) low-fat ricotta, about 2 cups
    (480 ml)

3 egg whites

1 Tbsp (15 ml) finely chopped fresh basil

1 Tbsp (15 ml) finely chopped fresh flat leaf
    parsley

3 cups (720 ml) Clean Marinara Sauce (see
    p. 276) or jarred Clean spaghetti sauce

¼ cup (60 ml) freshly grated Parmesan cheese

Preheat oven to 375°F (190°C).

Cook shell pasta according to package directions in salted water. Drain and spread out on a baking sheet in a single layer.

Meanwhile, finely crumble tempeh by grating on a stand grater or by pulsing in a food processor.

Heat olive oil in a large nonstick skillet on medium. Add onion and herbes de Provence, and cook until soft and translucent. Add crumbled tempeh, paprika, garlic powder and nutmeg, and season with salt and pepper. Increase heat and cook, stirring occasionally, until tempeh starts to brown. Transfer tempeh to a large bowl and add ricotta, egg whites, basil and parsley, and season with salt and pepper. Mix well.

Spread ½ cup (120 ml) marinara sauce on the bottom of a very large casserole dish or pan. Spoon ricotta mixture into shells, about 1½ Tbsp (22.5 ml) for each shell, and place the shells in prepared dish. Pour remaining marinara sauce over shells and sprinkle with Parmesan. Cover and bake for about 45 minutes until bubbling.

NUTRITIONAL VALUE PER SERVING:
Calories: 315 | Calories from Fat: 79 | Protein: 15 g | Carbs: 42 g | Total Fat: 9 g |
Saturated Fat: 3.5 g | Trans Fat: 0 g | Fiber: 3 g | Sodium: 463 mg | Cholesterol: 20 mg

Taco Night

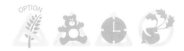

PREP: 20 minutes | **COOK:** 10 minutes | **YIELD:** 8 servings

Make taco night a family activity by getting the kids to assemble their own tacos! Tex Mex Beans and Tex Mex Rice (see p. 191) make perfect side dishes.

1 cup (240 ml) high-protein textured soy or vegetable protein (see Prep Tip at right)

1 cup (240 ml) low-sodium vegetable broth, boiling, gluten free if necessary

8 oz (225 g) tempeh

1 Tbsp (15 ml) extra virgin olive oil

1 cup (240 ml) finely chopped onion

1 tsp (5 ml) chili powder

1 tsp (5 ml) ground cumin

½ tsp (2.5 ml) garlic powder

1 chipotle pepper in adobo, minced (for less heat substitute ½ tsp / 2.5 ml smoked paprika)

1 Tbsp (15 ml) tomato paste

1 Tbsp (15 ml) Bragg's Liquid Aminos

Pinch sea salt

8 x 8- or 9-inch whole wheat flour tortillas or 16 x 5- or 6-inch corn tortillas

TACO FIXIN'S

Shredded lettuce

Chopped tomatoes

Chopped onion

Sliced or diced avocados

Chopped cilantro

Plain yogurt (omit for vegan)

Mexican hot sauce

In a bowl, stir together textured soy or vegetable protein and vegetable broth, and set aside. Pulse tempeh in a food processor until finely crumbled. In a large nonstick skillet, heat olive oil on medium. Add onion and cook, stirring occasionally, until soft and translucent, 3 to 5 minutes. Add the crumbled tempeh, rehydrated textured soy protein, chili powder, cumin, garlic powder, chipotle pepper (or paprika), tomato paste, Bragg's Liquid Aminos, ¼-½ cup (60-120 ml) water, and a pinch of sea salt. Stir mixture to combine and heat through.

Serve in warm tortillas topped with your favorite taco fixin's.

PREP TIP

Textured soy or vegetable protein is also known as TSP or TVP. It is made of defatted soy flour and can be found on shelves in the health food section. It does not need to be refrigerated since it comes dehydrated. To rehydrate, follow package directions. Generally, combine 1 cup (240 ml) TSP or TVP with 7/8 cup (207 ml) boiling water or broth, stir, and let sit for 5 to 10 minutes until soft.

NUTRITIONAL VALUE PER SERVING (1 X 8- OR 9-INCH WHOLE WHEAT TORTILLA FILLED WITH ½ CUP TACO FILLING OR 2 X 5- OR 6-INCH CORN TORTILLAS EACH FILLED WITH ¼ CUP TACO FILLING):
Calories: 190 | Calories from Fat: 39 | Protein: 14 g | Carbs: 32 g | Total Fat: 4 g | Saturated Fat: 0.5 g | Trans Fat: 0 g | Fiber: 11 g | Sodium: 509 mg | Cholesterol: 0 mg

Butternut Squash, Portobello Mushroom, Caramelized Onion and Hazelnut Pizza

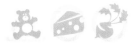

PREP: 60 minutes | **COOK:** 15-20 minutes | **YIELD:** 8 slices

These may seem like unlikely toppings for a pizza, but the combination is pure heaven, and it will make you feel like you're eating something truly gourmet.

1½ lbs (680 g) whole wheat pizza dough (store bought or see p. 277), at room temperature

½ butternut squash, about 1½ lbs (680 g), seeds scooped out

2 tsp (10 ml) extra virgin olive oil, divided

1 small clove garlic, chopped

1 tsp (5 ml) fresh thyme

Pinch freshly grated nutmeg

1 large yellow onion, halved and thinly sliced

¼ tsp (1.25 ml) herbes de Provence

2 Portobello mushrooms, stemmed, halved and sliced into ¼-inch thick pieces

½ cup (120 ml) Yogurt Cheese* (see p. 276)

¼ cup (60 ml) hazelnuts or filberts, coarsely chopped

Eat-Clean Cooking Spray (see p. 277)

Pinch each sea salt and freshly ground black pepper

Whole wheat flour or cornmeal, for dusting the pizza stone or baking sheet

Preheat oven to 425°F (215°C). Spray flesh of squash with Eat-Clean Cooking Spray and place flesh side down on a baking sheet. Bake until tender when pierced with a skewer, about 40 minutes. Remove and let cool until comfortable to handle. Scoop squash from skin and transfer to a food processor. Add 1 tsp (5 ml) olive oil, garlic, thyme, nutmeg and a pinch of salt and pepper. Blend until smooth.

Heat 1 tsp (5 ml) olive oil in a large skillet on medium high. Add onion and herbes de Provence. Cook until onions are starting to brown, about 3 minutes. Reduce heat to medium low and continue to cook, stirring occasionally, until thoroughly caramelized, 20 to 25 minutes. Remove from heat.

Heat a large skillet on medium and spray with Eat-Clean Cooking Spray. Add Portobello mushrooms in a single layer, spray tops with a little Eat-Clean Cooking Spray, and cook, stirring rarely, until soft and golden brown, 3 to 5 minutes. Season with a pinch of salt and pepper and remove from heat.

Stretch, roll out or toss the pizza dough into a shape that will cover a 15- or 16-inch pizza stone or round or large rectangular baking sheet. Sprinkle pizza stone or baking sheet with a little flour or cornmeal to prevent dough from sticking, and stretch dough over top. Spread squash purée onto dough, leaving ½-inch of crust at the edge. Top with mushrooms and caramelized onions. Dollop with yogurt cheese, and sprinkle with hazelnuts.

Place pizza in oven and bake until crust is golden brown at the edges, and pizza is cooked through, 15 to 20 minutes.

Transfer to a cutting board to cut into slices and serve.

TIME SAVER

The dough and toppings can be prepared up to two days ahead of time. When you're ready, just assemble and bake.

NOTE

*Yogurt Cheese must be made ahead of time.

NUTRITIONAL VALUE PER SLICE:
Calories: 299 | Calories from Fat: 66 | Protein: 9 g | Carbs: 51 g | Total Fat: 7 g | Saturated Fat: 0.5 g | Trans Fat: 0 g | Fiber: 6 g | Sodium: 435 mg | Cholesterol: 1 mg

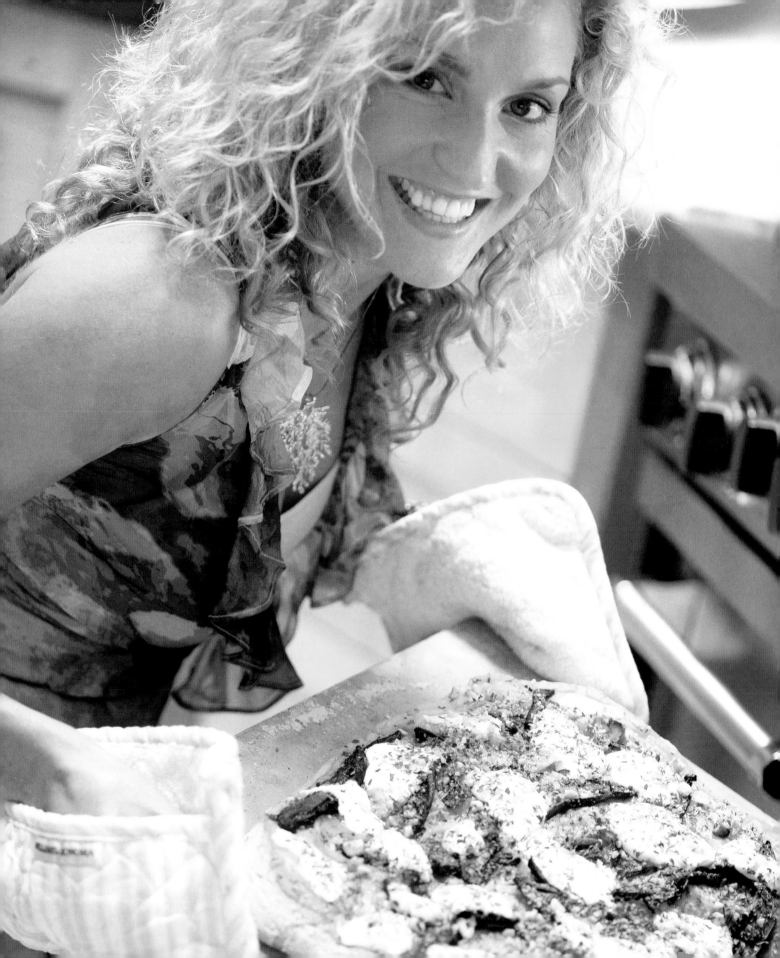

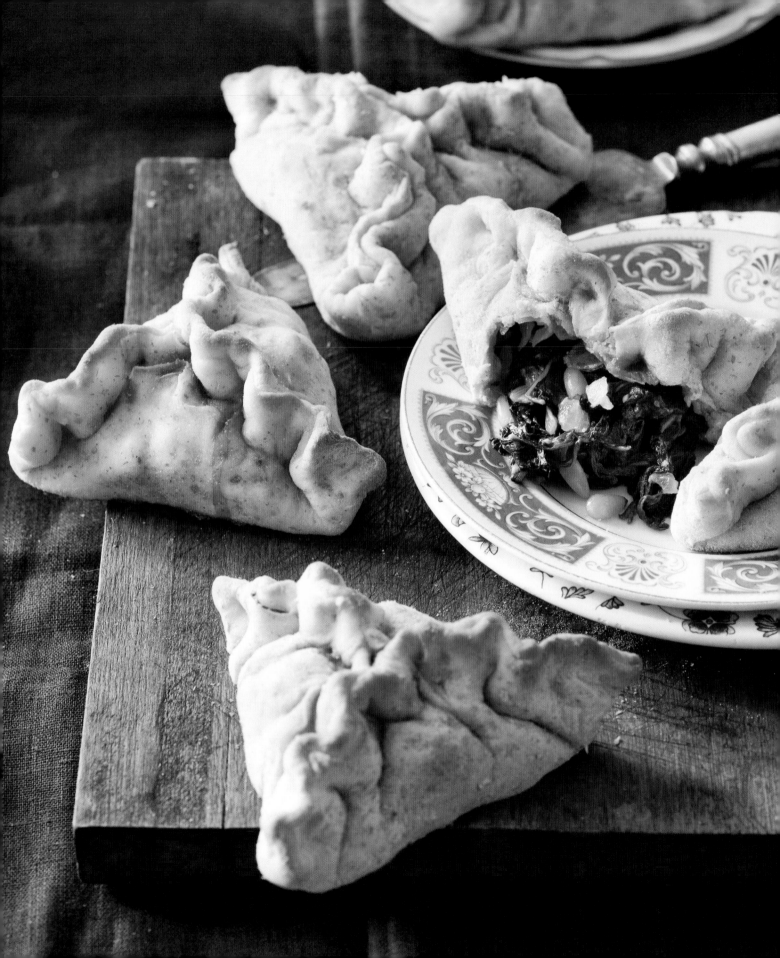

Lebanese Spinach Triangles

PREP: 30 minutes | **COOK:** 15 minutes | **YIELD:** 10 triangles

Middle Eastern cuisine provides some of the most delicious vegetarian options I have ever tasted. These fatayer are typically enjoyed as a meat pie, but the spinach version is tastier and healthier. The spices and ingredients all work together to create robust flavors you won't even realize are healthy. Perfect!

2 Tbsp (30 ml) extra virgin olive oil

½ yellow onion, finely chopped

1 lb (454 g) frozen chopped spinach, thawed and drained with all of the water squeezed out (see Prep Tip at right)

2 Tbsp (30 ml) fresh lemon juice

1 Tbsp (15 ml) toasted pine nuts

2 Tbsp (30 ml) chopped fresh parsley

2 tsp (10 ml) sumac (see Tosca's Tip at right)

¾ tsp (3.75 ml) sea salt

¼ tsp (1.25 ml) freshly ground black pepper

1 lb (454 g) whole wheat pizza dough, cut into 10 equal portions (store bought or see p. 277)

Eat-Clean Cooking Spray (see p. 277)

Place rack in lower third of oven, and preheat to 425°F (215°C).

Heat olive oil in a skillet on medium. Add onions and cook until soft and translucent but not brown, about 3 minutes. Scrape into a medium bowl. Add spinach, lemon juice, pine nuts, parsley, sumac, salt and pepper. Mix well. You should have about 2 cups (480 ml) of spinach filling.

Roll out each portion of dough into a ball, and then, using a rolling pin, roll out each ball into a five-inch circle. Place about 3 Tbsp (45 ml) of the spinach filling in the middle of the dough. Bring 3 edges up and pinch them together at the top, then continue pinching the edges together, making a triangle, until the pie is sealed. Spray a baking sheet with Eat-Clean Cooking Spray and place spinach triangle on the sheet. Repeat with remaining dough and spinach filling until all are used. Bake for about 15 minutes, or until lightly browned and heated through. Remove from oven and serve.

PREP TIP
To make sure the spinach is as dry as possible, you can squeeze it in some cheesecloth or press it in a colander.

TOSCA'S TIP
Sumac can be found in Middle Eastern or international grocery stores. If you can't find it, you can approximate the flavor by combining equal parts paprika and lemon pepper.

NUTRITIONAL VALUE PER TRIANGLE:
Calories: 144 | Calories from Fat: 38 | Protein: 4 g | Carbs: 22 g | Total Fat: 4 g |
Saturated Fat: 0.4 g | Trans Fat: 0 g | Fiber: 2 g | Sodium: 513 mg | Cholesterol: 0 mg

Miso Udon Noodle Bowl with Roasted Sweet Potato, Tofu and Sea Vegetables

PREP: 15 minutes | **COOK:** 30 minutes | **YIELD:** 5 servings

Noodle bowls are perfect for bringing a variety of different tastes together in one easy-to-prepare dish. Best of all, the sea vegetables provide tons of vitamins and minerals that work hard to nourish our bodies and keep them functioning at their best.

1 large sweet potato, peeled and diced into ½-inch pieces

1 Tbsp (15 ml) extra virgin olive oil

1 tsp (5 ml) grated ginger

12 oz (340 g) udon noodles

4 cups (950 ml) low-sodium mushroom broth, vegetable broth or a combination (my favorite)

2 Tbsp (30 ml) red miso

1 Tbsp (15 ml) low-sodium soy sauce or tamari

4 cups (950 ml) fresh baby spinach

1 Tbsp (15 ml) cut wakame (dried seaweed)

⅓ cup (80 ml) dried dulse (strips, not crumbled)

4 scallions, thinly sliced crosswise, divided

8 oz (225 g) firm tofu, drained and diced into ½-inch cubes

2 oz (57 g) enoki mushrooms, root ends trimmed

Sesame oil and sambal oelek, for flavor and to garnish

Preheat oven to 425°F (215°C). Place sweet potato on a baking sheet, and toss with olive oil and ginger. Place in oven to roast until golden brown and soft, 15 to 20 minutes.

In the meantime, cook udon noodles according to package directions, or follow this method: Bring 4 cups (950 ml) water to a rolling boil. Add noodles and stir well. As it begins to boil over, add 1 cup (240 ml) cold water and stir. Repeat. This will take about 10 minutes. As it begins to boil a third time, remove pot from heat, cover, and let sit for about 5 minutes. Drain and rinse with cold water.

To a large pot, add broth, 4 cups (950 ml) water, miso and soy sauce. Bring to a simmer and whisk to mix miso in with the broth. Stir in spinach, wakame, dulse and half of scallions. Add roasted sweet potato and tofu, and let simmer about 1 minute to heat through.

Divide noodles among 5 bowls. Ladle soup over noodles, about 2 cups (480 ml) per bowl, top with enoki mushrooms and remaining scallions. Serve with sesame oil, sambal oelek and more soy sauce, if desired.

NUTRITIONAL VALUE PER SERVING (EACH SERVING CONTAINS 2 CUPS SOUP AND ABOUT 2½ OZ NOODLES):
Calories: 228 | Calories from Fat: 66 | Protein: 8 g | Carbs: 31 g | Total Fat: 7 g | Saturated Fat: 1 g | Trans Fat: 0 g | Fiber: 4 g | Sodium: 403 mg | Cholesterol: 0 mg

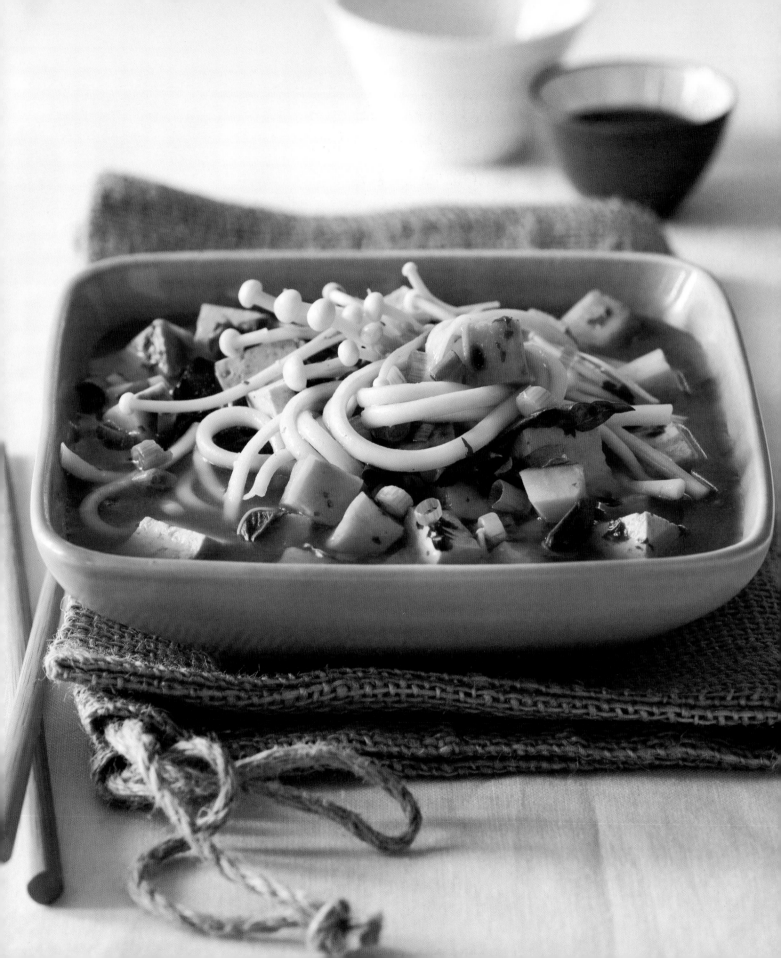

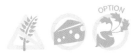

Greek Tempeh-Stuffed Peppers

PREP: 20 minutes | **COOK:** 55 minutes | **YIELD:** 4 stuffed peppers

You definitely don't have to sacrifice your love of Greek food when following a vegetarian lifestyle. Try these stuffed peppers full of veggies and spice and everything the Greeks think is nice!

8 oz (225 g) tempeh

1 Tbsp (15 ml) extra virgin olive oil

1 onion, finely chopped

2 large cloves garlic, minced

⅛ tsp (0.625 ml) red pepper flakes

¼ tsp (1.25 ml) ground allspice

¼ tsp (1.25 ml) ground cinnamon

½ tsp (2.5 ml) paprika

Pinch freshly grated nutmeg

1 baby zucchini, diced

1 x 15-oz (440 ml) BPA-free can no-salt-added diced tomatoes, drained and liquid reserved

¼ cup (60 ml) pitted kalamata olives, chopped

1 cup (240 ml) cooked brown rice

2 Tbsp (30 ml) chopped fresh parsley

1 Tbsp (15 ml) chopped fresh oregano

Sea salt and freshly ground black pepper, to taste

4 large bell peppers (red, orange, yellow or green)

4 tsp (20 ml) grated Parmigiano Reggiano cheese or nutritional yeast

Preheat oven to 400ºF (200ºC).

Finely grate tempeh or pulse in a food processor into little crumbles.

Heat olive oil in a large nonstick skillet on medium. Add onion and cook until soft and translucent. Add tempeh and garlic and cook, stirring occasionally, until tempeh starts to brown, about 3 minutes. Stir in spices. Add zucchini and cook until it starts to soften. Stir in tomatoes, olives, rice, parsley and oregano, and season with salt and black pepper.

Slice tops off peppers and remove all ribs and seeds. Cut a very thin slice from the base to help the pepper stand upright.

Place peppers in a baking dish and spoon tempeh mixture into peppers. Pour reserved tomato liquid plus ¼ cup (60 ml) water into the dish to surround peppers. Cover dish and bake for about 45 minutes. Remove cover, sprinkle the top of each pepper with 1 tsp (5 ml) cheese or nutritional yeast and continue baking until cheese is golden, about 10 minutes. Remove from oven and carefully transfer stuffed peppers to serving plates.

NUTRITIONAL VALUE PER PEPPER:
Calories: 314 | Calories from Fat: 115 | Protein: 15 g | Carbs: 37 g | Total Fat: 13 g |
Saturated Fat: 3 g | Trans Fat: 0 g | Fiber: 6 g | Sodium: 199 mg | Cholesterol: 1 mg

Israeli Couscous and Chickpeas with Eggplant, Red Peppers, Parsley and Mint

PREP: 20 minutes + overnight soaking of chickpeas | **COOK:** 1 hour | **YIELD:** 9 x 1-cup servings

Couscous is made of wheat flour, meaning it can cause tummy upset if you are gluten intolerant or suffer from celiac disease. If not, whip up this dish for a fabulous balance of grains and legumes. It's tasty, healthy and very unique.

1½ cups (360 ml) dried chickpeas

1 bay leaf

1 clove garlic, lightly smashed

1 eggplant, ends trimmed and diced into 1-inch pieces

1 red pepper, seeded and diced into 1-inch pieces

1 Tbsp (15 ml) extra virgin olive oil

¼ tsp (1.25 ml) each sea salt and freshly ground black pepper

1½ cups (360 ml) Israeli couscous

¼ cup (60 ml) pimento stuffed green olives, sliced

½ cup (120 ml) chopped flat leaf parsley

2 Tbsp (30 ml) chopped fresh mint

1 Tbsp (15 ml) capers, drained

DRESSING

2 Tbsp (30 ml) extra virgin olive oil

¼ cup (60 ml) freshly squeezed lemon juice

½ tsp (2.5 ml) ground cumin

¼ tsp (1.25 ml) turmeric

¼ tsp (1.25 ml) ground allspice

¼ tsp (1.25 ml) dried oregano, crumbed

¼ tsp (1.25 ml) dried mint, crumbled

¼ tsp (1.25 ml) each sea salt and freshly ground black pepper

Place chickpeas in a large container, cover with plenty of cold water, and let sit overnight. Drain and rinse. Transfer chickpeas to a large pot, cover with plenty of fresh, cold water and add bay leaf and garlic clove. Bring to a simmer and cook, partially covered, until tender, about 1 hour. Drain.

Meanwhile, heat oven to 425°F (215°C). On a sheet pan, toss together eggplant, red pepper, olive oil, salt and pepper to coat. Spread vegetables out in a single layer and place in oven to cook until tender and starting to brown, stirring once, about 20 minutes.

While chickpeas or veggies cook, combine Israeli couscous with 4 cups (950 ml) lightly salted water in a pot and heat on high until boiling. Reduce heat and simmer, uncovered, until tender, about 8 minutes. Drain. Do not rinse.

In a large bowl, add chickpeas, roasted eggplant, red peppers and Israeli couscous. Add green olives, parsley, mint and capers. In a small bowl, whisk together dressing ingredients and pour over the top. Toss to combine. Can be served hot, at room temperature or chilled.

PREP TIP

Israeli couscous is larger than your typical couscous. If you can't find it at your local grocer, try regular whole wheat couscous and follow the cooking times outlined on the package.

CHILL OUT

This dish will keep in the refrigerator for up to three days.

NUTRITIONAL VALUE PER SERVING:
Calories: 200 | Calories from Fat: 55 | Protein: 6 g | Carbs: 31 g | Total Fat: 6 g |
Saturated Fat: 1 g | Trans Fat: 0 g | Fiber: 3 g | Sodium: 69 mg | Cholesterol: 0 mg

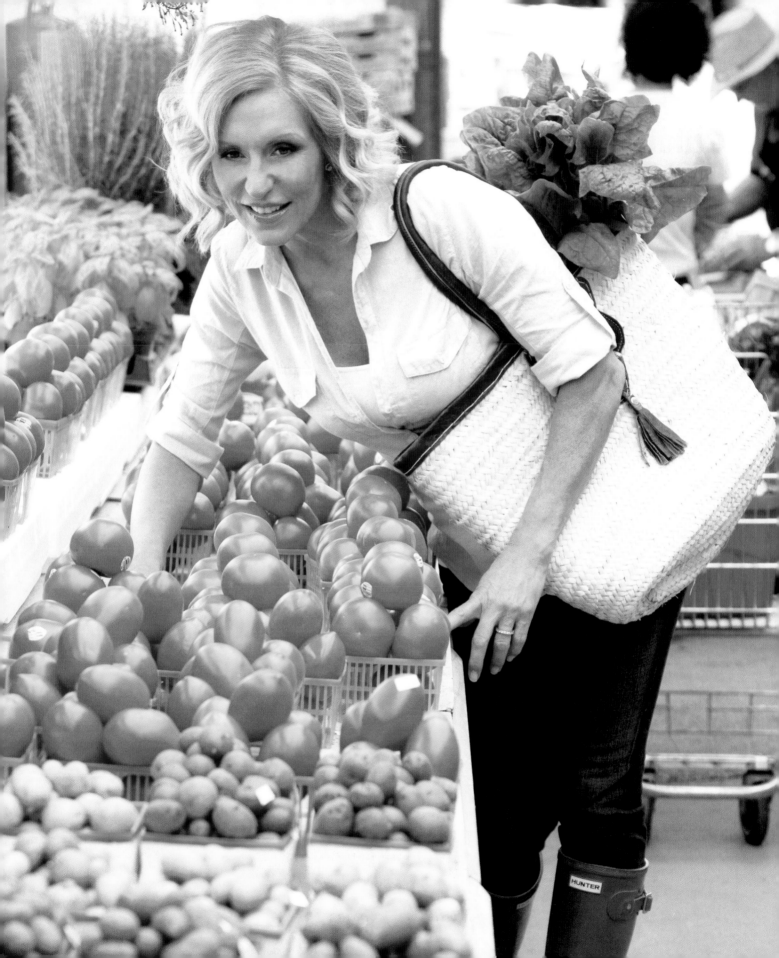

Late Summer Spelt with Crunchy Vegetables

PREP: 5 minutes + overnight soaking of spelt berries | **COOK:** 50 minutes | **YIELD:** 10 x 1-cup servings

Spelt is an excellent grain to incorporate into your vegetarian lifestyle. Popular in ancient European times, spelt is a species of wheat with 17% protein. Wow! So you're getting your carbs and protein in this dish, plus lots more. Talk about multitasking!

1½ cups (360 ml) spelt berries, soaked 8 hours or overnight, drained

½ lb (225 g) green beans, vine end trimmed

1 yellow bell pepper, seeded and thinly sliced into 2-inch strips

1 large carrot, peeled, quartered lengthwise and cut into small pieces

2 cups (480 ml) cherry or grape tomatoes, halved

2 green onions, chopped

¼ cup (60 ml) pimento stuffed green olives, sliced

2 Tbsp (30 ml) finely chopped fresh basil

2 Tbsp (30 ml) finely chopped fresh tarragon

2 Tbsp (30 ml) finely chopped fresh flat leaf parsley

Zest and juice of 1 large lemon

2 Tbsp (30 ml) best-quality extra virgin olive oil

½ tsp (2.5 ml) each sea salt and freshly ground black pepper

In a pot, combine the spelt berries and 6 cups (1.44 L) water and bring to a boil on high heat. Then reduce heat to simmer, covered, with the lid tilted, until tender but still chewy, about 50 minutes. Drain.

Meanwhile, steam green beans until tender-crisp, then run under cold water and drain. Transfer to a large bowl. Add yellow pepper, carrots, tomatoes, green onions and olives. Add cooked spelt and herbs. In a small bowl, whisk together lemon zest and juice, olive oil, salt and pepper, and pour overtop spelt. Toss to combine.

NUTRITIONAL VALUE PER SERVING:
Calories: 143 | Calories from Fat: 38 | Protein: 5 g | Carbs: 24 g | Total Fat: 4 g |
Saturated Fat: 0.5 g | Trans Fat: 0 g | Fiber: 4 g | Sodium: 64 mg | Cholesterol: 0 mg

Green Pea Risotto with Fresh Pea Shoots

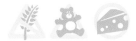

PREP: 10 minutes | **COOK:** 50 minutes | **YIELD:** 4 x ¾-cup servings

Risotto is a true gourmet meal. Luckily, this recipe doesn't require you to have the abilities of a master chef ... just excellent stirring skills (and maybe a bit of patience).

1¼ cups (300 ml) frozen petite peas

2 tsp (10 ml) extra virgin olive oil

¼ cup (60 ml) finely chopped shallots

1 clove garlic, minced

1 cup (240 ml) medium-grain brown rice, not rinsed

½ cup (120 ml) dry white wine (see note at right)

3 cups (710 ml) low-sodium vegetable broth, gluten free if necessary

½ cup (120 ml) Yogurt Cheese* (see p. 276)

1 Tbsp (15 ml) chopped fresh basil

¼ tsp (1.25 ml) each sea salt and freshly ground black pepper

½ cup (120 ml) snipped fresh pea shoots, to garnish (optional)

Place peas in a bowl and cover with boiling water. Let sit for about 1 minute, then drain and set aside.

Heat olive oil in a large skillet on medium. Add shallots and cook until soft but not brown, 1 or 2 minutes. Stir in garlic and cook until fragrant but not brown, about 1 minute. Add rice and stir for about 1 minute. Add white wine (or substitute), stir, and let liquid reduce by half. Add vegetable broth and stir to combine. Bring mixture to a gentle boil, then partially cover and reduce heat to gently simmer for about 45 minutes, stirring occasionally, until almost all of the broth is absorbed. Rice should be tender but still a little chewy. Remove from heat.

Transfer 1 cup (240 ml) peas to a food processor, and add Yogurt Cheese and basil. Blend until smooth. Scrape pea mixture into risotto, along with remaining ¼ cup (60 ml) peas and salt and pepper. Stir to combine. Serve in shallow bowls topped with pea shoots.

TOSCA'S TIP
When stirring the risotto, be sure not to leave the stove for too long. You might wind up with a sticky mess.

PREP TIP
If you don't want to use wine in this recipe, you can substitute it with ½ cup (120 ml) low-sodium vegetable broth plus 1 tsp (5 ml) white wine vinegar or lemon juice.

NOTE
*Yogurt Cheese must be made ahead of time.

NUTRITIONAL VALUE PER SERVING:
Calories: 182 | Calories from Fat: 31 | Protein: 7 g | Carbs: 24 g | Total Fat: 4 g |
Saturated Fat: 1 g | Trans Fat: 0 g | Fiber: 4 g | Sodium: 183 mg | Cholesterol: 1 mg

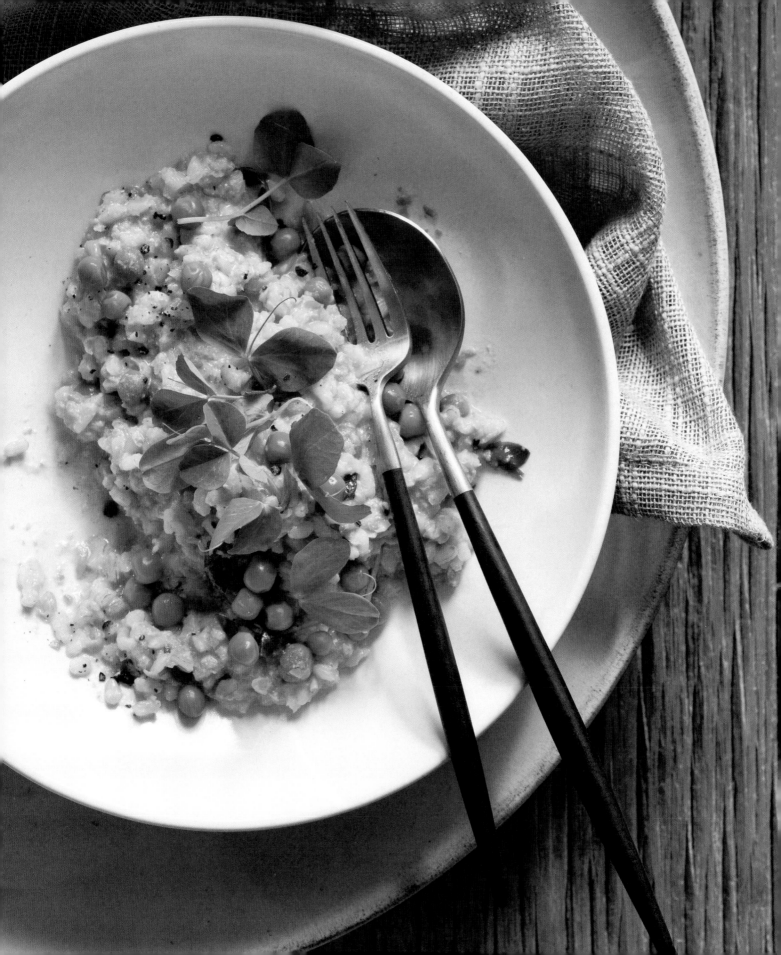

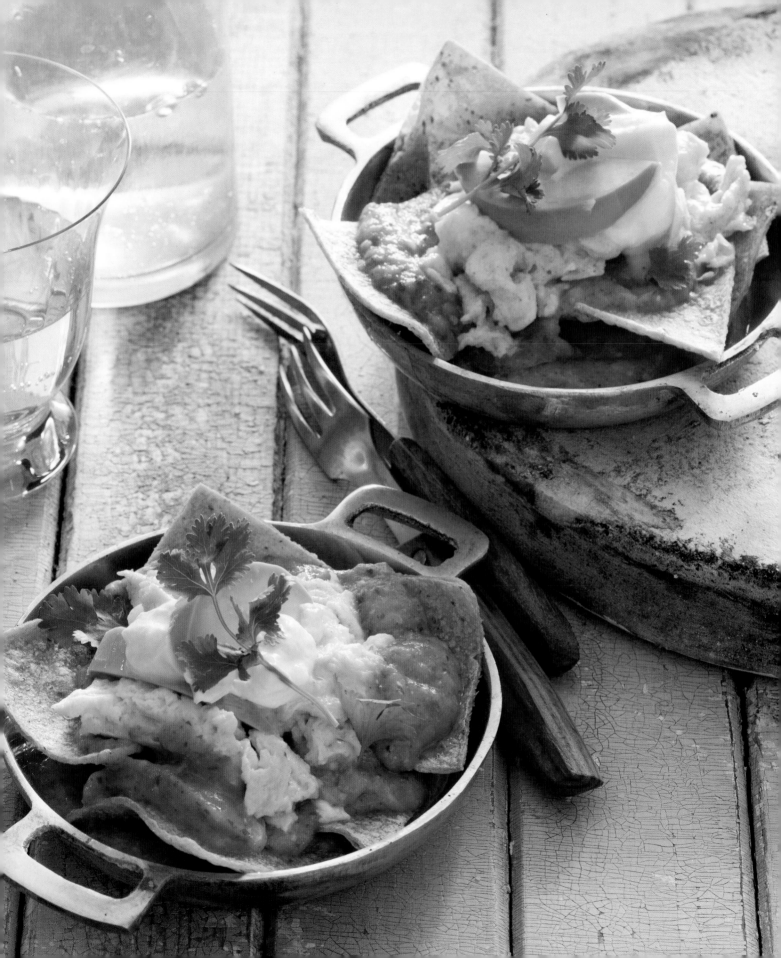

Chilaquiles

PREP: 20 minutes | **COOK:** 15 minutes | **YIELD:** 6 servings

In traditional chilaquile preparation there is a whole lot of fryin' goin' on! But in true Eat-Clean fashion, we've chosen to toast the tortillas. Is there a sacrifice on taste? No way!

½ lb (225 g) tomatillos, skins removed and quartered

½ yellow onion, cut into 6 pieces

1 jalapeño, stemmed, seeded (or leave seeds in for a spicier dish), and quartered

1 Anaheim pepper, stemmed, seeded and cut into 3-inch pieces

1 clove garlic, peeled and slightly smashed

½ cup (120 ml) cilantro including stems, roughly chopped, plus more cilantro leaves to garnish

½ cup (120 ml) water

Juice of ½ lime

1 avocado, pitted

½ tsp (2.5 ml) sea salt, divided

¼ tsp (1.25 ml) freshly ground black pepper

6 whole-grain sprouted corn tortillas, about 6 inches in diameter, cut into 4 wedges

4 whole eggs + 8 egg whites

¼ tsp (1.25 ml) each ground turmeric and ground cumin

Eat-Clean Cooking Spray (see p. 277)

½ cup (120 ml) nonfat Greek yogurt

Heat a large, dry cast-iron skillet on medium. Add tomatillos, onion, jalapeño, Anaheim pepper and garlic, and cook, stirring occasionally, until charred and slightly soft, 5 to 8 minutes. Transfer to a blender and add cilantro, water, lime juice, one-quarter of the avocado, ¼ tsp (1.25 ml) salt, and pepper. Blend until smooth.

Heat oven to 425°F (215°C). Spread tortilla wedges out on a baking sheet, and toast in oven for about 5 minutes.

Heat a large nonstick skillet on medium low. In a large bowl, beat eggs and egg whites with turmeric and cumin, and add remaining ¼ tsp (1.25 ml) sea salt. Spray skillet with Eat-Clean Cooking Spray, if necessary, and pour in eggs. Cook, stirring regularly, until eggs are set and cooked to your liking.

In a large baking dish, pour half of the tomatillo-pepper sauce. Lay toasted tortilla wedges over sauce, pour remaining sauce over tortillas, and add scrambled eggs. Slice remaining avocado and lay over eggs. Dollop with yogurt, and sprinkle with cilantro leaves. Serve hot.

NUTRITIONAL VALUE PER SERVING:
Calories: 225 | Calories from Fat: 87 | Protein: 14 g | Carbs: 21 g | Total Fat: 9 g | Saturated Fat: 2 g | Trans Fat: 0 g | Fiber: 3 g | Sodium: 299 mg | Cholesterol: 143 mg

Tandoori Tofu with Grilled Vegetables

PREP: 20 minutes + 2 hours | **COOK:** 25 minutes | **YIELD:** 4 servings

Masala literally means a spicy mixture. In this recipe, the combination works perfectly with tandoori tofu. Tandoori means food cooked in a tandoor, or cylindrical clay oven. You'll find lots of tandoori in Middle Eastern and South Asian cultures, but now you can bring it home with this very recipe!

1 cup (240 ml) plain low-fat yogurt

1 Tbsp (15 ml) tandoori masala spice (see Prep Tip at right)

1 lb (454 g) firm or extra-firm tofu, drained, liquid pressed out with a towel, and cut into 1-inch cubes

¼ tsp (1.25 ml) sea salt

1 baby zucchini, ends trimmed, halved lengthwise and cut into 1-inch pieces

½ onion, cut into wedges

1 cup (240 ml) cherry tomatoes

Eat-Clean Cooking Spray (see p. 277)

Pinch sea salt and freshly ground black pepper

Lemon wedges

In a large bowl or container, mix together yogurt, tandoori masala and salt. Stir in tofu making sure it is completely covered in yogurt marinade. Cover and refrigerate for about 2 hours.

Meanwhile, heat oven to 450°F (230°C). Heat a grill or grill pan on high and wipe with oil to prevent sticking.

Remove tofu from yogurt marinade and thread on skewers. Thread vegetables on separate skewers. Spray vegetables with a little Eat-Clean Cooking Spray and sprinkle with a pinch of salt and pepper. Grill tofu and vegetables 8 to 10 minutes, turning once or twice. Remove vegetables and set aside. Transfer tofu skewers to a baking sheet and brush with remaining yogurt marinade. Bake in oven 12 to 15 minutes until the marinade is dry. Remove tofu skewers from oven. Serve with grilled vegetables and a wedge of lemon to squeeze overtop.

TRY THIS!
Serve this with steamed brown rice to make a complete meal.

PREP TIP
Tandoori masala spice can be found in the international aisle of the grocery store. If you can't find it, you can make your own by combining ground turmeric, ginger, cardamom, mace, cumin, garlic powder, fenugreek, coriander, chilies, cinnamon and cloves.

EQUIPMENT TIP
If using wooden skewers, soak in water for about 20 minutes prior to grilling to prevent scorching.

NUTRITIONAL VALUE PER SERVING:
Calories: 135 | Calories from Fat: 52 | Protein: 13 g | Carbs: 10 g | Total Fat: 6 g | Saturated Fat: 2 g | Trans Fat: 0 g | Fiber: 2 g | Sodium: 176 mg | Cholesterol: 4 mg

Tofu Gyros with Tzatziki

PREP: 25 minutes | **COOK:** 10 minutes | **YIELD:** 4 servings

Gyros offer a simple, easy and tasty way to enjoy a complete Clean meal. Dill and mint make this a refreshing meal that will make you feel like you are dining by the sea in Greece.

TZATZIKI

1 medium or ½ large English cucumber, peeled, seeds scooped out, and grated

1 cup (240 ml) good quality low-fat Greek yogurt, strained, or Yogurt Cheese* (see p. 276)

1 small or ½ large clove garlic, squeezed through a garlic press

1 tsp (5 ml) finely chopped fresh mint

½ tsp (2.5 ml) finely chopped fresh dill

1 tsp (5 ml) fresh lemon juice

Pinch sea salt

1 lb (454 g) extra-firm tofu, drained

Eat-Clean Cooking Spray (see p. 277)

2 tsp (10 ml) Marvelous Mediterranean Seasoning (see p. 167)

1 Tbsp (15 ml) Bragg's Liquid Aminos

4 whole wheat pocketless pitas, warmed

2 cups (480 ml) shredded romaine lettuce

2 or 3 Roma tomatoes, sliced

Place grated cucumber in cheesecloth or a strainer lined with paper towels and squeeze out as much of the liquid as possible. Transfer to a bowl. Add yogurt, garlic, mint, dill, lemon juice and salt. Mix together and refrigerate to let flavors meld.

Meanwhile, cut tofu lengthwise into eight slices and lay on paper towels. Cover with more paper towels and press out the liquid. Repeat with fresh paper towels until tofu is as dry as possible, but still intact.

Heat a large nonstick skillet on medium high and spray with Eat-Clean Cooking Spray. Sprinkle half of Mediterranean seasoning over tofu slices and place in pan, seasoned side down. Sprinkle the tops of the tofu slices with remaining seasoning and spray with Eat-Clean Cooking Spray. Cook tofu slices until nicely browned on both sides, turning once, 5 to 10 minutes. Sprinkle Bragg's Liquid Aminos over the tofu slices, and shake the pan a little so all the liquid gets absorbed into tofu. Remove from heat.

To assemble gyros, place pita on a square of aluminum foil. Add two slices of tofu down the center of each pita, top with tzatziki, romaine lettuce and tomato slices. Roll up like a cone and secure the foil to hold gyro in shape.

CHILL OUT

If you have any leftover tzatziki, store it in the fridge for up to three days and serve with pita chips and crudités.

NOTE

*Yogurt Cheese must be made ahead of time.

NUTRITIONAL VALUE PER GYRO SANDWICH:
Calories: 272 | Calories from Fat: 54 | Protein: 24 g | Carbs: 30 g | Total Fat: 6 g | Saturated Fat: 1 g | Trans Fat: 0 g | Fiber: 6 g | Sodium: 638 mg | Cholesterol: 1 mg

Top Protein Sources

Protein is an *Eat-Clean Diet®* follower's constant companion. We eat a protein source at each of our five or six meals every day to keep our blood sugar stable and ensure our metabolism runs at a steady rate throughout the day. Vegetarians and vegans need to be extra aware of their protein sources to ensure they are eating complete proteins – and enough of them!

What is a complete protein? It is a source of protein that includes all of the essential amino acids. Essential amino acids are those the body cannot create, as it can the nonessential amino acids. They are absolutely necessary for growth and repair of body tissues (think skin, bone, muscle and organs), hormone and enzyme function. As you can see, these are some important building blocks for keeping us healthy and fit.

Unfortunately, most legumes, grains and vegetables do not provide a complete spectrum of essential amino acids. They contain some in adequate amounts, but some in inadequate amounts. This is why food combining and eating a variety of protein sources throughout the day is important for the vegetarian. Getting the complete array of essential amino acids daily can be more or less challenging depending on which animal products you choose to eat.

For example, lacto-ovo vegetarians have the benefit of getting a complete protein source from eggs and dairy products. Pescatarians are also at an advantage because they can eat fish, which boasts complete, bioavailable protein. Vegetarians who choose to avoid eggs, dairy or fish and individuals who practice a vegan diet have to be much more aware of the components and bioavailability of the protein they are putting in their body. Plant sources – except for hemp, soy, quinoa and some blue-green algaes such as spirulina – do not contain all of the essential amino acids in enough quantity. This means they must be combined with other plant sources to make them complete, or conversely you may choose to eat a large variety of protein sources throughout each day.

What Are You Risking?

So what's the risk of not getting enough protein? Muscle wasting, fatigue, osteoporosis, hormone imbalances, skin disorders, nervous dysfunction, brittle hair, abdominal bloating and pain, and more. The most commonly known protein deficiency disorder is kwashiorkor. This form of malnutrition is caused by a lack of complete protein sources causing wasting, edema and reduced intelligence, along with marasmus (from a combination of low energy supply and protein). It is most commonly seen in developing countries where famine runs rampant, especially in children. Kwashiorkor can happen to unaware vegetarians, too. For this reason, choosing to follow a vegetarian lifestyle means much more than simply choosing not to eat meat – it means adopting a heightened awareness of what you do eat!

Bioavailability:

Bioavailability of protein sources is also an important issue for vegetarians. Most plant sources of protein have a low bioavailability, meaning your body has a tough time using all the amino acids it's received after you have eaten. A common bioavailability issue is trypsin inhibition. Trypsin inhibitors are found in lima beans, soy beans and raw egg whites. They grasp hold of the amino acid trypsin and do not allow it to be used by the body. There goes one more amino acid! The best way to combat bioavailability problems such as this is to eat a wide variety of protein sources throughout the day.

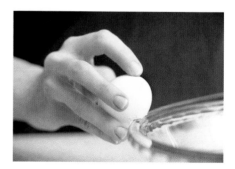

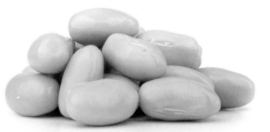

How Much is Enough?

The average woman (140 lbs) and man (180 lbs) requires 0.8 g of protein per kilogram of bodyweight, while strength and endurance athletes require closer to 1.1 g of protein per kilogram of body weight. Essentially, you are looking at a daily average of 46 grams of protein for women and 56 grams of protein for men. But don't get too hung up on the numbers – you are all unique and require varied amounts! Following the portions recommended in *The Eat-Clean Diet®* and in the correct combinations (a variety of proteins paired with complex carbs throughout the day) means you will meet your needs.

Protein Sources		
Complete Protein Sources	**Combined Protein Sources**	
• Egg whites • Soy protein isolate • Whey protein isolate • Quinoa • Hempseeds • Soy products (edamame, tofu, tempeh, miso) • Spirulina **Note:** quinoa, hemp and soy should still be eaten in combination with other proteins and whole grains, because their bioavailability is low.	• Pair legumes with nuts and seeds, grains, corn, and/or dairy or other animal sources. Example: falafel • Pair nuts & seeds with legumes, grains, corn, and/or dairy or other animal sources. Example: oatmeal with walnuts • Pair grains with legumes, nuts & seeds, corn, and/or dairy or other animal sources. Example: bean burrito	**Grains:** oats, millet, buckwheat, quinoa, amaranth and brown rice. **Legumes:** black beans, chickpeas, kidney beans, lentils, pinto beans and puy lentils. For more details on legumes please see p. 66. **Nuts and Seeds:** sunflower seeds, pumpkin seeds, almonds, walnuts, cashews and peanuts.

Scallops with Tarragon
Corn Supreme Sauce, p. 148

From the Sea

Scallops with Tarragon Corn Supreme Sauce

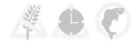

PREP: 20 minutes | **COOK:** 10 minutes | **YIELD:** 4 servings

Scallops are a quick and easy meal to prepare, but with this sauce, your guests will think you've been in the kitchen for hours. It's a win-win situation: You'll fool your dinner-mates into thinking you're a gourmet chef and you'll still have time to sneak in a good workout!

2 tsp (10 ml) extra virgin olive oil, divided

2 Tbsp (30 ml) chopped shallots

1 clove garlic, minced

¾ cup (180 ml) frozen sweet yellow corn

1 cup (240 ml) low-sodium, gluten-free
    vegetable broth

2 pinches each sea salt and freshly ground
    black pepper, divided

1 tsp (5 ml) chopped fresh tarragon leaves

1 lb (454 g) large (U-10) sea scallops, drained

Pinch curry powder

Heat olive oil in a saucepan on medium, and cook shallots and garlic for about 1 minute until soft, but not brown. Add corn and vegetable broth and simmer for about 3 minutes, or until corn is heated through. Pour sauce into a blender and blend until very smooth, or leave it a little chunky if you prefer. Pour sauce back into the pan and stir in salt, pepper and tarragon. Set aside to keep warm while you prepare the scallops.

Pat scallops thoroughly dry on both sides with a paper towel. In a small bowl, mix together curry powder, salt and pepper. Sprinkle half of spice mixture over the scallops. Heat remaining 1 tsp (5 ml) olive oil in a nonstick skillet on medium. Place scallops in skillet, seasoned side down. Sprinkle remaining spice mixture overtop. Let scallops cook for about 2 minutes without moving. Turn them over, and cook 1 to 2 minutes longer. Do not overcook scallops or they will be tough. Remove scallops from heat. To serve, divide sauce among four plates, spreading it out in little pools, and place scallops on top.

NUTRITIONAL VALUE PER SERVING (4 OZ SCALLOPS WITH ¼ CUP SAUCE):
Calories: 198 | Calories from Fat: 39 | Protein: 1 g | Carbs: 12 g | Total Fat: 3 g |
Saturated Fat: 0.5 g | Trans Fat: 0 g | Fiber: 2 g | Sodium: 444 mg | Cholesterol: 60 mg

Poached Halibut in Lemon Caper Broth

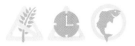

PREP: 10 minutes | **COOK:** 13 minutes | **YIELD:** 4 servings

If you're not a fish lover, white fish species are great choices for you. Try this dish; with its mild lemon flavor and easy preparation, you might just become a convert!

1½ cups (360 ml) low-sodium, gluten-free vegetable broth

½ cup (120 ml) dry white wine

1 heaping tsp (7 or 8 ml) finely chopped shallots

½ tsp (2.5 ml) Dijon mustard

1 Tbsp (15 ml) capers, drained

1 lb (454 g) wild halibut filet, skin removed, filet kept in one piece

Pinch each sea salt and freshly ground black pepper

1 Tbsp (15 ml) fresh lemon juice

1 tsp (5 ml) finely chopped fresh dill

In a large skillet or sauté pan, whisk together vegetable broth, wine, shallots, Dijon mustard and capers. Bring to a simmer over medium-high heat. Season the top of the halibut with a pinch of salt and pepper, and place in the broth. Mostly cover the pan, reduce heat to a gentle simmer and poach fish until opaque in the center, about 10 minutes. The fish will still be soft to the touch at the thickest part.

Gently place halibut on a plate and cover to keep warm. Bring broth to a vigorous simmer for about 3 minutes on medium-high heat to reduce slightly. Remove pan from heat, stir in lemon juice and dill, and season with additional salt and pepper, if desired. To serve, divide halibut into four portions and place in shallow bowls. Ladle broth around the halibut, and garnish with a sprig of fresh dill.

NUTRITIONAL VALUE PER SERVING:
Calories: 193 | Calories from Fat: 31 | Protein: 30 g | Carbs: 2 g | Total Fat: 3 g |
Saturated Fat: 0.5 g | Trans Fat: 0 g | Fiber: 0.3 g | Sodium: 311 mg | Cholesterol: 47 mg

Tri-Color Pasta with Tuna, Spinach and Artichoke Hearts

PREP: 15 minutes | **COOK:** 12 minutes | **YIELD:** 8 x 2-cup servings

This fresh and wholesome dish can be easily adapted to suit a variety of audiences. Sub in brown rice pasta to make it gluten free or try tri-colored bowties to give it a fun twist for the kids (what a great way to get them to eat their spinach!).

12 oz (340 g) tri-color pasta (such as farfalle, penne or shells)

15 oz (425 g) no-salt-added solid white albacore tuna in water, drained

8 cups (1.9 L) fresh baby spinach

1 x 13- to 14-oz (385 to 414 ml) BPA-free can quartered artichoke hearts in water, drained

1½ cups (360 ml) cherry or grape tomatoes, halved

½ cup (120 ml) chopped pepperoncini

½ cup (120 ml) chopped fresh basil

¼ cup (60 ml) chopped fresh dill

1 lemon, zested and juiced

1 Tbsp (15 ml) extra virgin olive oil

½ tsp (2.5 ml) each sea salt and freshly ground black pepper

Bring a large pot of water to boil, add the pasta and stir. Cook according to package directions until al dente. Drain, reserving ¼ cup (60 ml) of the cooking water. Transfer pasta to a large bowl and add remaining ingredients. Add reserved cooking water, and toss to combine. Can be served warm, at room temperature or cold.

CHILL OUT
This dish will keep in the refrigerator for up to two days.

ON THE GO
This dish travels well! Why not double the recipe and have planned leftovers?

NUTRITIONAL VALUE PER SERVING:
Calories: 280 | Calories from Fat: 37 | Protein: 20 g | Carbs: 38 g | Total Fat: 4 g |
Saturated Fat: 1 g | Trans Fat: 0 g | Fiber: 4 g | Sodium: 338 mg | Cholesterol: 30 mg

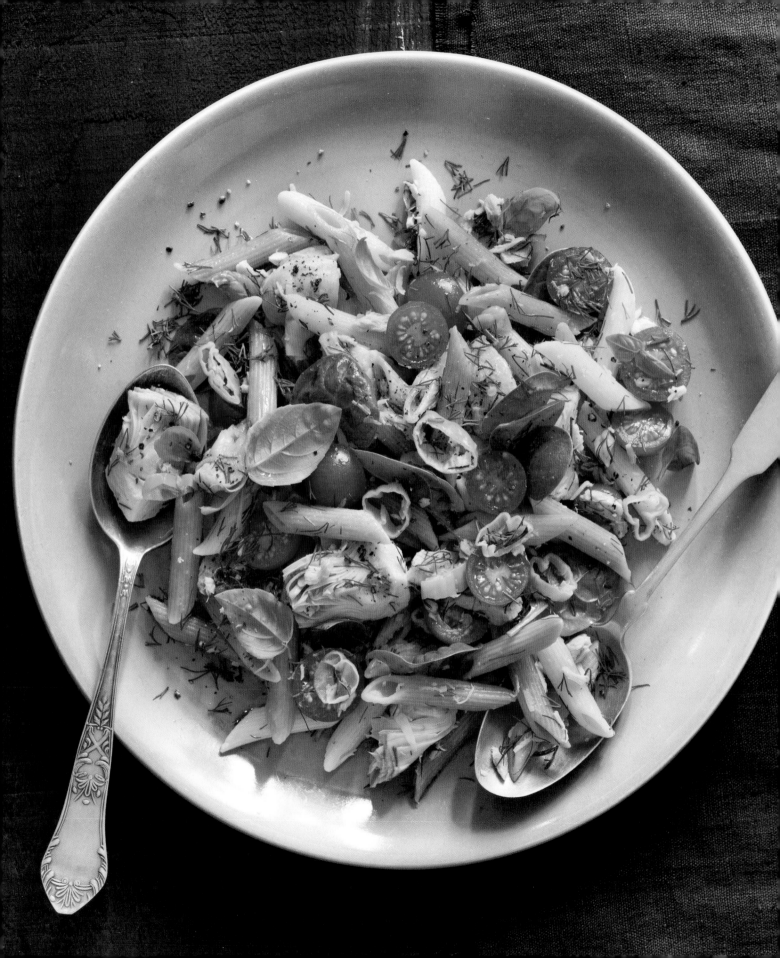

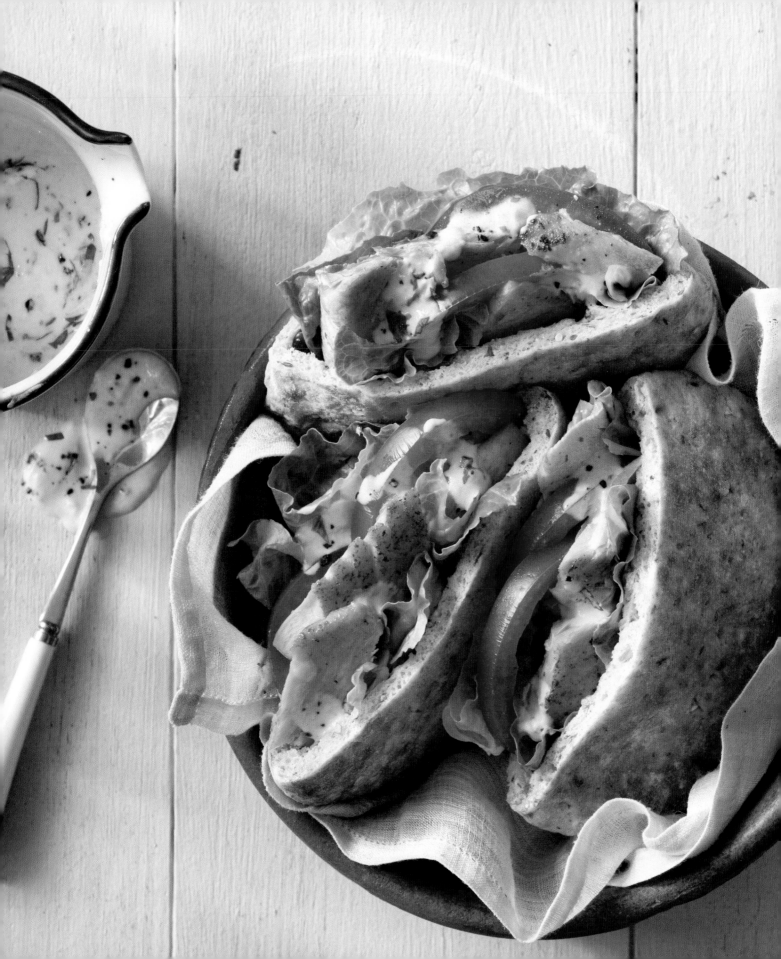

Clean Salmon Caesar Pita Pockets

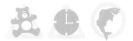

PREP: 20 minutes | **COOK:** 6-10 minutes | **YIELD:** 4 servings

Salmon? Yum! Caesar? Double yum! Pita pockets? Now we're talking. This simple dish has it all in a handy, portable pocket. Yum, yum, yum!

CLEAN HERBED CAESAR DRESSING

½ cup (120 ml) plain, low-fat yogurt

1 large clove garlic

¼ tsp (1.25 ml) anchovy paste or
    minced anchovy

1 handful basil leaves

1 Tbsp (15 ml) Dijon mustard

1 Tbsp (15 ml) fresh lemon juice

Dash hot sauce, such as Tabasco

Pinch each sea salt and freshly ground
    black pepper

1 tsp (5 ml) extra virgin olive oil

4 x 4-oz (113 g) wild salmon filets, skin and
    pin bones removed

Pinch each sea salt and freshly ground
    black pepper

4 whole wheat pitas, halved to create "pockets"

4 cups (950 ml) romaine lettuce, cut into
    1-inch pieces

2 to 3 tomatoes, sliced

Add all dressing ingredients to a food processor or blender and whirl until thoroughly blended. Transfer to a bowl or container and set aside. You will have extra dressing, which will keep in the fridge for up to one week.

Heat olive oil in a large nonstick skillet on medium high. Season salmon with a pinch of salt and pepper and place in skillet. Cook for about 3 minutes on each side for medium-rare to medium, or longer for more well done. Salmon that is left a little pink in the center (medium-rare to medium) will be more moist and tender and is safe to eat, but cook to your desired doneness. When salmon is finished cooking, remove and transfer to a cutting board.

Stuff pita pockets with romaine and tomato slices. Cut salmon filets in half, and nestle them into pitas. Drizzle 1 to 2 Tbsp (15 to 30 ml) dressing into each pita pocket. Serve immediately.

TIME SAVER
Sandwiches can be made ahead of time, but wait to drizzle them with dressing until just before eating.

NUTRITIONAL VALUE PER PITA SANDWICH:
Calories: 394 | Calories from Fat: 159 | Protein: 32 g | Carbs: 45 g | Total Fat: 11 g |
Saturated Fat: 2 g | Trans Fat: 0 g | Fiber: 7 g | Sodium: 410 mg | Cholesterol: 64 mg

Calamari Parsley Salad

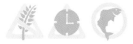

PREP: 20 minutes | **COOK:** 1-2 minutes | **YIELD:** 6 x 1-cup servings

This recipe was inspired by my travels in Turkey. It's very much like tabouleh, but contains no bulgur.

1 tsp + 1 Tbsp (5 ml + 15 ml) extra virgin olive oil, divided

1 lb (454 g) squid tubes and tentacles, tubes cut into ½-inch-thick rings

1 bunch curly parsley, washed and dried, chopped by hand or in a food processor, about 4 cups (950 ml)

2 vine-ripened tomatoes, diced

2 finely chopped scallions

¼ cup (60 ml) finely chopped fresh mint

Juice of 1 lemon

½ tsp (2.5 ml) sambal oelek (chili garlic sauce)

¼ tsp (1.25 ml) each sea salt and freshly ground black pepper

Heat 1 tsp (5 ml) olive oil in a nonstick skillet on high. Drain liquid from squid and pat it dry with a paper towel. Add squid to hot skillet and sauté for 1 to 2 minutes until just opaque. Do not overcook or it will be tough and rubbery. Transfer squid to a large metal bowl and place in refrigerator, uncovered, to cool.

In the meantime, prepare parsley, tomatoes, scallions and mint, and add to a large bowl. In a small bowl, whisk together the lemon juice, sambal oelek, salt and pepper, and remaining 1 Tbsp (15 ml) olive oil. Remove cooled squid from the fridge, drain any liquid, and add to parsley and other ingredients in the large bowl. Pour lemon dressing over top and toss to combine.

CHILL OUT
This salad will keep in the refrigerator for up to two days.

PREP TIP
When cooking squid, cook it either for 1 to 2 minutes, or for a very long time. Anything in between will make it rubbery and tough.

NUTRITIONAL VALUE PER SERVING:
Calories: 189 | Calories from Fat: 80 | Protein: 16 g | Carbs: 13 g | Total Fat: 9 g | Saturated Fat: 2 g | Trans Fat: 0 g | Fiber: 2 g | Sodium: 97 mg | Cholesterol: 43 mg

Penang Curry with Tofu and Pineapple

PREP: 25 minutes | **COOK:** 10 minutes | **YIELD:** 6 x 1½-cup servings

Penang – the namesake of this dish – is a Malaysian state known as the food capital. It takes many influences from its neighbors, including this curry dish bursting with sweet pineapple and spicy red curry paste. So if you can't make it to Penang for some delicious street fare, whip up this curry and let it take you on a taste adventure to the other side of the world.

1 x 13- to 14-oz (385 to 414 ml) BPA-free can light coconut milk

1 Tbsp (15 ml) red curry paste, or more for spicier sauce

1 Tbsp (15 ml) natural peanut butter

2 tsp (10 ml) gluten-free Asian fish sauce (see tip at right)

1 Tbsp (15 ml) pure honey

½ tsp (2.5 ml) sea salt

1 carrot, sliced into thin half moons

1 cup (240 ml) shredded red or green cabbage

½ yellow onion, thinly sliced

2 cups (480 ml) broccoli florets

12 oz (340 g) extra-firm tofu, drained, liquid pressed out, and cut into 1-inch cubes

½ fresh pineapple, cut into bite-sized pieces, or 2 cups (480 ml) canned pineapple chunks, drained

Juice of 1 large lime

½ cup (120 ml) Thai basil leaves

1 tomato, cut into 8 wedges

Steamed brown rice

In a large high-sided pan, whisk together coconut milk, red curry paste, peanut butter, Asian fish sauce, honey and sea salt. Bring mixture to a simmer on medium heat, whisking until curry paste and peanut butter are blended in. Add carrot, cabbage, onion and broccoli. Cook for about 3 minutes or until veggies start to soften. Add tofu and pineapple and cook until heated through, about 3 minutes. Stir in lime juice, basil leaves and tomato. Serve over steamed brown rice.

PREP TIP
Fish sauce can go by different names depending on where it is from. In Thailand it is known as nam pla and in Vietnam it is known as nuoc mam. Many brands contain wheat, so if you avoid gluten make sure to find a brand that does not.

NUTRITIONAL VALUE PER SERVING:
Calories: 202 | Calories from Fat: 84 | Protein: 8 g | Carbs: 24 g | Total Fat: 9 g | Saturated Fat: 5 g | Trans Fat: 0 g | Fiber: 3 g | Sodium: 271 mg | Cholesterol: 0 mg

Miso Soy Broiled Salmon
with Salad Greens and Snap Peas

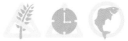

PREP: 15 minutes | **COOK:** 3-5 minutes | **YIELD:** 4 servings

Broiled salmon offers a texture like no other, and as an added bonus, this recipe is extremely easy to prepare. Who needs fish sticks when you can have delicious, nutritious salmon like this in no time?

4 x 4-oz (113 g) wild salmon filets, pin
  bones removed

1 clove garlic, minced

1½ Tbsp (22.5 ml) natural salt- and sugar-free
  rice vinegar

1½ Tbsp (22.5 ml) low-sodium tamari

1 tsp (5 ml) miso

2 tsp (10 ml) Sucanat or other unrefined sugar

1 Tbsp (15 ml) sesame oil

8 cups (1.9 L) mixed greens, lightly packed

1 cup (240 ml) shredded carrots

½ English cucumber, chopped

1 avocado, pitted and sliced

1 cup (240 ml) stringless sugar snap peas

2 tsp (10 ml) sesame seeds, to garnish

Position oven rack in the second-highest position from top, and set broiler to low.

Place salmon filets, skin side down, on an aluminum foil-lined baking sheet. Sprinkle garlic on top of salmon.

In a small bowl, whisk together rice vinegar, tamari, miso, Sucanat and sesame oil.

Place greens, carrots and cucumber in a large bowl. Pour half of the miso soy dressing over salad, toss and divide among four plates or individual salad bowls. Pour the other half of the dressing over salmon filets. Spoon or brush sauce onto filets to make sure they're coated well.

Place salmon under broiler and cook for about 3 minutes for medium-rare or about 5 minutes for medium-well. Remove from oven and use a metal spatula to separate salmon from its skin, and place on top of salad greens. Arrange avocado slices and snap peas around salmon, and garnish with sesame seeds. Serve immediately.

NUTRITIONAL VALUE PER SERVING:
Calories: 322 | Calories from Fat: 132 | Protein: 31 g | Carbs: 16 g | Total Fat: 15 g |
Saturated Fat: 3 g | Trans Fat: 0 g | Fiber: 7 g | Sodium: 435 mg | Cholesterol: 62 mg

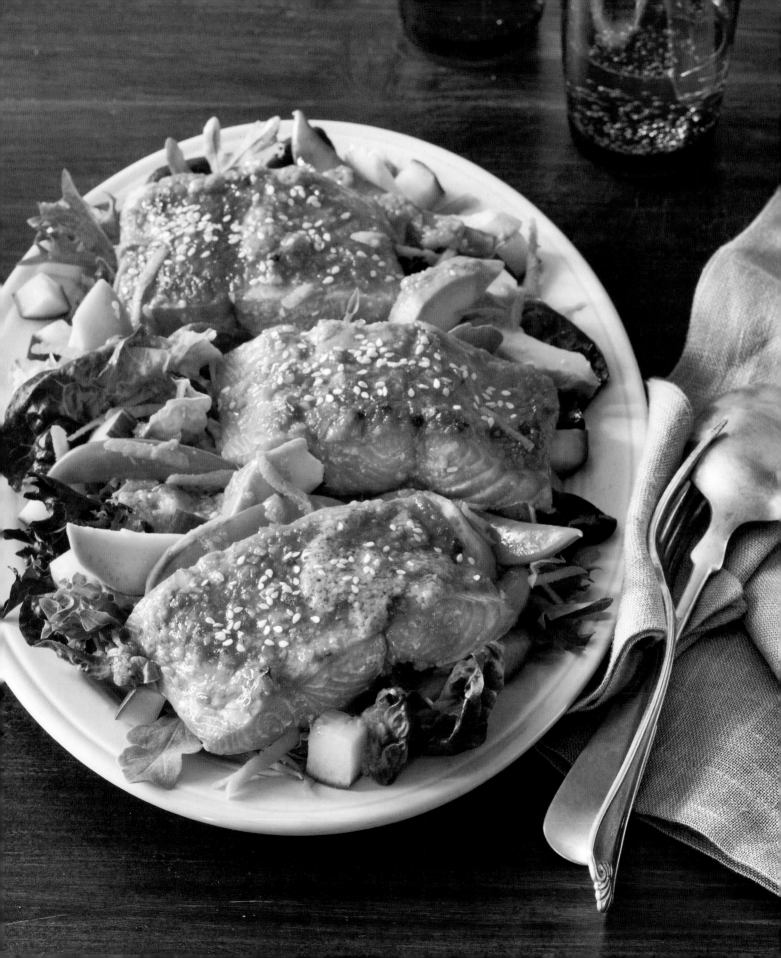

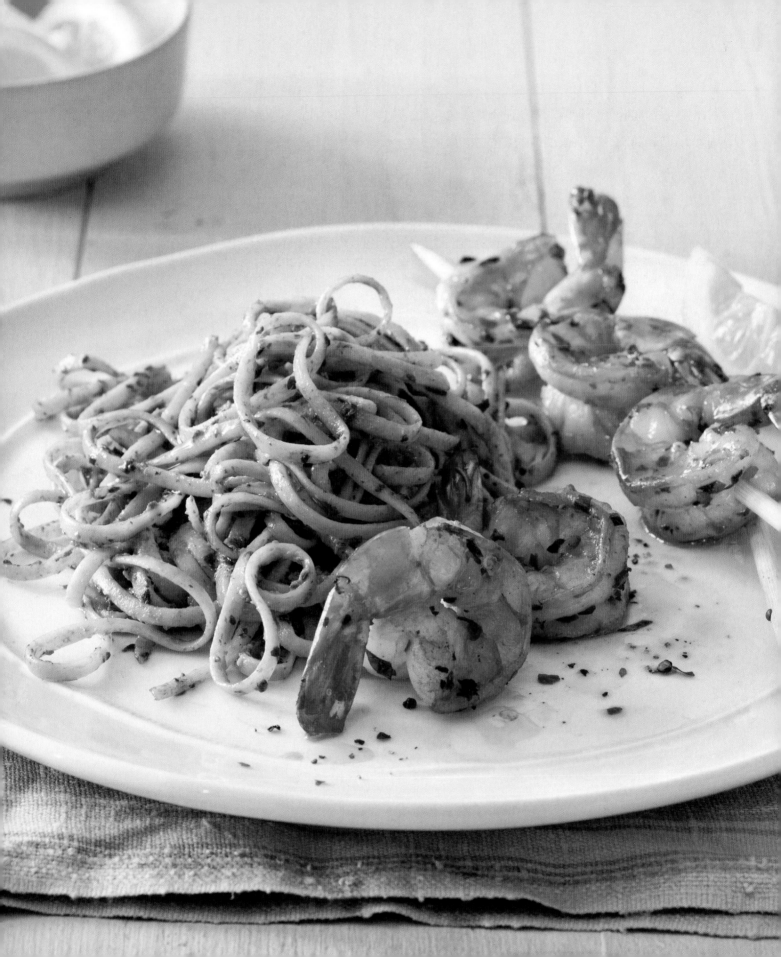

Herb-Grilled Shrimp Skewers with Avocado Linguini

PREP: 20 minutes | **COOK:** 10 minutes | **YIELD:** 6 servings

This recipe is perfect for a weeknight meal because the shrimp cook fast, and the pasta sauce doesn't require any cooking at all. Also, cooking the shrimp in their shells not only speeds up the prep time, but also ensures they are more flavorful and juicy. Just peel them as you eat them.

12 oz (340 g) whole wheat linguini

1½ lbs (680 g) large shrimp, shells on, deveined

1 Tbsp (15 ml) extra virgin olive oil

1 Tbsp (15 ml) freshly squeezed lemon juice

1 Tbsp (15 ml) cilantro, minced

1 Tbsp (15 ml) basil, minced

¼ tsp (1.25 ml) red pepper flakes

SAUCE

2 avocados, pitted and peeled

1 Tbsp (15 ml) extra virgin olive oil

1 lemon, zested and juiced

4 cups (950 ml) spinach, packed

½ cup (120 ml) cilantro

½ cup (120 ml) basil

2 cloves garlic

¼ tsp (1.25 ml) each sea salt and freshly
    ground black pepper

Bring a large pot of water to boil on high heat. Add a pinch of salt, if desired, and cook linguini until tender, but still firm to the bite. Scoop out ¼ cup (60 ml) of the cooking liquid, then drain the pasta and transfer to a large bowl.

In the meantime, in a bowl, toss the shrimp with olive oil, lemon juice, cilantro, basil, red pepper flakes and a pinch of salt and pepper until coated. Thread shrimp on metal or wooden skewers (if using wooden skewers, soak for about 20 minutes prior to using to prevent scorching).

To make suace, add to a food processor avocados, olive oil, lemon zest and juice, spinach, cilantro, basil, garlic, salt and pepper. Pulse-chop until chunky. While processor is running, stream in reserved pasta water 1 Tbsp (15 ml) at a time until mixture resembles a chunky sauce. You may not need to use all of the water. Pour sauce over pasta and toss to coat.

Heat a grill or grill pan to high. Grill shrimp for about 3 minutes, turn, and grill 2 to 3 minutes longer until opaque and curled.

NUTRITIONAL VALUE PER SERVING:
Calories: 341 | Calories from Fat: 137 | Protein: 28 g | Carbs: 22 g | Total Fat: 15 g |
Saturated Fat: 2 g | Trans Fat: 0 g | Fiber: 7 g | Sodium: 68 mg | Cholesterol: 33 mg

Rex Sole with Gingered Petite Vegetables and Shiitake Mushrooms

PREP: 30 minutes | **COOK:** 20 minutes | **YIELD:** 4 servings

Sole features a mild flavor that pairs well with light vegetables, and for a treat, a glass of white wine. Offer this as a simple summer meal and your dinner guests will definitely not be disappointed.

1 tsp (5 ml) safflower oil

20 oz (567 g) rex sole, bones intact, it's okay to have the skin on (see tip at right)

Pinch each sea salt and freshly ground black pepper

1 Tbsp (15 ml) extra virgin olive oil, divided

1 Tbsp (15 ml) freshly grated ginger, divided

1 large leek, white and light green parts only, rinsed well, halved and thinly sliced crosswise

½ lb (225 g) shiitake mushrooms, stemmed and thinly sliced

2 large cloves garlic, minced, divided

1 medium zucchini, ends trimmed, cut into fat "matchsticks" or petite "French fries"

1 cup (240 ml) shredded carrots

1 Tbsp (15 ml) low-sodium tamari

1 tsp (5 ml) sesame oil

1 Tbsp (15 ml) black sesame seeds

Heat safflower oil in a large nonstick skillet on medium. Season both sides of fish with a pinch of salt and pepper. It's okay if the skin is still on the fish, because it will crisp up and come off during cooking. Place fish in pan one piece at a time and circle it around in the oil a few times before settling the fish in. This will help prevent it from sticking. Let fish cook without disturbing it for about 3 minutes, then flip and cook for about 3 more minutes or until cooked through and lightly browned. Remove from pan and set aside. You can remove the skin at this point, or leave it on and eat it.

Use a paper towel to wipe out skillet and return to stove on medium heat. Add half of olive oil and half of ginger. Cook for about 1 minute or until fragrant. Add sliced leeks and mushrooms, and sauté until soft and starting to brown, about 3 minutes. Stir in half the minced garlic and cook for 1 minute longer. Transfer to a bowl and return skillet to heat. Add remaining olive oil and ginger, and cook for about 1 minute. Add zucchini and carrots and sauté until tender, about 3 minutes. Stir in remaining garlic and cook for about 1 minute longer. Add reserved leek and mushroom mixture. Remove skillet from heat and stir in tamari, sesame oil, sesame seeds, and season with salt and pepper, if desired. Mound sautéed vegetables on a platter or divide among four plates, and place sole on top of vegetables. The flesh will easily slide off the bones using a knife and fork, but do take care to avoid eating the bones.

PREP TIP
If rex sole is unavailable, you can substitute 16 oz (454 g) skinless boneless Pacific Dover sole.

NUTRITIONAL VALUE PER SERVING (5 OZ REX SOLE AND ¾ CUP VEGETABLES):
Calories: 297 | Calories from Fat: 83 | Protein: 36 g | Carbs: 15 g | Total Fat: 10 g |
Saturated Fat: 1 g | Trans Fat: 0 g | Fiber: 5 g | Sodium: 195 mg | Cholesterol: 17 mg

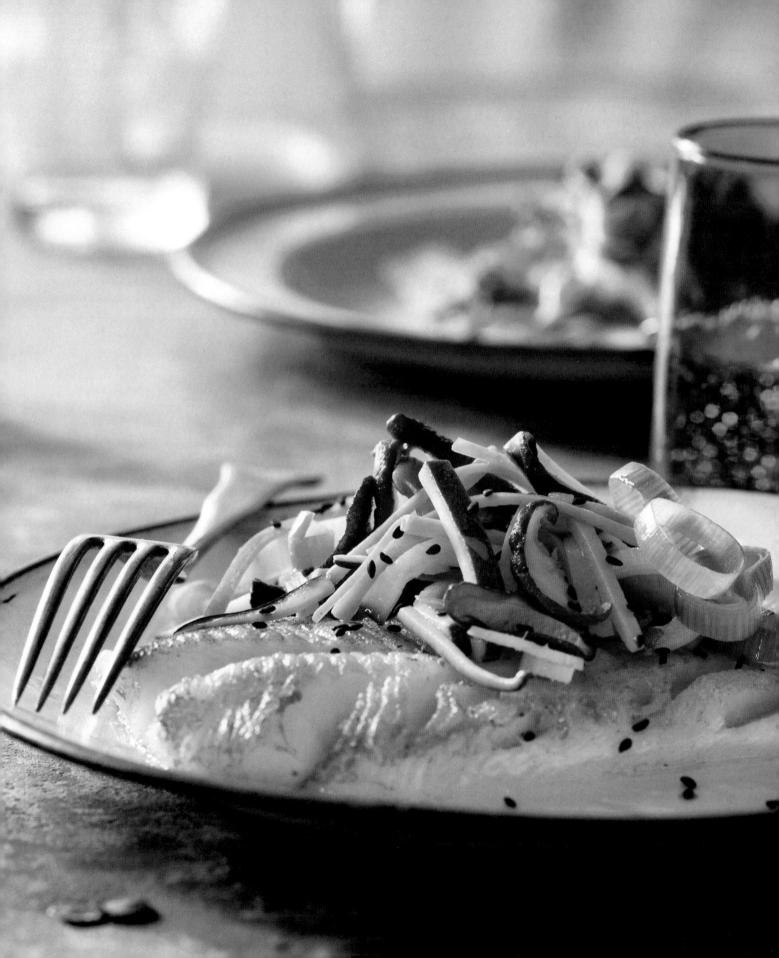

Jacked Jill

Who says you need to eat meat to build muscles? I picked the brain of Jill Holland, *Eat-Clean Diet* Ambassador, former vegan and now pescatarian, who gave me the inside scoop on finding balance, staying motivated and how she got that amazing physique!

When it comes to Eating Clean as a vegetarian, Jill Holland knows where it's at! She's been fine-tuning her exercise and nutrition plan for the past 18 years! She's also an awesome *Eat-Clean Diet* Ambassador who helps spread the word on our online forums (see sidebar) and at events across North America. If you've ever come out to see me at a fitness show, chances are you've seen Jill working the booth, chatting with fans and just being her super-energetic, kind and helpful self.

So, what made Jill give up meat in the first place? She says it was "by choice, not by protest." She was a young working professional with little interest in cooking and more interest in enjoying a social life. For her, foregoing meat was just easier than going through the preparations of thawing, marinating, cooking and so on.

A Rocky Start

Jill is the first to admit that her initial foray into the vegetarian lifestyle wasn't the Cleanest. "I just cut out the meat, leaving me as a really lousy vegetarian who was eating processed foods." Luckily, though, an "aha!" moment helped her realize it was time to say goodbye to frozen dinners. She started chopping up fresh veggies and tossing them in the fridge to grab and go when she headed off to work.

Although this transition was Cleaner, Jill's mostly raw, vegan lifestyle still left her with little in the way of balance. Her hectic schedule made it difficult for her to ensure she was getting enough nutrition to maintain her high activity levels. She decided to introduce fish and eggs into her diet to round things out. "I work best when I have guidelines to follow," Jill says. "Becoming vegetarian gave me boundaries and made me feel kind of unique. I especially love that it greatly increased the volume of food I could eat."

Challenges and Choices

Although it's a lot easier for Jill to eat at restaurants now that she has expanded her diet to include some animal products, she still likes to check the menu online and plan ahead. "I try to morph into any scenario so as not to draw unnecessary attention to my choices," Jill says of her dining-out strategy. "If necessary, I'll take an easily portable and discreet protein source with me. I emphasize discreet as I would never want my choices to be anyone else's consequence."

When it comes to the challenges of living as a vegetarian in what can sometimes feel like a meat-centered world, Jill knows she is fortunate to have a family that is so supportive. She doesn't mind when people are curious about her vegetarian lifestyle and will willingly answer neutral questions in meaningful conversations. "As I don't flaunt my choice of vegetarianism, I don't entertain negative comments either."

Getting Ripped

After adopting a vegetarian lifestyle, Jill quickly became interested in fitness and joined her local gym. Of the transition,

---

VEGGIE TECH

Jill uses the iPhone app Lose It to keep track of her daily food intake, but she stresses that she doesn't obsess over the numbers and listens to her body instead.

Find Jill and many other supportive and knowledgeable *Eat-Clean Diet*® followers (including vegetarians!) on The Kitchen Table (**eatcleandiet.com/kitchentable**) and on the *Eat-Clean Diet* Facebook page.

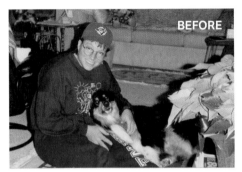
BEFORE

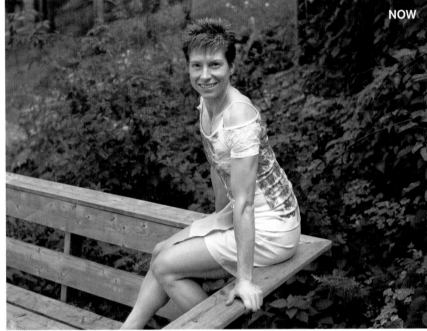
NOW

Name: Jill Holland

Age: 40

Occupation: Computer technician and systems administrator

Location: Kitchener, Ontario, Canada

On being vegetarian: "It's become my lifestyle, and I can't imagine not doing this!"

she says, "It creates a whole package. When you start to see positive changes happening in your body there's a curiosity of what could be, as well as an excitement for feeling whole." She even went on to become an aerobics instructor, but these days she focuses on building her sculpted muscles with the help of a personal trainer who keeps her motivated, challenged and accountable.

When you're as fit as Jill is, protein is an essential part of your day. Jill feels better in the gym because eating a semi-vegetarian diet ensures that she is getting her daily doses of omega-3 fatty acids and high-quality proteins. She doesn't combine proteins, but simply relies on the basics of eggs, fish and Clean protein powder (Again, convenience is important to our busy gal!).

Supplements

When it comes to her nutrient levels, Jill is vigilant. She takes a multivitamin each day, a calcium supplement and omega-3 fatty acids. She expresses the importance of being a responsible vegetarian. "It isn't a decision to take lightly because you have to be so careful that you are varying your diet to get enough of what you need. Do your research and find out what you need to replace," she says. (See p. 240 for info about important nutrients for vegetarians.)

Jill also visits her doctor on a regular basis to test her iron, vitamin B12 and calcium levels, and for the most part her numbers are off the charts! Aside from sitting down with her copies of The *Eat-Clean Diet*, Jill also meets with a nutritionist on occasion to make any necessary adjustments.

The Quotable Ms. Holland

On motivation:

"I love striving for super-health and fitness, but being able to help others to even a basic level of health and wellness is what really pushes me."

On cravings:

"I can count on one hand the number of times in almost 19 years that I would crave anything to do with meat. I do, however, crave my raw veggies!"

On Eating Clean:

"Eating Clean is an easy stress-free lifestyle. It's not meant to tie you to journals and scales but rather to listen to the signals that your body is sending you. Eat unprocessed foods, and enjoy the tastes and flavors that come out in the fresh unaltered states. Be creative!"

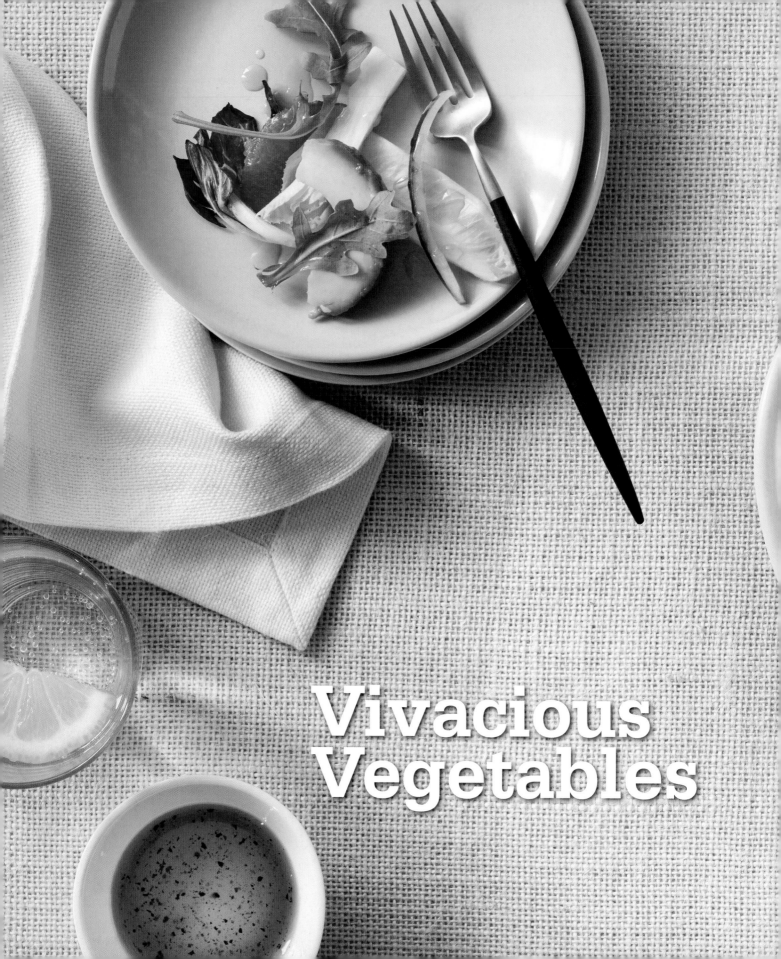

Vivacious Vegetables

Bitter Greens with
Pomelo and Avocado, p. 166

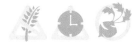

Bitter Greens with Pomelo and Avocado

PREP: 20 minutes | **COOK:** 0 minutes | **YIELD:** 6 x 1½-cup servings

Pomelo is a citrus fruit native to Southeast Asia. I've included it here as a balancing flavor against the bitterness of arugula, radicchio and endive. With the addition of avocado you've got a smooth, exciting and oh-so-good-for-you side dish!

2 cups (480 ml) baby arugula

½ head radicchio, cored and cut into
   bite-sized pieces

1 Belgian endive, stalk end trimmed ½-inch,
   and cut into 1-inch pieces

¼ small red onion, thinly sliced

1 pomelo, or large red grapefruit

1 tsp (5 ml) red wine vinegar

2 tsp (10 ml) lemon juice

1 Tbsp (15 ml) extra virgin olive oil

½ tsp (2.5 ml) brown rice syrup, yacon syrup
   or pure honey

¼ tsp (1.25 ml) sea salt

Pinch freshly ground black pepper

1 avocado, pitted and diced into 1-inch pieces

Add arugula, radicchio, endive and red onion to a large salad bowl.

To prepare pomelo, cut off the top and bottom to expose the pink flesh of the fruit. Stand pomelo on one of the cut ends, and cut down the side of the fruit to remove peel and pith. Using a paring knife, cut in between the membranes to remove pomelo segments. Cut each segment into small, bite-sized pieces and add to the bowl of greens.

In a small bowl, whisk together vinegar, lemon juice, olive oil, syrup or honey, salt and pepper, and pour over salad. Toss to combine. Add avocado, and gently toss again. Serve immediately.

NUTRITIONAL VALUE PER SERVING:
Calories: 74 | Calories from Fat: 50 | Protein: 1.3 g | Carbs: 6 g | Total Fat: 6 g |
Saturated Fat: 1 g | Trans Fat: 0 g | Fiber: 3 g | Sodium: 48 mg | Cholesterol: 0 mg

Marvelous Mediterranean Seasoning

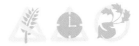

PREP: 10 minutes | **COOK:** 0 minutes | **YIELD:** ¼ cup

I know this list of ingredients seems daunting, but you probably already have many of these items in your spice rack – and the combination of flavors is fantastic! Need proof? Try it on Tofu Gyros (see p. 143) and taste how it takes them to the next level. And just think, once you've mixed the spices together, the seasoning is ready to use whenever you like!

2 tsp (10 ml) sweet paprika

2 tsp (10 ml) dried oregano, crumbled

2 tsp (10 ml) sea salt

1½ tsp (7.5 ml) garlic powder

1 tsp (5 ml) dried parsley, crumbled

½ tsp (2.5 ml) onion powder

½ tsp (2.5 ml) ground cumin

½ tsp (2.5 ml) ground cinnamon

½ tsp (2.5 ml) black pepper

½ tsp (2.5 ml) fennel seeds, coarsely ground in mortar and pestle or spice grinder

¼ tsp (1.25 ml) white pepper

¼ tsp (1.25 ml) anise seeds, coarsely ground in mortar and pestle or spice grinder

¼ tsp (1.25 ml) ground allspice

⅛ tsp (0.625 ml) ground coriander

⅛ tsp (0.625 ml) freshly grated nutmeg

Place all ingredients in an airtight container and shake to combine. Store in a cool, dry place.

TRY THIS!
Try a sprinkle of this seasoning on vegetables, tempeh or fish before grilling or roasting.

NUTRITIONAL VALUE PER 1-TSP SERVING:
Calories: 5 | Calories from Fat: 1 | Protein: 0.2 g | Carbs: 1 g | Total Fat: 0.1 g |
Saturated Fat: 0 g | Trans Fat: 0 g | Fiber: 0.5 g | Sodium: 157 mg | Cholesterol: 0 mg

Forbidden Black Quinoa

PREP: 15 minutes | **COOK:** 30 minutes | **YIELD:** 5 x 1-cup servings

Intrigued? You should be! This quinoa has a unique flavor that will keep you coming back for more. In fact, it's so good you might want to keep it your little secret. Shhh!

1 tsp (5 ml) extra virgin olive oil

2 tsp (10 ml) whole cumin seeds

½ onion, finely chopped

1 jalapeño, seeds and ribs removed, thinly sliced into half circles

2 cherry peppers, seeds and ribs removed, thinly sliced into half circles

1 Tbsp (15 ml) fresh ginger, finely grated

2 cloves garlic, minced

1½ cups (360 ml) black quinoa*, rinsed and drained

2¼ cups (540 ml) low-sodium vegetable broth or water

¼ tsp (1.25 ml) ground coriander

¼ tsp (1.25 ml) ground turmeric

⅛ tsp (0.625 ml) ground cloves

1 stick cinnamon

1 bay leaf

½ cup (120 ml) chopped cilantro

In a medium pot with lid, heat olive oil on medium. Add cumin seeds and stir in oil until fragrant. Add onion, jalapeño, cherry peppers, ginger and garlic, and cook, stirring occasionally, until soft, about 3 minutes. Add remaining ingredients, except for cilantro. Stir to combine.

Increase heat and bring to a boil, then reduce heat and simmer, covered, for about 20 minutes or until all water is absorbed and quinoa is plump. Remove from heat and keep covered for 5 minutes to allow all water to absorb. Remove cinnamon stick and bay leaf and discard. Stir in cilantro and serve.

NOTE:
*Can't find black quinoa? White or red quinoa will work too.

NUTRITIONAL VALUE PER SERVING:
Calories: 223 | Calories from Fat: 38 | Protein: 8 g | Carbs: 38 g | Total Fat: 4 g | Saturated Fat: 0.4 g | Trans Fat: 0 g | Fiber: 5 g | Sodium: 71 mg | Cholesterol: 0 mg

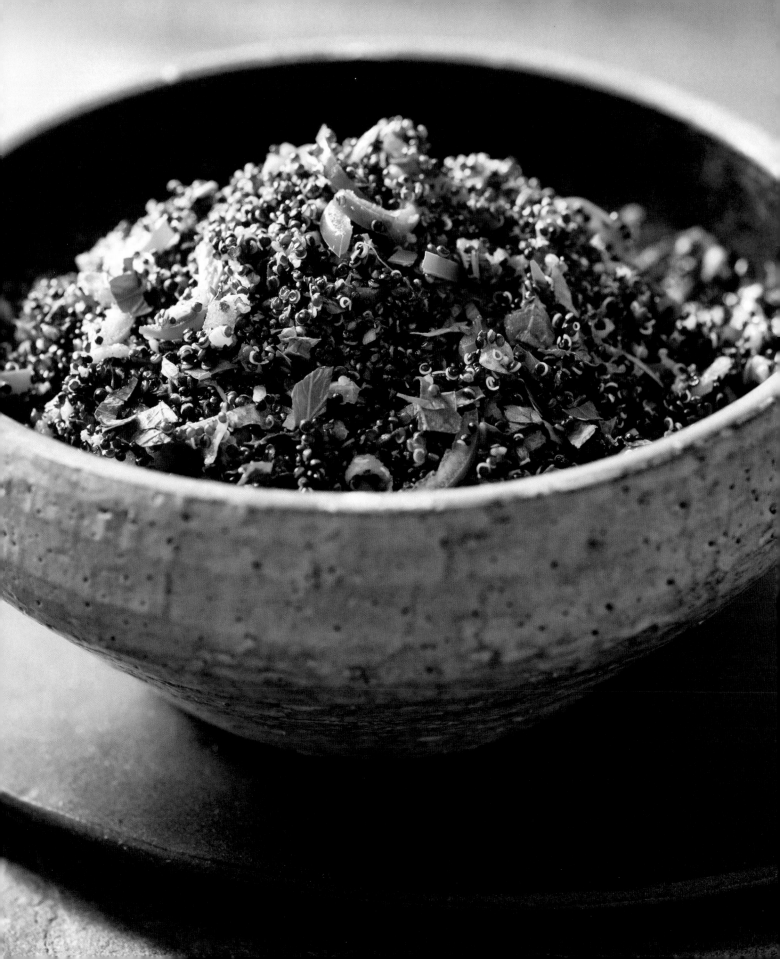

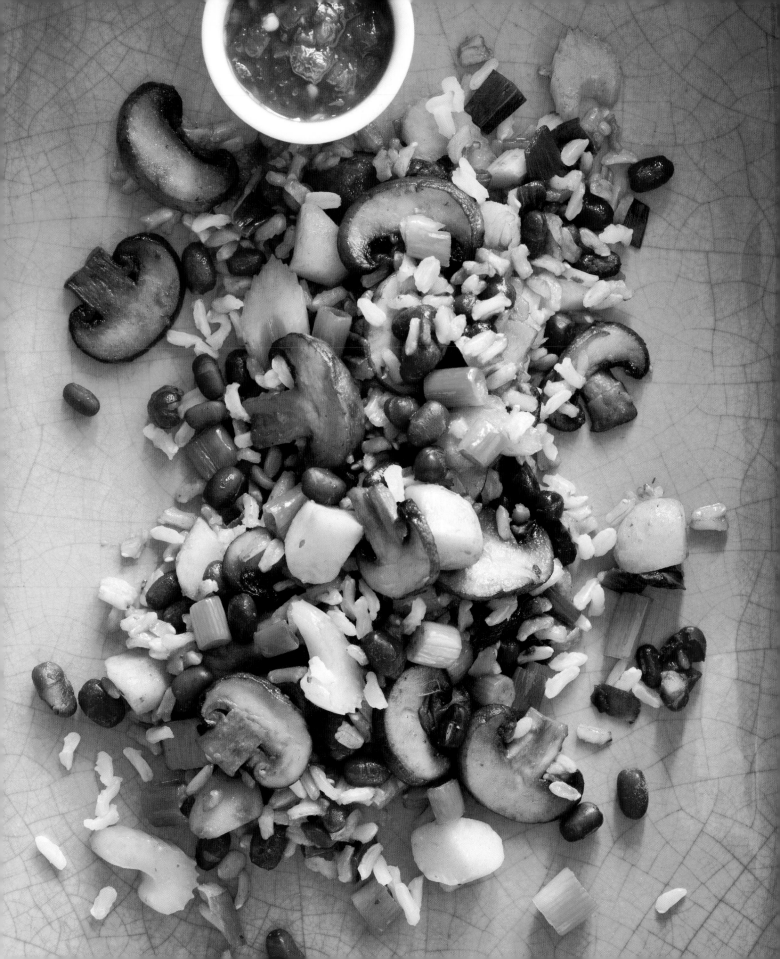

Adzuki Beans and Brown Rice with Mushrooms and Water Chestnuts

PREP: 15 minutes | **COOK:** 50 minutes | **YIELD:** 11 x 1-cup servings

Adzuki beans are native to Asia. They are typically eaten in sweet desserts, but here we have paired them with mushrooms and water chestnuts for a more savory flavor. This is the perfect side dish for grilled tofu. Give it a try!

1½ cups (360 ml) dried adzuki beans, rinsed and picked through

1 cup (240 ml) long-grain brown rice, rinsed

2 tsp (10 ml) sesame oil, divided

½ lb (225 g) cremini mushrooms, thinly sliced

2 ribs celery, thinly sliced crosswise

6 scallions, thinly sliced crosswise

1 x 5-oz (150 ml) BPA-free can sliced water chestnuts, drained, peeled and chopped

1 Tbsp (15 ml) low-sodium tamari

½ tsp (2.5 ml) each sea salt and freshly ground black pepper

Bring adzuki beans and 5 cups (1.2 L) water to a boil over high heat. Reduce heat and simmer, covered, until beans are tender but still firm enough to hold their shape, about 50 minutes. Drain.

Bring rice and 2 cups (480 ml) water to a boil, then reduce heat and simmer, covered, until cooked through, about 50 minutes. Remove from heat and fluff with a fork.

In the meantime, heat a wok or large skillet thoroughly on medium. When hot, add sesame oil, mushrooms and celery, and cook until soft, about 3 minutes. Transfer to a large bowl. Add cooked adzuki beans, brown rice, scallions, water chestnuts and tamari, and season with salt and pepper. Toss to combine. Serve with extra tamari and hot Asian-style chili sauce, if desired.

CHILL OUT
Leftovers from this recipe, which are delicious by the way, will last in the fridge for up to three days.

TRY THIS!
For a variation on this recipe, you can make bean and rice cakes by pressing the mixture into patties and pan-frying or roasting them in Eat-Clean Cooking Spray.

NUTRITIONAL VALUE PER SERVING:
Calories: 125 | Calories from Fat: 13 | Protein: 5 g | Carbs: 24 g | Total Fat: 1.5 g |
Saturated Fat: 0.1 g | Trans Fat: 0 g | Fiber: 4 g | Sodium: 122 mg | Cholesterol: 0 mg

Red Lentil Dal with Spinach

PREP: 15 minutes | **COOK:** 30-40 minutes | **YIELD:** 4 x 1-cup servings

Dal is a popular dish of Indian origin resembling a thick stew made of split pulses (dried lentils, beans or peas). Lentils provide the important proteins needed in a vegetarian or vegan diet. And pairing dal with rice or pocketless pita gives you just what you need for a complete Clean meal. Scoop it up!

1 tsp (5 ml) extra virgin olive oil

2 tsp (10 ml) whole cumin seeds

½ tsp (2.5 ml) whole fenugreek seeds

1 cup (240 ml) red lentils, picked through and rinsed

½ onion, finely chopped

2 Tbsp (30 ml) grated fresh ginger

2 cloves garlic, finely chopped

1 tsp (5 ml) ground turmeric

Chili pepper, to taste

½ tsp (2.5 ml) sea salt

4 cups (950 ml) baby spinach

1 Tbsp (15 ml) fresh lemon juice

In a large heavy-bottomed pot or Dutch oven, heat olive oil on medium high. Add cumin and fenugreek seeds and toast until fragrant, about 1 minute. Add red lentils, onion, ginger, garlic, turmeric, chili pepper, 4 cups (950 ml) water and salt. Stir to combine, bring to a boil, and then reduce heat to simmer. Skim and discard foam that floats to the top as lentils cook. Once foam no longer forms, stir lentils and cook uncovered until they are so tender that they fall apart, about 30 to 40 minutes.

Turn off heat and stir in spinach and lemon juice. Ladle into shallow bowls and serve.

TRY THIS!
Delicious accompaniments include brown rice, yogurt, cilantro and whole grain pita bread.

NUTRITIONAL VALUE PER SERVING:
Calories: 99 | Calories from Fat: 15 | Protein: 6 g | Carbs: 17 g | Total Fat: 2 g | Saturated Fat: 0.2 g | Trans Fat: 0 g | Fiber: 6 g | Sodium: 159 mg | Cholesterol: 0 mg

Roasted Exotic Mushrooms

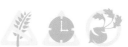

PREP: 15 minutes | **COOK:** 10-15 minutes | **YIELD:** 6 x ½-cup servings

Mushrooms! Hearty, delicious and totally aromatic. Enough said!

1 lb (454 g) mixed exotic mushrooms, such as black trumpet, oyster and porcini, brushed clean and cut or pulled apart into large bite-sized pieces

Eat-Clean Cooking Spray (see p. 277)

1 tsp (5 ml) finely chopped rosemary

Pinch each sea salt and freshly ground black pepper

2 Tbsp (30 ml) shallots, chopped

1 clove garlic, chopped

Preheat oven to 425˚F (220˚C). Place prepared mushrooms on a baking sheet, spray with Eat-Clean Cooking Spray and season with rosemary and a pinch of salt and pepper. Roast in oven for 5 minutes, then remove and stir in shallots and garlic. Place back in oven to cook for 5 to 10 minutes more, until mushrooms are browned at edges and cooked through, and shallots and garlic are soft. Check every few minutes to ensure garlic does not burn.

NUTRITIONAL VALUE PER SERVING:
Calories: 36 | Calories from Fat: 3 | Protein: 3 g | Carbs: 6 g | Total Fat: 0.03 g | Saturated Fat: 0 g | Trans Fat: 0 g | Fiber: 3 g | Sodium: 53 mg | Cholesterol: 0 mg

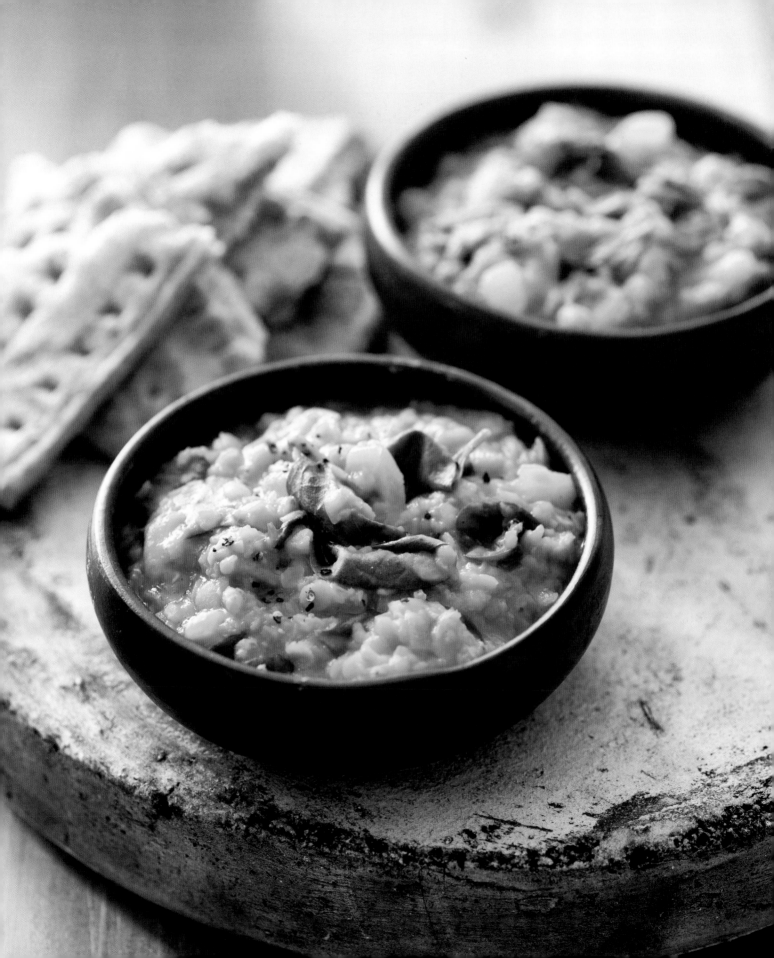

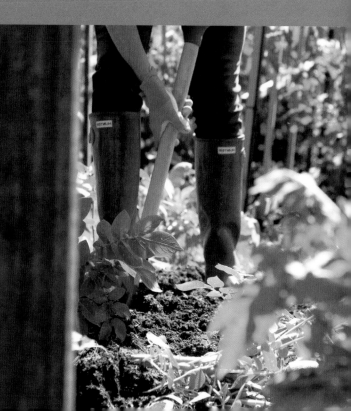

"Grow it, pick it, clean it, eat it! As Rule #32 in my book *Just the Rules* states, growing your own veggies is relaxing, rewarding and good for you."

Autumn Harvest Wild Rice

PREP: 20 minutes | **COOK:** 55 minutes | **YIELD:** 11 x 1-cup servings

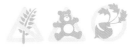

Transform this dish into a main course simply by adding a source of protein. Choose from eggs, fish or tofu. I always enjoy supper-in-a-bowl dishes.

1 cup (240 ml) wild rice, rinsed and drained

½ cup (120 ml) long-grain brown rice, rinsed and drained

Pinch sea salt

1 delicata squash, washed well, halved, seeds scooped out, and cut into bite-sized pieces

1 apple, cored and diced

3 ribs celery, sliced crosswise

1 ear corn, husked

3 tsp (15 ml) extra virgin olive oil, divided

½ tsp (2.5 ml) finely chopped fresh sage

½ tsp (2.5 ml) finely chopped fresh rosemary

Freshly ground black pepper, to taste

½ cup (120 ml) chopped pecans

¼ cup (60 ml) shelled pumpkin seeds (pepitas)

½ cup (120 ml) dried cranberries

½ cup (120 ml) chopped flat leaf parsley

1 tsp (5 ml) Dijon mustard

2 Tbsp (30 ml) apple cider vinegar

2 Tbsp (30 ml) extra virgin olive oil

Sea salt and freshly ground black pepper, to taste

In a medium saucepan, combine wild and brown rice with 3 cups (710 ml) water and a pinch sea salt. Bring to a boil, cover and reduce heat to simmer for 45 minutes. Remove from heat and let stand 10 minutes. Fluff with a fork. If any water remains, place back on heat to simmer a few minutes until water has evaporated.

Preheat oven to 425°F (220°C) and position two racks close to center. Place squash on one baking sheet and apple, celery and corn on another, with corn off to the side. Drizzle 2 tsp (10 ml) olive oil over squash, and add sage, rosemary and a pinch of salt and pepper. Toss to coat. Drizzle remaining 1 tsp (5 ml) oil over apple, celery and corn, and season with a pinch of salt and pepper. Rub oil over corn to coat. Toss apple and celery, then spread out in a single layer and place in oven. Check apple, celery and corn after 10 minutes, and remove when tender but not mushy. Cook squash until soft and golden brown.

Cut kernels from corn cob into a large bowl. Add apples, celery and squash. Add cooked rice, pecans, pumpkin seeds, cranberries and parsley.

In a small bowl, whisk together Dijon mustard, vinegar and olive oil with a pinch of salt and pepper, and pour over rice. Gently toss to combine.

Can be served immediately, or refrigerated and served chilled.

NUTRITIONAL VALUE PER SERVING:
Calories: 182 | Calories from Fat: 87 | Protein: 3 g | Carbs: 22 g | Total Fat: 10 g |
Saturated Fat: 1 g | Trans Fat: 0 g | Fiber: 3 g | Sodium: 56 mg | Cholesterol: 0 mg

Parsnip Fries

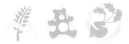

PREP: 20 minutes | **COOK:** 12-15 minutes | **YIELD:** 6 x 1-cup servings

Who doesn't love a good fry? I know for a lot of new *Eat-Clean Diet* followers ditching fries can be a little challenging. To them I say, "Don't despair!" There are so many ways to Clean up your fries that you won't feel an ounce of guilt after munching on a healthy handful. What could be better than that?

¼ tsp (1.25 ml) each curry powder, paprika, chili powder, onion powder, garlic powder and ground celery seed

¼ tsp (1.25 ml) each sea salt and freshly ground black pepper

2 lbs (908 g) parsnips, peeled and trimmed, cut into "French fry" shapes, about 3 inches long and ½-inch squared around

Eat-Clean Cooking Spray (see p. 277)

Preheat oven to 425˚F (220˚C). In a small bowl, mix together spices, salt and pepper. Place parsnips on a baking sheet and spray evenly with Eat-Clean Cooking Spray so spice mixture will stick. Sprinkle spice mixture on parsnips and toss to coat evenly. Spread in a single layer and bake 12 to 15 minutes or until golden brown and cooked through.

NUTRITIONAL VALUE PER SERVING:
Calories: 114 | Calories from Fat: 6 | Protein: 2 g | Carbs: 27 g | Total Fat: 0.1 g |
Saturated Fat: 0 g | Trans Fat: 0 g | Fiber: 6 g | Sodium: 55 mg | Cholesterol: 0 mg

THE EAT-CLEAN DIET VEGETARIAN COOKBOOK

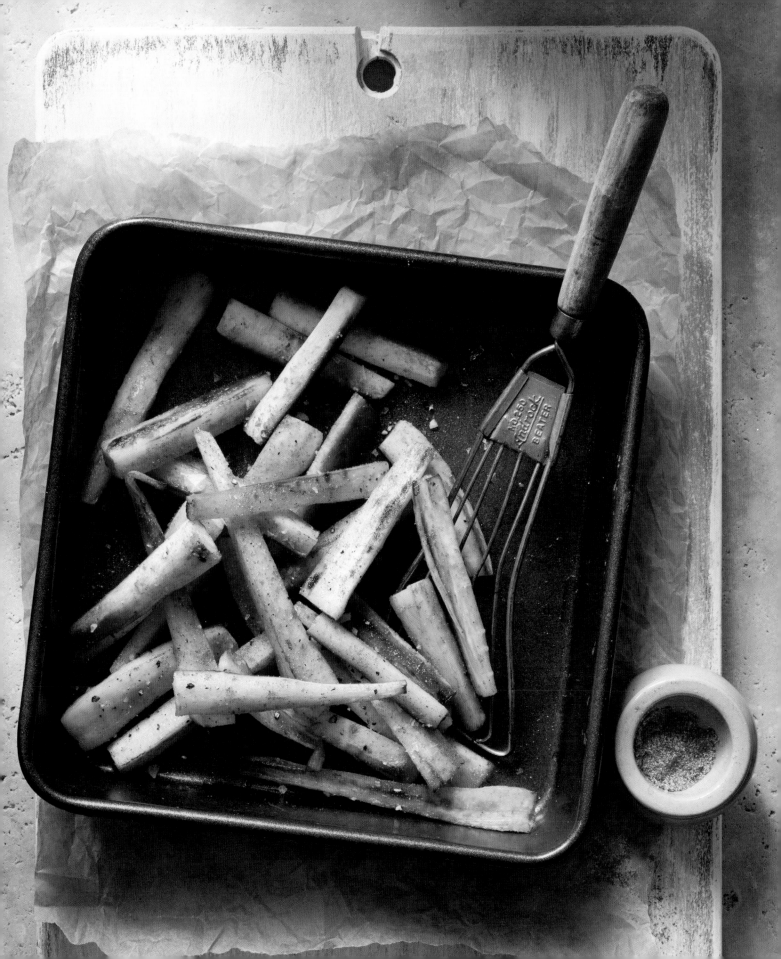

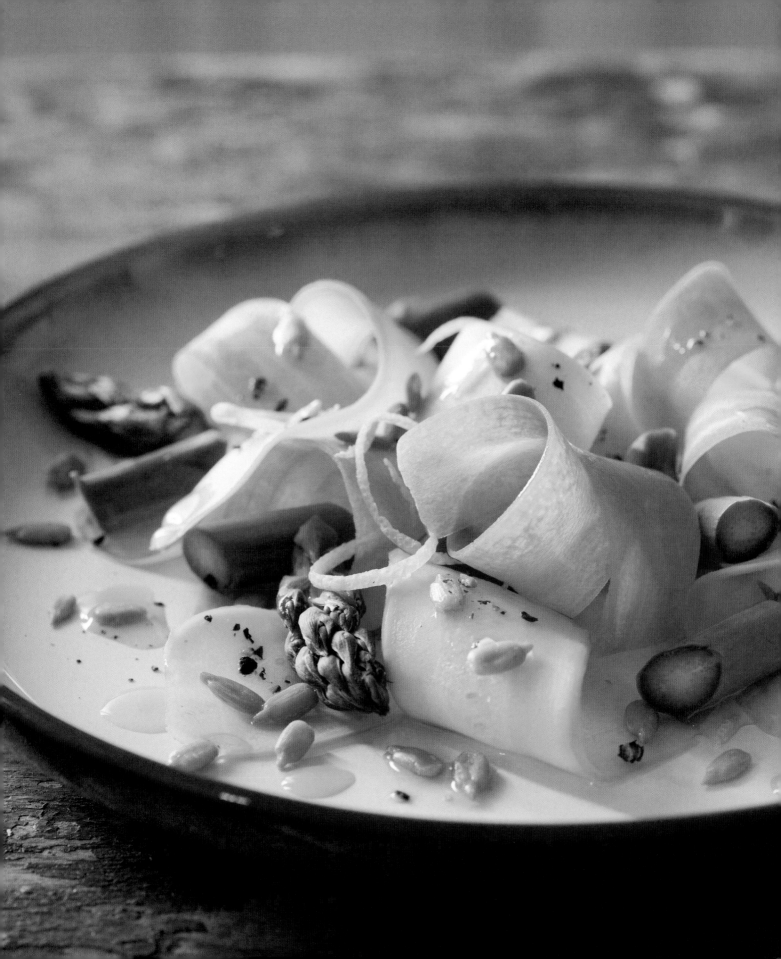

Summer Vegetable Crudi

PREP: 20 minutes | **COOK:** 0 minutes | **YIELD:** 5 x 1-cup servings

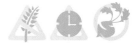

This is an Italian version of crudités, meaning raw vegetables. This dish takes the raw vegetables and turns them into bite-sized pieces and ribbons, then tosses them with a summery lemon vinaigrette. Eating the vegetables raw preserves their vital nutrients.

½ bunch baby asparagus, about ½ lb (225 g),
    stalk ends trimmed

2 baby yellow or "crookneck" squash,
    about ½ lb (225 g) each, ends trimmed

1 large carrot, peeled and trimmed

1 tsp (5 ml) lemon zest

Juice of ½ lemon

2 tsp (10 ml) extra virgin olive oil

Pinch each sea salt and freshly ground
    black pepper

2 Tbsp (30 ml) unsalted shelled sunflower seeds

Cut asparagus into ½-inch pieces on the diagonal. Using a vegetable peeler, peel squash and carrot lengthwise into ribbons. Add all prepared vegetables to a salad bowl.

In a small bowl, whisk together lemon zest and juice, olive oil, salt and pepper, and pour over vegetables. Gently toss to combine. Sprinkle with sunflower seeds and serve.

NUTRITIONAL VALUE PER SERVING:
Calories: 65 | Calories from Fat: 34 | Protein: 1 g | Carbs: 6 g | Total Fat: 4 g |
Saturated Fat: 0.5 g | Trans Fat: 0 g | Fiber: 3 g | Sodium: 59 mg | Cholesterol: 0 mg

Braised Baby Bok Choy

PREP: 10 minutes | **COOK:** 5 minutes | **YIELD:** 4 servings

Though this dish is called Braised Baby Bok Choy, it's more like a quick simmer – just long enough to make the bok choy tender.

1 Tbsp (15 ml) extra virgin olive oil

2 cloves garlic, minced

1 lb (454 g) baby bok choy, washed and
    drained, halved lengthwise

½ cup (120 ml) low-sodium vegetable broth

1 Tbsp (15 ml) low-sodium tamari

½ tsp (2.5 ml) dried crumbled dulse seaweed

½ tsp (2.5 ml) sesame oil

Heat olive oil in a very large skillet on medium high. Stir in garlic and cook until fragrant but not brown, about 1 minute.

Nestle in the baby bok choy, cut side down, and add vegetable broth and tamari. Sprinkle dulse over the top, and drizzle with sesame oil. Cover and simmer for 5 minutes until just tender.

NUTRITIONAL VALUE PER SERVING:
Calories: 58 | Calories from Fat: 37 | Protein: 2 g | Carbs: 4 g | Total Fat: 4 g |
Saturated Fat: 0.6 g | Trans Fat: 0 g | Fiber: 1.5 g | Sodium: 240 mg | Cholesterol: 0 mg

Red Quinoa Pilaf

PREP: 15 minutes | **COOK:** 30 minutes | **YIELD:** 6 x ⅔-cup servings

This dish pops with color. Pair it with tofu or eat it on its own for a great-tasting, high-protein, high-fiber meal!

1 tsp (5 ml) extra virgin olive oil

¼ red bell pepper, finely chopped

¼ yellow onion, finely chopped

2 cloves garlic, minced

1 cup (240 ml) red quinoa*

1¾ cups (420 ml) low-sodium vegetable broth

1 tsp (5 ml) finely chopped fresh thyme or ½ tsp (2.5 ml) dried

½ tsp (2.5 ml) finely chopped fresh rosemary

Pinch each sea salt and freshly ground black pepper

Heat olive oil in a medium lidded pan on medium heat. Add red pepper, onion and garlic and cook, stirring occasionally, until onion is translucent, about 5 minutes. Add quinoa, broth, thyme, rosemary, salt and pepper. Stir to combine. Increase heat to bring to a boil, and then reduce to a simmer. Cover and cook until liquid is absorbed and quinoa is plump, about 20 minutes. Remove from heat and let sit 5 minutes. Uncover and fluff with a fork.

NOTE:
*Can't find red quinoa? White will do.

NUTRITIONAL VALUE PER SERVING:
Calories: 57 | Calories from Fat: 13 | Protein: 2 g | Carbs: 9 g | Total Fat: 1.5 g | Saturated Fat: 0.1 g | Trans Fat: 0 g | Fiber: 1.5 g | Sodium: 83 mg | Cholesterol: 0 mg

Puréed Watercress

PREP: 5 minutes | **COOK:** 10 minutes | **YIELD:** 4 x ½-cup servings

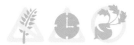

This watercress is not your typical side dish of greens. In fact, it has a peppery kick that will wake you up and keep you reaching for another spoonful to accompany your meal. Enjoy!

1 small russet potato, about ½ lb (225 g), peeled and cut into 1-inch pieces

3-4 large bunches watercress, about 1½ lbs (680 g), root ball removed and discarded, and cress washed well

1 Tbsp (15 ml) extra virgin olive oil

¼ tsp (1.25 ml) sea salt

Pinch white pepper

Place potato pieces in a very large pot filled with cold water. Place on stove over high heat, bring to a boil and add a generous pinch of salt. Cook until potato is tender when pierced with a knife, 8 to 10 minutes. Add watercress and cook barely 1 minute until bright green. Drain both into a colander and use a rubber spatula or the back of a spoon to press out as much water as possible.

Transfer to a food processor and whirl until it forms a purée. Add olive oil, salt and pepper, and whirl again until thoroughly combined.

NUTRITIONAL VALUE PER SERVING:
Calories: 78 | Calories from Fat: 33 | Protein: 5 g | Carbs: 9 g | Total Fat: 4 g | Saturated Fat: 0.5 g | Trans Fat: 0 g | Fiber: 1 g | Sodium: 128 mg | Cholesterol: 0 mg

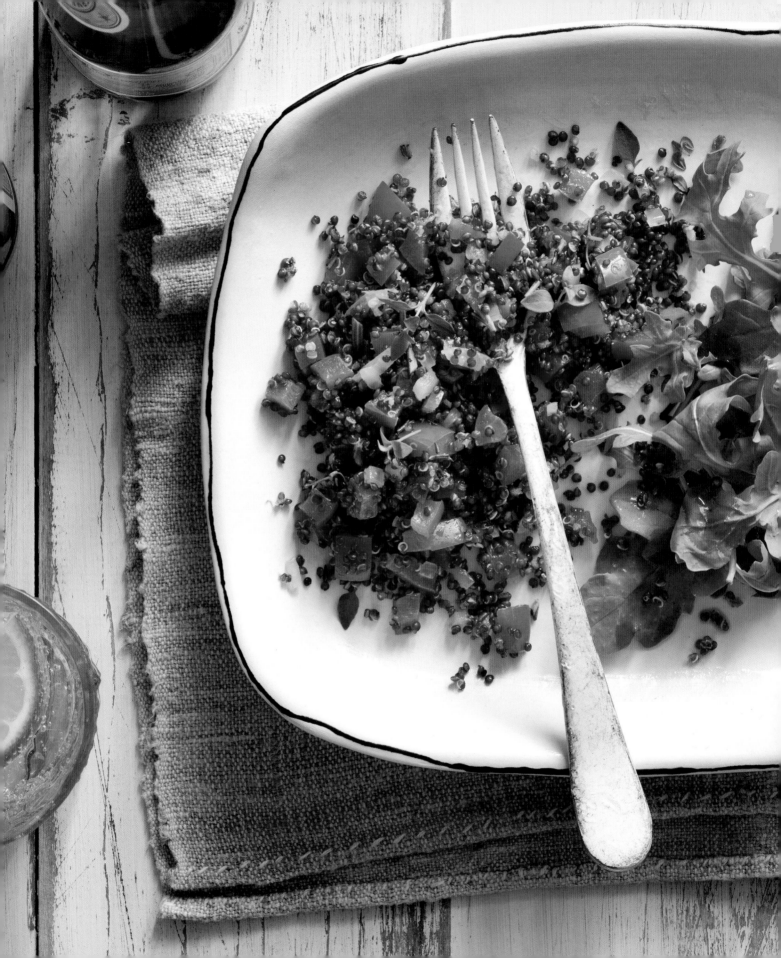

Yakisoba

PREP: 25 minutes | **COOK:** 20 minutes | **YIELD:** 8 x 1-cup servings

Yakisoba literally means "fried buckwheat noodles;" soba means buckwheat. I've chosen to pan-fry the noodles in healthy oil and serve them up with tons of veggies!

2 Tbsp (30 ml) low-sodium tamari

1 Tbsp (15 ml) rice vinegar

1 Tbsp (15 ml) Sucanat or other unrefined sugar

½ tsp (2.5 ml) sesame oil

8 oz (225 g) Chinese or Japanese
　　buckwheat noodles

1 Tbsp (15 ml) grapeseed oil, or other
　　high-heat Clean oil

1 yellow or white onion, thinly sliced

1 Tbsp (15 ml) grated ginger

2 ribs celery, thinly sliced crosswise

4 cups (950 ml) shredded red or
　　purple cabbage

1 cup (240 ml) shredded carrot

8 oz (225 g) sliced bamboo shoots, drained

2 green onions, green parts only, chopped

1-2 Tbsp (15-30 ml) sesame seeds

In a small bowl, stir together tamari, rice vinegar, Sucanat and sesame oil until Sucanat is dissolved. Set aside.

Cook noodles according to package instructions, drain and set aside.

Heat a large wok or cast-iron skillet thoroughly on high until almost smoking. Add oil and onion and cook, stirring occasionally, until soft and slightly charred, about 3 minutes. Stir in ginger. Add celery, cabbage, carrot and bamboo shoots, and use metal tongs or two wok spatulas to fold in vegetables and toss together. Cook until vegetables are soft and reduced in volume, folding and tossing occasionally, 3 to 5 minutes.

Add cooked noodles and pour reserved bowl of sauce on top. Toss to combine noodles with vegetables and coat all ingredients with sauce. Continue to cook until noodles are heated through. Mound Yakisoba in bowls and top with chopped green onions and sesame seeds.

TRY THIS!
Serve with hot Asian chili sauce, if desired.

PROTEIN POWER!
Add tofu to this side dish and it becomes a complete, Clean vegan meal!

NUTRITIONAL VALUE PER SERVING:
Calories: 104 | Calories from Fat: 28 | Protein: 3 g | Carbs: 17 g | Total Fat: 3 g | Saturated Fat: 0.5 g | Trans Fat: 0 g | Fiber: 2 g | Sodium: 207 mg | Cholesterol: 0 mg

Puttanesca Sauce

PREP: 15 minutes | **COOK:** 35 minutes | **YIELD:** 10 x ¾-cup servings

The direct translation of puttanesca isn't pleasant so I will spare you the details, but the taste of this sauce certainly is something to enjoy. Puttanesca sauce is a little spicy, a little salty and a little tangy. Sounds pleasant to me!

1¼ cups (300 ml) dried textured soy protein (see note at right)

1⅛ cup (241 ml) boiling water or low-sodium, gluten-free vegetable broth

2 x 28-oz (828 ml) BPA-free cans no-salt-added whole plum tomatoes

1 Tbsp (15 ml) extra virgin olive oil

½ onion, finely chopped

4 cloves garlic, minced

1 Tbsp (15 ml) tomato paste

¼ cup (60 ml) packed pitted kalamata olives, chopped

1 Tbsp (15 ml) capers, drained and rinsed

½ tsp (2.5 ml) dried Italian herbs

¼ tsp (1.25 ml) red pepper flakes

Pinch sea salt and freshly ground black pepper

Place textured soy protein in a bowl and pour boiling water or broth overtop. Stir, and let sit 5 minutes to rehydrate.

Place tomatoes in a large bowl and use your hands to squish them into bite-sized pieces.

Heat olive oil in a Dutch oven or large pot on medium. Add onion and cook until soft and translucent, but not brown, about 3 minutes. Stir in garlic and cook for 1 minute. Stir in tomato paste, and then add squished tomatoes. Add olives, capers, Italian herbs, red pepper flakes and rehydrated textured soy protein. Stir to combine, and increase heat to bring sauce to a vigorous simmer. Partially cover pot, reduce heat and let simmer gently, stirring once or twice, about 30 minutes.

When sauce has finished cooking, taste and season with a pinch of salt and pepper, if desired. Serve over your favorite whole-grain pasta, quinoa or steamed brown rice.

PREP TIP
Textured soy protein is also known as TSP or TVP, and is normally found in the health food aisle or bulk section of your grocery store.

NUTRITIONAL VALUE PER SERVING:
Calories: 90 | Calories from Fat: 29 | Protein: 7 g | Carbs: 11 g | Total Fat: 3 g | Saturated Fat: 0.2 g | Trans Fat: 0 g | Fiber: 4 g | Sodium: 74 mg | Cholesterol: 0 mg

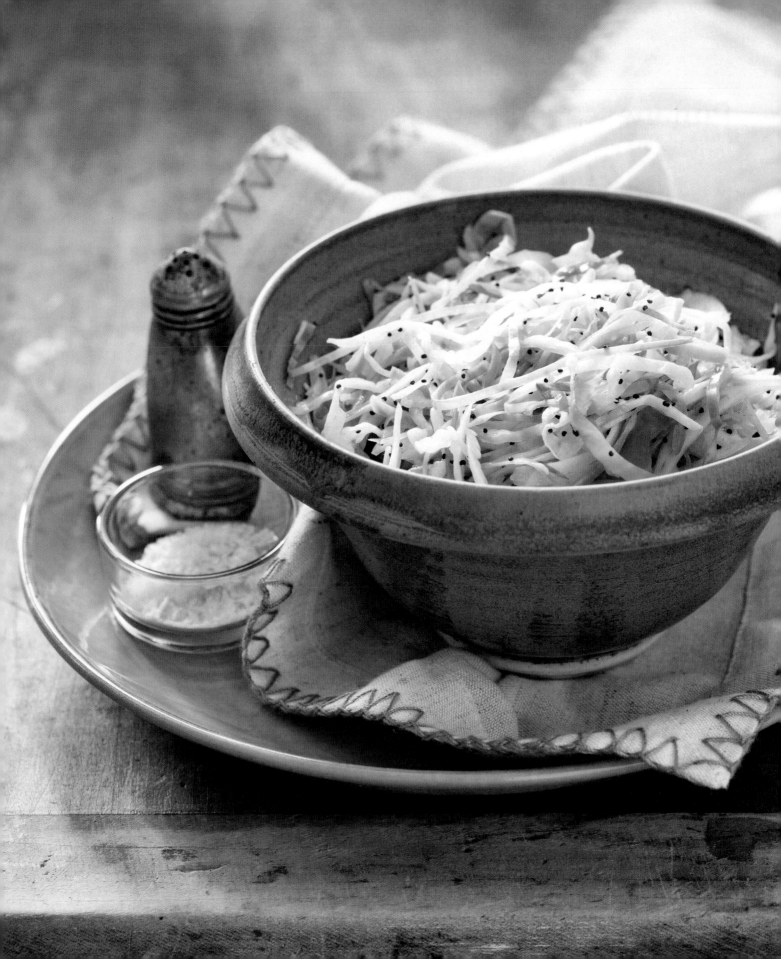

Croatian Cabbage Slaw

PREP: 10 minutes active, 3 hours inactive | **COOK:** 0 minutes | **YIELD:** 6 x 1-cup servings

I had this salad once at a Croatian friend's house. I loved it so much I went home and made a huge Eat-Clean batch … and I then discovered that this salad really cleans out your insides!

½ head green cabbage, shredded or very thinly
    sliced, about 8 cups (1.9 L)
1 Tbsp (15 ml) safflower oil or light olive oil
¼ cup (60 ml) distilled white vinegar
½ tsp (2.5 ml) sea salt
¼ tsp (1.25 ml) freshly ground black pepper
1-2 Tbsp (15-30 ml) chia seeds

In a large bowl, combine cabbage, safflower oil, vinegar, salt and pepper. Using your hands, mix ingredients together and squeeze cabbage to help it break down. Cover and refrigerate until chilled, at least 3 hours or overnight. When ready to serve, mix in the chia seeds.

CHILL OUT
This slaw will keep in the fridge up to three days. Just make sure you add the chia seeds right before serving, otherwise they will swell up and become gelatinous.

NUTRITIONAL VALUE PER SERVING:
Calories: 58 | Calories from Fat: 27 | Protein: 2 g | Carbs: 7 g | Total Fat: 3 g |
Saturated Fat: 0.2 g | Trans Fat: 0 g | Fiber: 3 g | Sodium: 97 mg | Cholesterol: 0 mg

Smoked Paprika Roasted Fingerling Potatoes

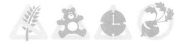

PREP: 10 minutes | **COOK:** 25 minutes | **YIELD:** 8 x ¾-cup servings

Roasted potatoes are a family favorite in my house. They produce a delicious smell that draws everyone to the dinner table with eager appetites. I love the smoky quality given to these potatoes by the paprika. They're a breeze to prepare and I can assure you your kids' plates will be as clean as the meal!

2 lbs (908 g) purple and white fingerling
    potatoes, halved lengthwise

1 yellow onion, halved and sliced

2 Tbsp (30 ml) extra virgin olive oil

2 tsp (10 ml) smoked paprika

½ tsp (2.5 ml) garlic powder

½ tsp (2.5 ml) onion powder

1 tsp (5 ml) sea salt

½ tsp (2.5 ml) freshly ground black pepper

¼ cup (60 ml) scallions, green part
    only, chopped

Preheat oven to 425°F (220°C). Place potatoes and onion on a baking sheet. Drizzle with olive oil, and sprinkle with paprika, garlic and onion powder, salt and pepper. Toss to combine, and turn as many of the potatoes cut side down as possible. Roast in oven until golden brown on outside, and tender and cooked through on inside, 20 to 25 minutes. Remove from oven, stir in scallions and serve warm.

NUTRITIONAL VALUE PER SERVING:
Calories: 96 | Calories from Fat: 32 | Protein: 2 g | Carbs: 15 g | Total Fat: 4 g | Saturated Fat: 0.5 g | Trans Fat: 0 g | Fiber: 3 g | Sodium: 126 mg | Cholesterol: 0 mg

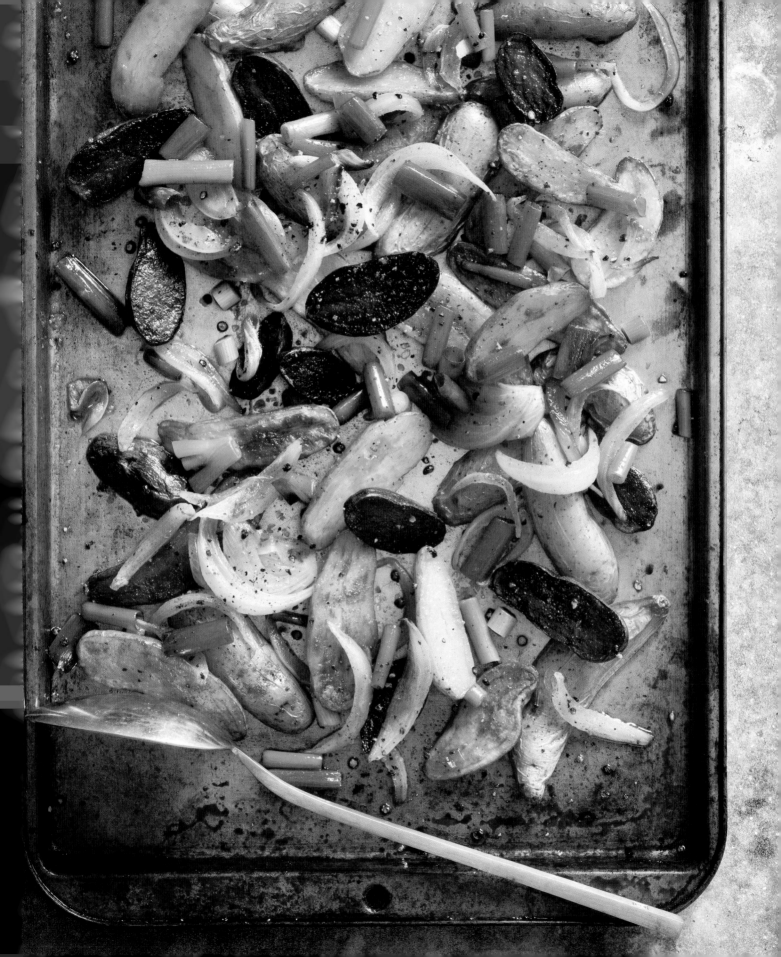

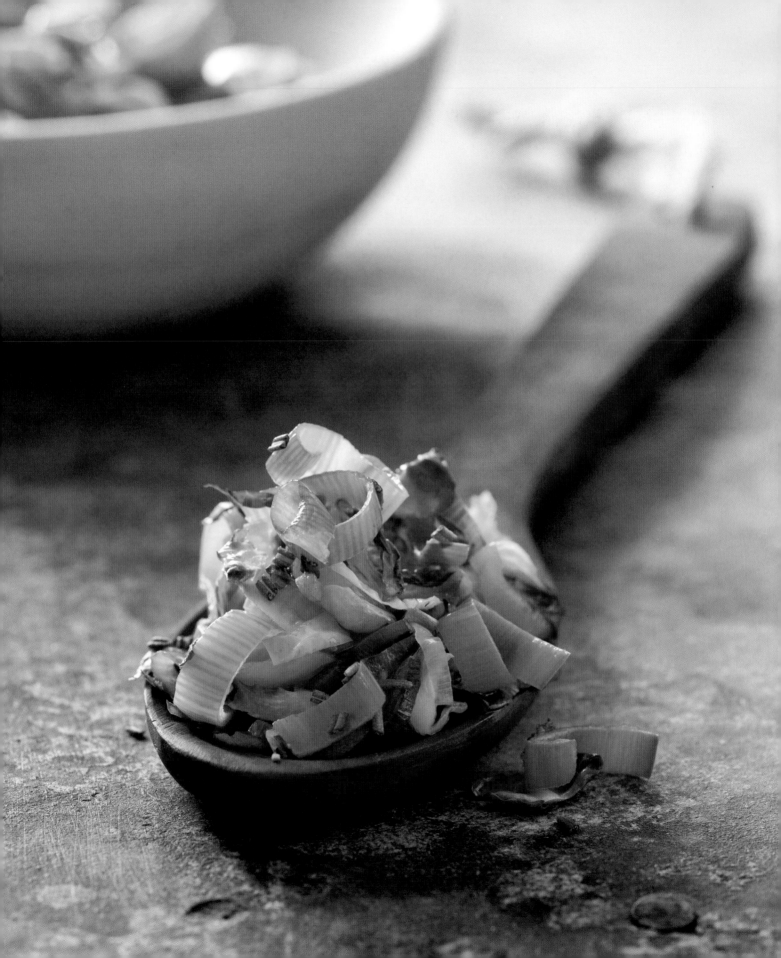

Golden Brussels and Leeks

PREP: 20 minutes | **COOK:** 20 minutes | **YIELD:** 7 x ½-cup servings

The definition of fast food is roasted vegetables. Chop 'em, dress 'em and pop 'em in the oven. In just 20 minutes, you've got an elegant side that is the perfect complement to a wide variety of mains.

1 lb (454 g) Brussels sprouts, trimmed with outer leaves removed, thinly sliced

2 large leeks, white and light green parts only, rinsed well, thinly sliced

1 Tbsp (15 ml) extra virgin olive oil

1 tsp (5 ml) herbes de Provence

¼ tsp (1.25 ml) each sea salt and freshly ground black pepper

Preheat the oven to 425°F (220°C). Toss all ingredients together on a baking sheet and spread out in a single layer. Roast in oven for about 20 minutes, stirring halfway through, or until soft and caramelized.

NUTRITIONAL VALUE PER SERVING:
Calories: 61 | Calories from Fat: 21 | Protein: 3 g | Carbs: 11 g | Total Fat: 2 g |
Saturated Fat: 0.3 g | Trans Fat: 0 g | Fiber: 3 g | Sodium: 55 mg | Cholesterol: 0 mg

Collards Southern Style

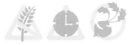

PREP: 10 minutes | **COOK:** 15 minutes | **YIELD:** 6 x 1-cup servings

Collard greens – they may drum up images of deep-fried Southern fare or you may be totally unfamiliar with them. Whatever the case, I urge you try them in this lightened-up recipe. Don't worry… you're in for a tasty treat (and not a cardiac arrest!).

2 large bunches collard greens, about 2 lbs (908 g)

1 Tbsp (15 ml) extra virgin olive oil

3 cloves garlic, minced

¼ tsp (1.25 ml) sea salt

1 cup (240 ml) low-sodium, gluten-free vegetable broth

⅛ tsp (0.625 ml) liquid smoke (about 5 drops)

½ tsp (2.5 ml) unsulfured blackstrap molasses

Trim collard stems, halve lengthwise and then cut crosswise into two-inch pieces. Wash, drain and spin them dry in a salad spinner until water is free of dirt and silt.

Heat olive oil in a very large skillet on medium high. Add garlic and cook 30 seconds until just fragrant. Add half the greens and use tongs to fold them into garlic and oil. Cook until they start to wilt. Add remainder of greens and sea salt, and use tongs to fold them in toward the bottom of the pan. Cook until they start to wilt as well.

Add vegetable broth, liquid smoke and molasses, and stir to combine. Cover and simmer until tender, about 10 minutes.

NUTRITIONAL VALUE PER SERVING:
Calories: 82 | Calories from Fat: 21 | Protein: 6 g | Carbs: 12 g | Total Fat: 2 g |
Saturated Fat: 0.3 g | Trans Fat: 0 g | Fiber: 6 g | Sodium: 345 mg | Cholesterol: 0 mg

Cuban Black Beans

PREP: 20 minutes + overnight soaking of beans | **COOK:** 1 hour 40 minutes | **YIELD:** 5 x 1-cup servings

The black beans in this side dish not only impart a satisfying texture but they also pair perfectly with the bold Cuban spices. Onions and bell peppers add a crunch to juxtapose the softness of the beans, and lime juice gives it all a perfectly tangy finish. Pair this dish with fish, tofu or a side of rice and you'll feel like you're suddenly on vacation!

1 lb (454 g) dried black beans

1 Tbsp (15 ml) extra virgin olive oil

1 yellow or white onion, finely chopped

1 green bell pepper, seeded and
       finely chopped

4 cloves garlic, minced

½ tsp (2.5 ml) sea salt

½ tsp (2.5 ml) freshly ground black pepper

2 cups (480 ml) low-sodium, gluten-free
       vegetable broth

1 tsp (5 ml) ground cumin

½ tsp (2.5 ml) dried oregano

1 bay leaf

1 tsp (5 ml) balsamic vinegar

Juice of 1 lime

Cover dried beans with plenty of water and let stand, covered, overnight or for at least 8 hours. To speed up the process, bring them to a boil, remove from heat, let stand covered for 1 hour, then drain.

Heat olive oil in a large pot or Dutch oven on medium. Add onion and green pepper and cook until onion is translucent, 8 to 10 minutes. Using a mortar and pestle (if you don't have one, see Prep Tip below), mash garlic, sea salt and black pepper into a paste. Stir garlic paste into onion-green pepper mixture and cook until fragrant but not brown, 1 or 2 minutes.

Add drained beans, vegetable broth, 1 cup (240 ml) water, cumin, oregano and bay leaf. Bring to a boil, and then reduce heat to simmer, covered with the lid tilted, until beans are tender, about 1½ hours. Occasionally skim the foam that appears on surface and discard it. If liquid cooks down so beans are no longer covered, add ½ cup (120 ml) water at a time. The beans should be thick, not soupy.

When beans are cooked, remove bay leaf and discard. Transfer 1 cup (240 ml) of beans to a food processor and blend until smooth. Return blended beans to the pot, Stir in balsamic vinegar and lime juice. Cover, remove from heat and let sit 10 minutes. Taste, and make any adjustments to seasoning with salt, pepper or more lime juice.

TRY THIS!
Serve over steamed brown rice, garnished with a sprinkle of finely chopped white or yellow onion and chopped cilantro.

PREP TIP
If you don't have a mortar and pestle, just use the side of a chef's knife to press the minced garlic into a paste.

NUTRITIONAL VALUE PER SERVING:
Calories: 370 | Calories from Fat: 39 | Protein: 20 g | Carbs: 64 g | Total Fat: 4 g |
Saturated Fat: 1 g | Trans Fat: 0 g | Fiber: 15 g | Sodium: 158 mg | Cholesterol: 0 mg

THE EAT-CLEAN DIET VEGETARIAN COOKBOOK

Tex-Mex Rice

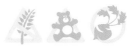

PREP: 10 minutes | **COOK:** 70 minutes | **YIELD:** 8 x ¾-cup servings

This makes a great side dish for Taco Night (see p. 127) or any time you're craving a rice dish with a kick. It also pairs perfectly with Tex-Mex Beans (see below) for a complete meal.

2 cups (480 ml) low-sodium, gluten-free
    vegetable broth

1 heaping Tbsp (17 or 18 ml) tomato paste

1 Tbsp (15 ml) extra virgin olive oil

½ yellow onion, finely chopped

2 cups (480 ml) long-grain brown rice

2 cloves garlic, minced

½ tsp (2.5 ml) chili powder

¼ tsp (1.25 ml) sea salt

In a small pot, combine vegetable broth, 1¾ cups (420 ml) water and tomato paste. Bring to a gentle simmer and stir once or twice to dissolve tomato paste.

Heat olive oil in a medium heavy-bottomed pot with lid. Add onion and cook until translucent, about 3 minutes. Add brown rice and stir to coat in oil. Cook, stirring, until almost starting to brown, 2 or 3 minutes. Stir in garlic and cook until fragrant, about 1 minute. Add simmering broth mixture, chili powder and salt. Stir once, cover, and reduce heat to simmer gently until liquid is absorbed and rice is cooked through, about 50 minutes. Remove from heat and let sit, covered, for 10 minutes. Fluff with a fork and serve.

NUTRITIONAL VALUE PER SERVING:
Calories: 200 | Calories from Fat: 27 | Protein: 4 g | Carbs: 38 g | Total Fat: 3 g |
Saturated Fat: 0.5 g | Trans Fat: 0 g | Fiber: 2 g | Sodium: 70 mg | Cholesterol: 0 mg

Tex-Mex Beans

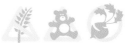

PREP: 10 minutes + overnight soaking of beans | **COOK:** 1 hour 40 minutes | **YIELD:** 10 x ½-cup servings

Here's a Clean version of refried beans that aren't actually fried. When combined with Tex-Mex Rice (see above) you've got a protein-rich meal. They also make a great side dish for Taco Night (see p. 127).

1 lb (454 g) dry pinto beans, picked through,
    soaked overnight and drained

1 bay leaf

½ onion, intact

1 Tbsp (15 ml) extra virgin olive oil

¼ onion, very finely chopped

1 clove garlic, finely minced

½ tsp (2.5 ml) ground cumin

½ tsp (2.5 ml) chili powder

½ tsp (2.5 ml) smoked paprika

½ tsp (2.5 ml) sea salt

Place drained beans in a large pot and add enough cold, fresh water to cover by 2 inches. Add bay leaf and onion half. Bring beans to a boil, cover pot with a tilted lid to allow steam to escape and simmer until very tender, stirring occasionally, about 1½ hours. Remove bay leaf and drain beans, reserving 1 cup (240 ml) cooking liquid.

In a large skillet or pot, heat olive oil on medium. Add chopped onion and cook until very soft and translucent, then add minced garlic and cook until soft, but not brown. Stir in cumin, chili powder and smoked paprika. Add drained beans, sea salt and half of reserved cooking liquid. Reduce heat to low, mash beans with a potato masher (use those arm muscles!) and stir. Continue to mash and stir beans, adding more liquid if needed, until you achieve desired consistency. Beans should be "loose" but not soupy.

NUTRITIONAL VALUE PER SERVING:
Calories: 174 | Calories from Fat: 18 | Protein: 10 g | Carbs: 30 g | Total Fat: 1 g |
Saturated Fat: 0.2 g | Trans Fat: 0 g | Fiber: 7 g | Sodium: 53 mg | Cholesterol: 0 mg

Roasted Spaghetti Squash with Hazelnuts and Crispy Sage

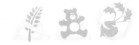

PREP: 10 minutes | **COOK:** 45 minutes | **YIELD:** 5 x 1-cup servings

In my opinion, spaghetti squash is a sorely overlooked gourd. Let's change that. It is the perfect replacement for pasta noodles, making it appropriate for gluten-free *Eat-Clean Diet* fans everywhere. Preparing it with hazelnuts and sage gives it a warm and toasty flavor that is both satisfying and healthy.

Eat-Clean Cooking Spray (see p. 277)

1 spaghetti squash, about 4-4½ lbs (1.8-2 kg), halved lengthwise, seeds scooped out

½ cup (120 ml) hazelnuts

1 Tbsp (15 ml) extra virgin olive oil

5 sage leaves

1 Tbsp (15 ml) real maple syrup

1 tsp (5 ml) unsulfured blackstrap molasses

¼ tsp (1.25 ml) freshly grated nutmeg

¼ tsp (1.25 ml) each sea salt and freshly ground black pepper

¼ cup (60 ml) chopped Italian parsley

Preheat oven to 350°F (177°C). Spray a baking sheet with Eat-Clean Cooking Spray and place squash cut side down on sheet. Place in oven to roast until a skewer can pierce the skin and pass through the flesh without resistance, 30 to 45 minutes. Remove from oven and let cool until comfortable enough to handle. Use a fork to pull out strands from spaghetti squash and transfer strands to a large bowl.

Place hazelnuts on a baking sheet and toast in oven for 5 minutes. Remove to cool slightly, and then coarsely chop. Set aside.

Heat olive oil in a small skillet on medium. Add sage leaves and "fry" in olive oil for 1 minute. Remove with a fork and transfer to a paper towel. Remove skillet from heat and stir in maple syrup, molasses, nutmeg, salt and pepper. Use a rubber spatula to scrape mixture over squash. Add chopped hazelnuts and parsley, and toss to thoroughly combine.

Mound spaghetti squash in shallow bowls and top each with a crispy sage leaf.

NUTRITIONAL VALUE PER SERVING:
Calories: 217 | Calories from Fat: 98 | Protein: 5 g | Carbs: 30 g | Total Fat: 11 g |
Saturated Fat: 1 g | Trans Fat: 0 g | Fiber: 7 g | Sodium: 118 mg | Cholesterol: 0 mg

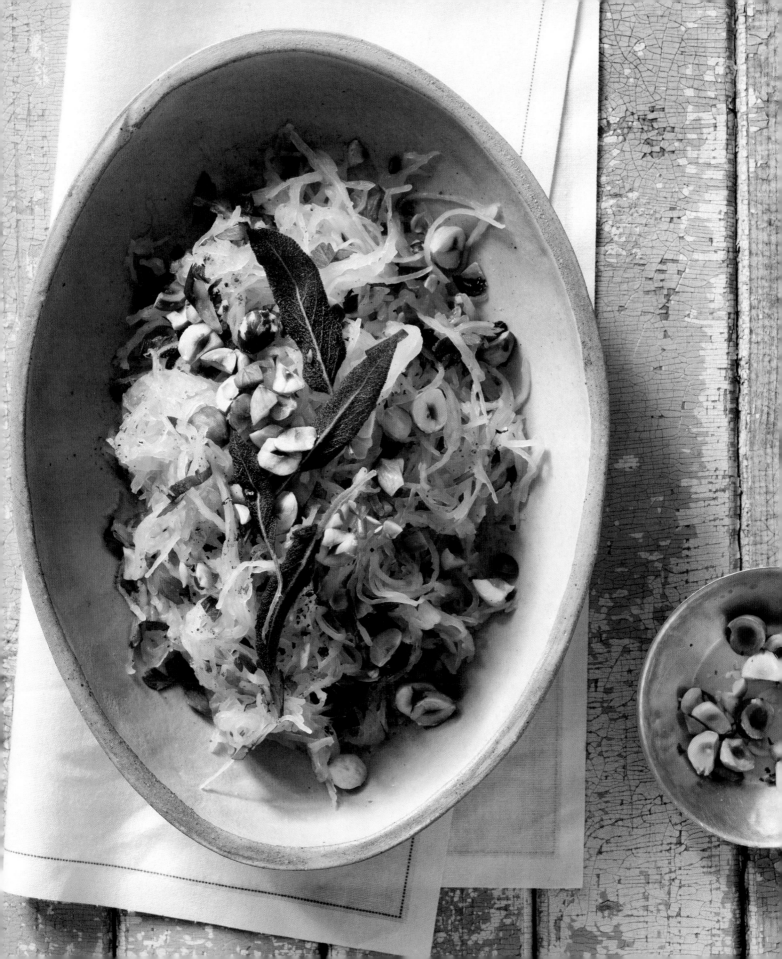

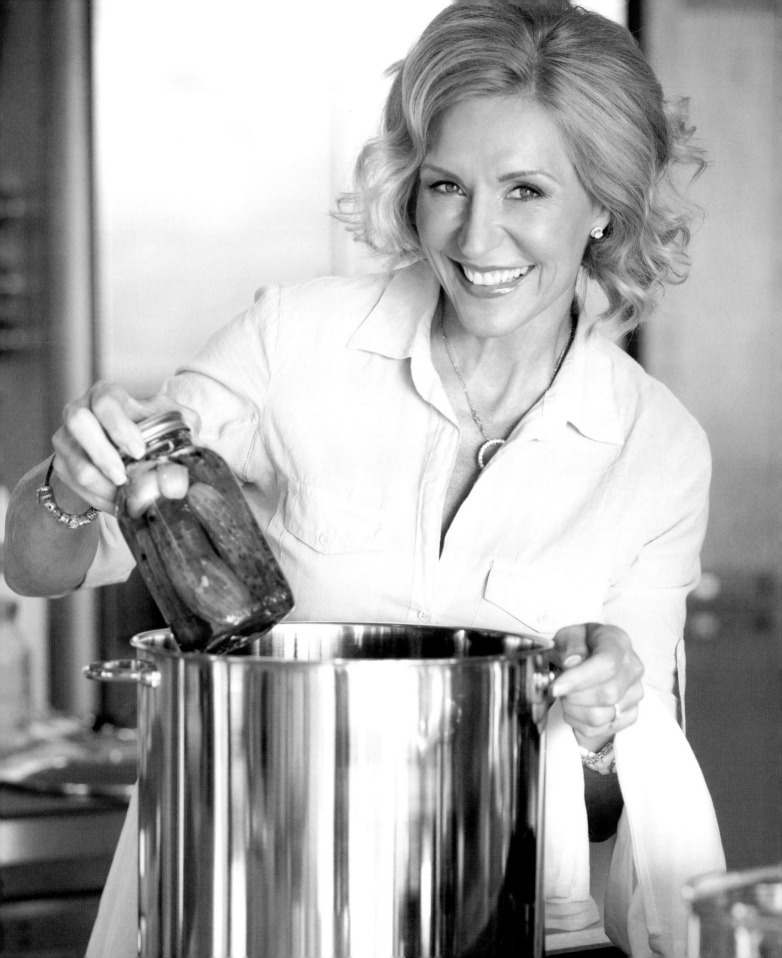

Vietnamese Fresh-Pickled Vegetables

PREP: 20 minutes active, 1 hour inactive (minimum) | **COOK:** 0 minutes | **YIELD:** 12 x ½-cup servings

Pickling is an amazing way to enhance food. It's simple, healthy and you wind up with a whole new way of enjoying your veggies. Yum!

3 cups (710 ml) all-natural salt- and sugar-free rice vinegar

3 Tbsp (45 ml) brown rice syryp or yacon syrup

1 tsp (5 ml) sea salt

1 large daikon radish, peeled and trimmed

2 carrots, peeled and trimmed

½ English cucumber

½ small white onion, thinly sliced

2 green jalapeño peppers, stemmed, quartered lengthwise and seeded

2 red jalapeño peppers, stemmed, quartered lengthwise and seeded

In a large bowl, whisk together vinegar, syrup and salt until salt is dissolved.

Using a mandoline slicer or sharp chef's knife, thinly slice daikon, carrots and cucumber into rounds. Add daikon, carrots, cucumber, onion and jalapeños to vinegar mixture. Stir to combine, and then press vegetables down to submerge in brine. Cover and refrigerate for at least 1 hour, and several hours if possible, to develop flavors. To serve, remove vegetables from brine. Delicious on sandwiches, added to salads or as a flavorful side dish.

CHILL OUT
These veggies will keep in the refrigerator for one week.

NUTRITIONAL VALUE PER SERVING:
Calories: 13 | Calories from Fat: 1 | Protein: 0.3 g | Carbs: 4 g | Total Fat: 0.1 g |
Saturated Fat: 0 g | Trans Fat: 0 g | Fiber: 0.4 g | Sodium: 91 mg | Cholesterol: 0 mg

Pickling And Preserving

I did not grow up in a household where pickling and preserving food was a custom. My mother did freeze all of the produce my father grew in his vegetable garden and she made applesauce, which also went into the freezer along with a myriad of berries. I developed an interest in the preservation of food when I spent a summer on a farm through a high school learning program. The beans, carrots, onions and berries that flew through my fingers numbered in the millions I am sure, but I had such a good time doing it and felt my work was worthwhile. Soon enough I was canning my own produce and enjoying the bounty of summer long through the winter months. I still enjoy keeping food this way and find time to preserve summer's abundance no matter how heavy my schedule because I know for sure what went into each jar of food. I like preserving food in jars because where I live we often experience power failures. If all my food was in a freezer I would be in trouble every time we went black.

More and more people are going back to preserving food for themselves and their families. It is a way of taking more of our food supply back into our own hands. This gives us a feeling of accountability and responsibility regarding food that we don't get from a drive-thru. Growing, preserving and eating local, fresh, in-season food is a powerful and positive contribution you can make in this environmentally stressed world. When this spark is ignited in you as it was in me you feel a greater sense of hope and power in the food decision-making part of your life. It feels downright good.

The proliferation of canning and preserving food was a positive outcome of World War I. Americans were asked to assist in the war effort by growing their own food in what was known as a Victory Garden. What grew in those mighty gardens fed a nation not just during the summer months but through the winter as well, thanks to the science of food preservation.

So many people are getting back to this old way of doing things that there are now community canning groups that gather strangers together to put up the shared harvest from each other's gardens. Experienced and newbie canners alike join in the work, helping to reduce the boredom of doing it on your own and the costs of equipment all while learning a valuable new skill. You will never have to ask the question "What do I do with all this zucchini?" again. Look for a community kitchen online at www.communitykitchens.com.

Preservation Techniques

Heat Processing

Preserving foods is as simple as baking but the results last up to a year. Home canning is called heat processing and is accomplished in one of two ways: in a boiling water bath or in a pressure canner. Properly prepared foods are placed in sterile glass jars, usually Mason jars, sealed with a sterile rubber ring and lid and placed in a boiling water bath or a pressure cooker. Recipes for canning various foods – even meats – provide clear instructions on how exactly to accomplish the task. It can be a bit unnerving the first time you do it but once you start to hear the unmistakable "pinging" of jars sealing themselves you will be hooked.

As a general rule foods high in natural acids like tomatoes are best in the hot water bath system while foods low in natural acids like beans and asparagus are better in a pressure canner.

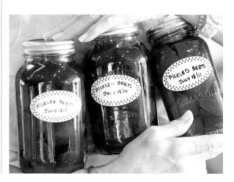

Pickling

Another time-honored method of preserving foods is to pickle them in a solution of vinegar and salt. The pickling process preserves food through fermentation, whereby lactic acid is produced when vinegar and salt are added to the food. The added acidity of the vinegar elevates the otherwise low acid levels of the food, ensuring its preservation. Often when foods are fermented their nutritional value is elevated because the lactic acid helps to liberate nutrients from the starting food. The most commonly pickled food is small cucumbers.

When pickling foods in your own kitchen you have absolute control over what goes in the jar with respect to the ingredients. There is no better way to keep it clean!

Sauerkraut

Fermentation is yet another way to preserve food. Kefir is really just a fermented food inoculated with a few hundred thousand healthy bacteria that do the job of preserv-

ing! This simple method of food keeping is used to create one of the world's most interesting preserved foods – sauerkraut. The homemade version of this German staple is far superior to anything purchased from a store. And you can do it too.

Sauerkraut and kimchi, the Korean version of pickled cabbage, have recently been found to supply enormous health benefits, particularly in the fight against cancer. Making your own may be a fun and easy way to ramp up your own health. The basic recipe asks for only two ingredients: salt and cabbage. The cabbage is shredded, doused with salt and then packed into a large porcelain or ceramic crock. A weight is placed on top of the mixture and the whole thing is covered. Friendly bacteria create lactic acid, helping to preserve food during the fermentation period, which can last up to a week. Eating fermented foods like sauerkraut and kimchi is an age-old tradition and a powerful ally in improving your health. Try it in your kitchen today.

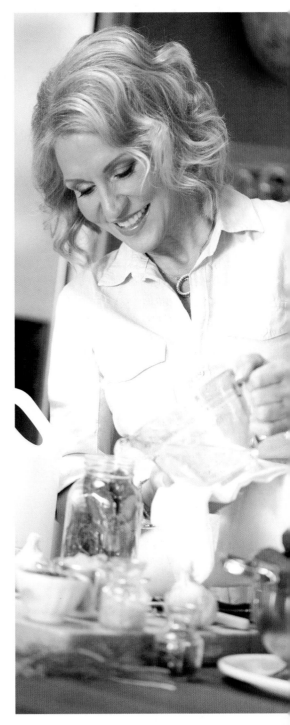

"Growing, preserving and eating local, fresh, in-season food is a powerful and positive contribution you can make in this environmentally stressed world."

Fast Foods

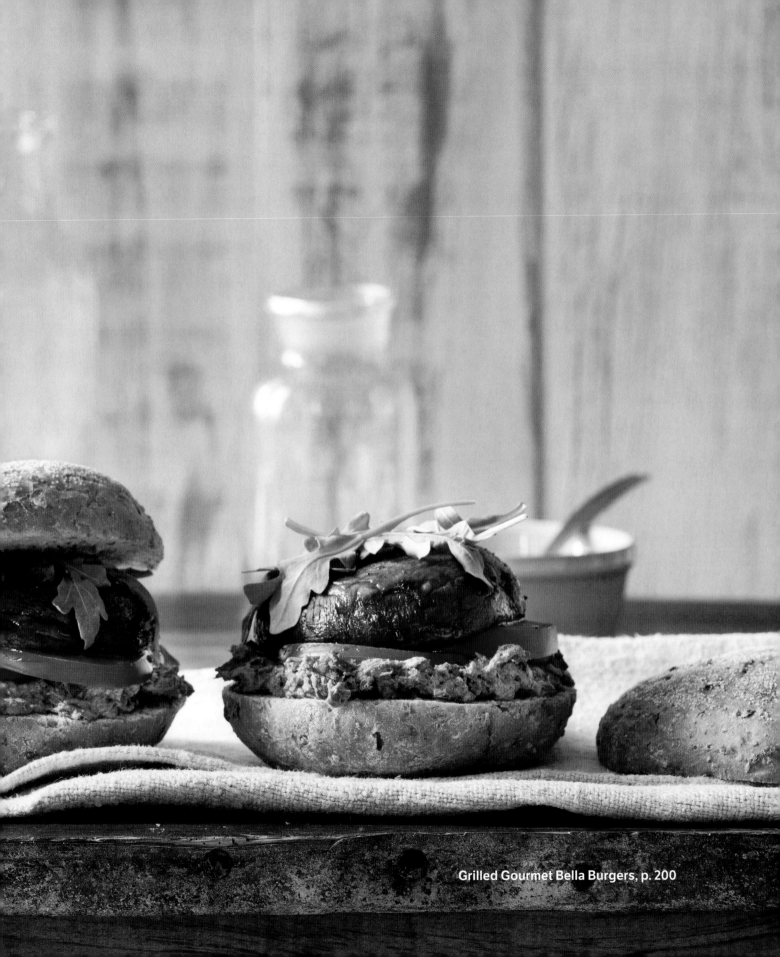

Grilled Gourmet Bella Burgers, p. 200

Grilled Gourmet Bella Burgers

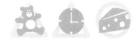

PREP: 20 minutes | **COOK:** 10 minutes | **YIELD:** 4 burgers

A vegetarian classic, Portobello mushroom burgers are as hearty as their beef counterparts. In fact, I know more carnivores who love to sink their teeth into these burgers than vegetarians. P.S. The spread is a must!

SUN-DRIED TOMATO BASIL SPREAD

½ cup (120 ml) Yogurt Cheese* (see p. 276) or plain, low-fat Greek yogurt

1 Tbsp (15 ml) Dijon mustard

¼ cup (60 ml) sun-dried tomatoes, not in oil, rehydrated in hot water and drained

1 handful basil leaves

1 clove garlic

¼ tsp (1.25 ml) each sea salt and freshly ground black pepper

Eat-Clean Cooking Spray (see p. 277)

4 large Portobello mushrooms, stemmed and wiped clean

Sea salt and freshly ground black pepper, to taste

4 whole-grain rolls or buns, big enough to fit the mushroom caps, split and toasted

2 cups (480 ml) baby arugula

2 vine-ripened tomatoes, thinly sliced

Place all Sun-dried Tomato Basil Spread ingredients in a food processor and whirl until thoroughly blended. Spread will be a little chunky. Scrape into a small bowl and refrigerate until ready to use.

Heat a grill or grill pan to medium high and spray with Eat-Clean Cooking Spray. Spray gill side of mushroom caps with Eat-Clean Cooking Spray and season with a pinch of salt and pepper. Place mushrooms gill side down on grill and cook 5 minutes. Spray tops of mushrooms with Eat-Clean Cooking Spray and season with salt and pepper, and then flip. Gently place a cast-iron skillet or heavy pan on top of mushrooms and heat until cooked through, another 3 minutes. Remove from grill.

To build burgers, spread both sides of rolls with Sun-dried Tomato Basil Spread and add arugula, mushrooms and tomato slices to bottom half. Place other halves on top and serve.

NOTE
*Yogurt Cheese must be made ahead of time (if using).

NUTRITIONAL VALUE PER BURGER:
Calories: 234 | Calories from Fat: 55 | Protein: 11 g | Carbs: 37 g | Total Fat: 6 g |
Saturated Fat: 1 g | Trans Fat: 0 g | Fiber: 7 g | Sodium: 537 mg | Cholesterol: 1 mg

Cucumber and Watercress Tea Sandwiches

PREP: 25 minutes | **COOK:** 0 minutes | **YIELD:** 16 servings

Perfect for a ladies' lunch, these tea sandwiches are light enough for a lazy afternoon meal but full of healthy and satisfying ingredients. Ahhh!

½ cup (120 ml) strained low-fat Greek yogurt or Yogurt Cheese* (see p. 276)

6 oz (170 g) soft goat cheese, room temperature

½ cup (120 ml) packed watercress leaves, chopped

¼ cup (60 ml) grated carrots, about ½ large carrot

1 Tbsp (15 ml) finely chopped fresh chives

Pinch sea salt

16 thin slices whole wheat, rye or pumpernickel bread

1 seedless cucumber, very thinly sliced

Drain any liquid from top of yogurt. (Tip: You can save it for a smoothie or drink it! You want the yogurt as thick as possible.)

In a bowl, thoroughly mix together yogurt and goat cheese. Stir in watercress, carrots, chives and sea salt until well combined.

Spread goat cheese mixture on each slice of bread. Arrange cucumber slices in a single layer on half of bread slices (you may have extra). Place remaining bread slices over cucumber, cheese mixture side down. Carefully cut off crusts (save them for snacks, or discard). Cut each sandwich in half diagonally, and then in half again to create four triangular tea sandwiches.

Arrange tea sandwiches very close together on a serving platter.

CHILL OUT
If not serving immediately, cover sandwiches with a damp paper towel, then wrap with plastic wrap, and store in refrigerator.

NOTE
*Yogurt Cheese must be made ahead of time.

NUTRITIONAL VALUE PER SERVING (2 SANDWICH QUARTERS):
Calories: 104 | Calories from Fat: 29 | Protein: 6 g | Carbs: 14 g | Total Fat: 3 g |
Saturated Fat: 2 g | Trans Fat: 0 g | Fiber: 2 g | Sodium: 186 mg | Cholesterol: 4 mg

Kimchi Fried Rice
(Kimchi Bokkeumbap)

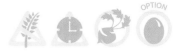

PREP: 15 minutes | **COOK:** 15 minutes | **YIELD:** 4 x 1-cup servings

This dish is a great way to use up leftover rice and odds and ends of vegetables you have in your refrigerator. Just use a combination of vegetables you already have, and be sure to cook the rice the day before so that it's cold and dry, otherwise you'll have mush. You might have to make a special trip to the store to buy kimchi, a spicy Korean favorite made with fermented cabbage, but it is well worth the trip!

2 Tbsp (30 ml) safflower oil

3 cloves garlic, chopped

3 scallions, cut into 1-inch pieces

2 cups (480 ml) vegetables, diced into ½-inch
  pieces (see Try This! tip at right)

4 oz (113 g) firm tofu, drained and liquid pressed
  out, diced into ½-inch pieces

3 cups (710 ml) cooked, day-old, refrigerated
  brown rice

1 cup (240 ml) kimchi, drained and liquid
  pressed out, chopped

1 tsp (5 ml) sesame oil

½ tsp (2.5 ml) sea salt

Heat a 9- or 10-inch cast-iron skillet or very large wok thoroughly on medium high. Once skillet is nearly smoking, add oil, garlic, scallions and vegetables. Stir vegetables in oil and cook until softened, 1 or 2 minutes. Add tofu and cook 1 more minute. Stir in rice, getting as much rice to touch bottom of skillet as possible. Allow to cook, without stirring, until rice starts to brown and get crunchy on the bottom of the skillet. Stir and repeat until all rice is browned as much possible, without burning, and has developed crispy, crunchy bits, about 8 minutes total. Stir in kimchi, sesame oil and salt, and heat through. Remove from heat and mound in bowls. Serve with chili paste or chili sauce, and low-sodium tamari.

TRY THIS!
When it comes to the mix of veggies for this dish, take my word for it, anything goes. Bell peppers, zucchini, yellow squash, mushrooms, broccoli, carrots, celery, bamboo shoots, baby corn, bok choy and kale – toss 'em in!

PROTEIN POWER
If you're an ovo vegetarian, you can top the fried rice with a sunny-side-up egg, allowing the diner to break up the yolk and mix it in with the rice, as is traditional in Korean cuisine.

NUTRITIONAL VALUE PER SERVING (WITHOUT EGG):
Calories: 347 | Calories from Fat: 129 | Protein: 11 g | Carbs: 44 g | Total Fat: 15 g |
Saturated Fat: 2 g | Trans Fat: 0 g | Fiber: 6 g | Sodium: 366 mg | Cholesterol: 0 mg

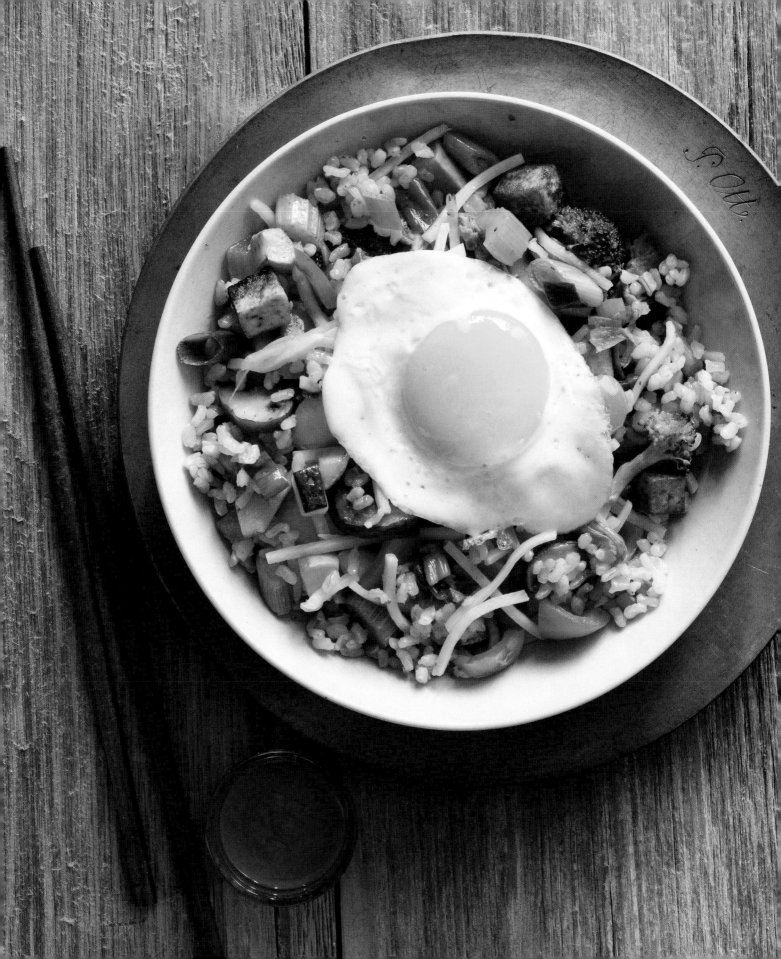

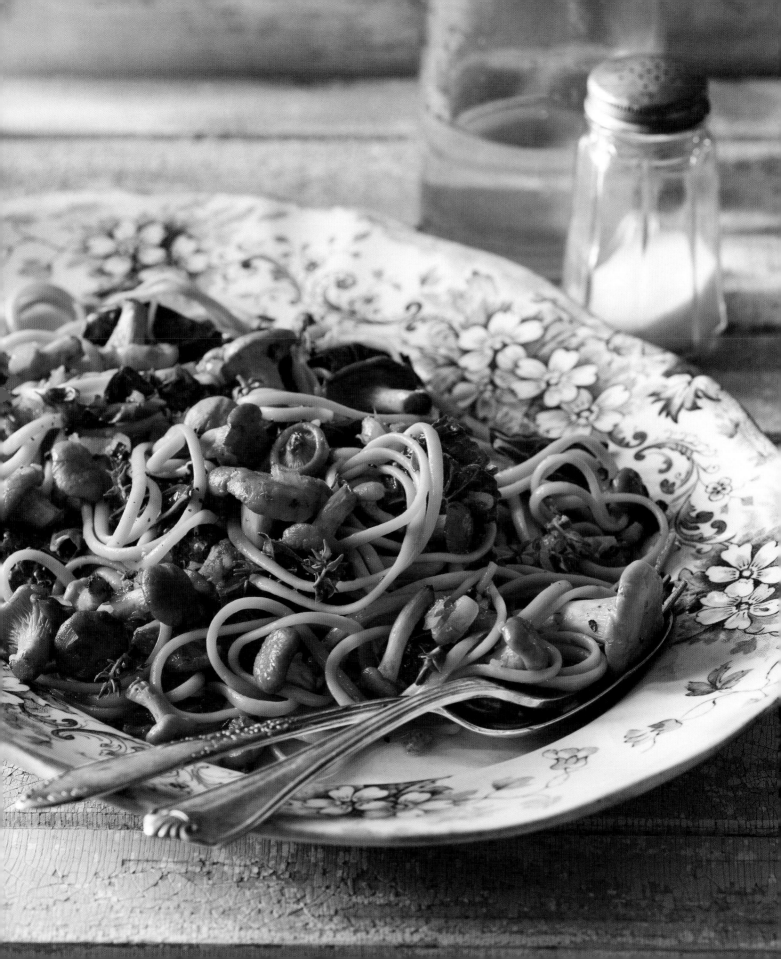

Spinach Fettuccini with Golden Chanterelles and Lacinato Kale

PREP: 20 minutes | **COOK:** 10 minutes | **YIELD:** 5 x 2-cup servings

Lacinato kale, aka Tuscan kale, boasts blue-green leaves and a sweeter taste than its curly cousin. Paring this mild kale with golden chanterelles creates a dish that is as visually appealing as it is tasty. A word of warning: Wow your guests with a meal this good and you might have them knocking on your door unannounced!

1 x 12-oz (340 g) package fresh spinach fettuccini, made without eggs

3 tsp (15 ml) extra virgin olive oil, divided

1 bunch lacinato kale*, about 8 oz (225 g), cut crosswise into 1-inch strips

1 lb (454 g) golden chanterelle mushrooms, brushed thoroughly to remove any dirt and cut into large bite-sized pieces

1 clove garlic, minced

1 tsp (5 ml) minced shallot

1 tsp (5 ml) minced fresh thyme

½ tsp (2.5 ml) each sea salt and freshly ground black pepper

Cook fettuccini according to package directions. Drain, reserving ¼ cup (60 ml) cooking water, and set aside.

In the meantime, in a very large skillet, heat 1 tsp (5 ml) olive oil on medium high. Add kale and cook until wilted, about 2 minutes. Transfer kale to a bowl and return skillet to heat. Add remaining 2 tsp (10 ml) olive oil to skillet and add mushrooms in a single layer. Let cook without moving for several minutes to brown on bottom. Once mushrooms are browned, stir in garlic, shallot and thyme, and continue cooking mushrooms until soft and cooked through, about 2 more minutes.

Add cooked pasta and kale to skillet, season with salt and pepper and toss to combine. Stir in reserved pasta cooking water a little at a time until sauce reaches desired consistency. Serve mounded in large pasta bowls.

If you have access to truffle-infused olive oil, add a few drops on top of each serving.

OPTION
*If you can't find lacinato kale, use red kale.

NUTRITIONAL VALUE PER SERVING:
Calories: 333 | Calories from Fat: 47 | Protein: 14 g | Carbs: 58 g | Total Fat: 6 g | Saturated Fat: 1 g | Trans Fat: 0 g | Fiber: 4 g | Sodium: 52 mg | Cholesterol: 12 mg

Korean Pancakes with Kimchi and Scallions

PREP: 10 minutes | **COOK:** 20 minutes | **YIELD:** 4 x 10-inch pancakes

These savory pancakes, called pajeon (prounounced "pa-jun"), contain scallions and almost anything else you'd like to add. The kimchi, a cabbage-based Korean dish, gives them a spicy, fermented dimension that I'm sure you'll enjoy.

DIPPING SAUCE

2 Tbsp (30 ml) low-sodium soy sauce

2 tsp (10 ml) rice vinegar

½ tsp (2.5 ml) sesame oil

½ tsp (2.5 ml) Korean hot pepper flakes or powder

½ cup (120 ml) whole wheat flour

½ cup (120 ml) brown rice flour

1 egg + 2 egg whites

1 tsp (5 ml) Sucanat or other unrefined sugar

1 tsp (5 ml) dried and crumbled dulse seaweed

1 tsp (5 ml) sesame seeds

1 bunch scallions, finely chopped

Eat-Clean Cooking Spray (see p. 277)

½ cup (120 ml) kimchi, drained, divided

In a small bowl, whisk together soy sauce, rice vinegar, sesame oil and Korean hot pepper flakes. Set aside.

In a separate bowl, whisk together flours, egg and egg whites, Sucanat, dulse seaweed and sesame seeds. Stir in scallions.

Heat a 9- or 10-inch nonstick skillet thoroughly on medium and spray with Eat-Clean Cooking Spray. Pour ½ cup (120 ml) batter into pan and place a few pieces of kimchi on top. Cook until browned on bottom, about 3 minutes. Using a large rubber spatula, flip and cook until pancake is cooked through, about 1 minute longer. Transfer pancake to a baking sheet.

Use a paper towel to wipe out skillet, spray with Eat-Clean Cooking Spray and repeat with another ½ cup (120 ml) batter and more kimchi until all are used. Cut each pancake into eighths, and serve with dipping sauce.

NUTRITIONAL VALUE PER PANCAKE:
Calories: 191 | Calories from Fat: 35 | Protein: 8 g | Carbs: 31 g | Total Fat: 4 g |
Saturated Fat: 1 g | Trans Fat: 0 g | Fiber: 4 g | Sodium: 579 mg | Cholesterol: 53 mg

Mediterranean Panini

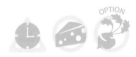

PREP: 10 minutes | **COOK:** 4-6 minutes | **YIELD:** 2 servings

Who wouldn't want to dine on delicious panini complete with sun-dried tomatoes, olives, mozzarella, spinach and toasted bread? Best of all, these quality ingredients provide the nutrients the body needs to function at its best. Just writing this is making me hungry! I hope you're ready to dig in!

4 slices rustic whole grain bread

4 Tbsp (60 ml) Sun-Dried Tomato Olive Tapenade (see p. 55) or store-bought Clean olive tapenade

4 oz (113 g) fresh mozzarella, thinly sliced

1 medium tomato, sliced

1 cup (240 ml) baby spinach

Preheat panini press, or heat a grill pan on medium low. Spread 1 Tbsp (15 ml) tapenade on each slice of bread and place mozzarella slices over tapenade. On bottom half of each sandwich, lay tomato slices, top with spinach and close sandwich.

If using a panini press, place sandwiches inside, close lid and cook until inside is hot and cheese is melted.

If using a grill pan, place sandwiches in pan, and place a skillet on top to gently press them down. Cook until bread has grill marks and cheese is starting to melt, about 2 or 3 minutes. Turn over, place skillet back on panini and cook until inside is hot and cheese is completely melted, 2 or 3 minutes longer. Serve immediately.

NUTRITIONAL VALUE PER PANINI:
Calories: 345 | Calories from Fat: 131 | Protein: 24 g | Carbs: 32 g | Total Fat: 14 g | Saturated Fat: 7 g | Trans Fat: 0 g | Fiber: 6 g | Sodium: 797 mg | Cholesterol: 36 mg

Hot and Comforting Couscous with Arugula

PREP: 10 minutes | **COOK:** 5 minutes | **YIELD:** 4 x 1-cup servings

This is my ultimate comfort food. When it's cold and wet outside, I whip up a batch of this creamy couscous and suddenly I have a big smile on my face. The cooking method is a little different than the way you usually cook couscous; you cook this dish like you'd cook polenta, which is how it gets its creamy, comforting texture.

1 cup (240 ml) whole wheat couscous

½ cup (120 ml) 1% low-fat milk, plain, unsweetened soy milk or other plain unsweetened milk substitute

1 oz (28 g) freshly grated Parmigiano Reggiano, or vegan nutritional yeast

¼ tsp (1.25 ml) sea salt

4 cups (950 ml) arugula, lightly packed

In a medium heavy-bottomed saucepan, bring 3 cups (710 ml) water to boil on high. Stir in couscous and reduce heat to simmer. Cook, stirring regularly, until most of the water is absorbed, about 5 minutes. Remove from heat and stir in milk, Parmigiano Reggiano and salt. Fold in arugula until wilted. Serve hot.

NUTRITIONAL VALUE PER SERVING:
Calories: 172 | Calories from Fat: 19 | Protein: 9 g | Carbs: 32 g | Total Fat: 2 g | Saturated Fat: 0 g | Trans Fat: 0 g | Fiber: 4 g | Sodium: 30 mg | Cholesterol: 1 mg

Mediterranean Breeze Bowl with Lemon Garlic Tahini Sauce

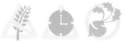

PREP: 5 minutes | **COOK:** 15 minutes | **YIELD:** 4 servings

… because it's a breeze to make and it makes you feel like you're sitting at a Mediterranean seaside café when you eat it! The pepperoncini adds a delightful spicy, pickled kick.

1 cup (240 ml) quinoa

½ tsp (2.5 ml) ground turmeric

½ tsp (2.5 ml) ground cumin

½ tsp (2.5 ml) dried oregano

2 cloves garlic

¼ tsp (1.25 ml) sea salt

Zest and juice of ½ large lemon

¼ cup (60 ml) tahini (sesame seed paste)

3 Tbsp (45 ml) low-sodium, gluten-free
vegetable broth or water

4 cups (950 ml) fresh baby spinach

2 cups (480 ml) shredded purple cabbage

2 cups cooked or 1 x 15-oz (440 ml) BPA-free
can no-salt-added organic chick peas,
drained and rinsed under hot water

½ cup (120 ml) deli-style sliced golden Greek
pepperoncini, drained

In a small pot with lid, combine quinoa, turmeric, cumin, oregano and 2 cups (480 ml) water. Bring to a boil on high heat, cover and reduce heat to simmer until all water is absorbed and quinoa is plump, 10 to 15 minutes. Fluff, cover and set aside.

On a cutting board, mince garlic, then sprinkle sea salt over minced garlic and use side of a chef's knife to press it into a paste. Scrape paste into a bowl, add lemon zest and juice, tahini and vegetable broth. Whisk together until smooth.

Divide ingredients among four bowls, layering spinach, cabbage, quinoa and then chick peas. Drizzle with sauce and top with sliced pepperoncini.

ON THE GO
Can be assembled ahead of time and packed in a container to go. The ingredients will hold up very well and not get soggy. When ready to eat, simply stir together.

NUTRITIONAL VALUE PER SERVING:
Calories: 282 | Calories from Fat: 96 | Protein: 11 g | Carbs: 37 g | Total Fat: 10 g |
Saturated Fat: 1 g | Trans Fat: 0 g | Fiber: 8 g | Sodium: 231 mg | Cholesterol: 0 mg

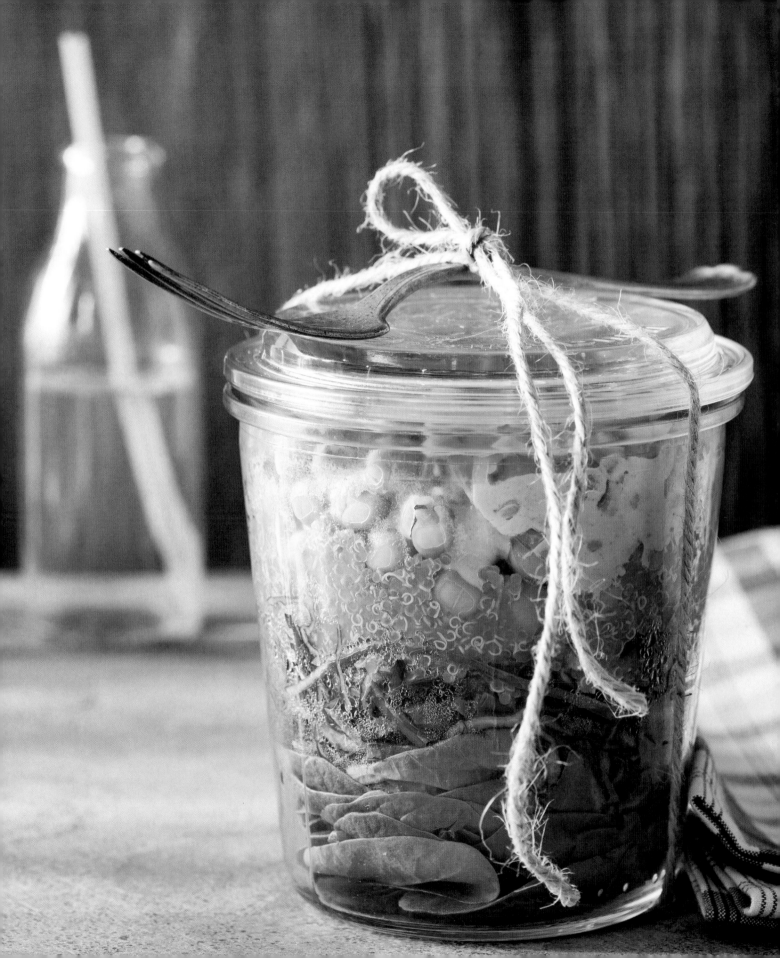

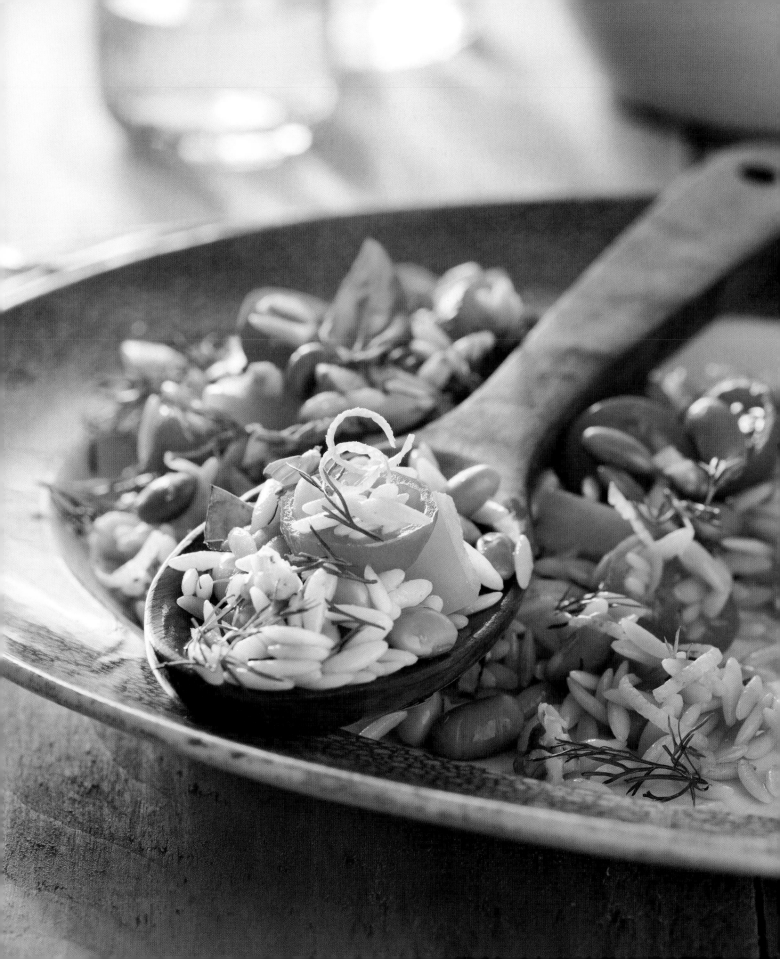

Lemon Orzo with Edamame, Orange Peppers and Cherry Tomatoes

PREP: 15 minutes | **COOK:** 8 to 10 minutes | **YIELD:** 5 x 1-cup servings

Orzo is the Italian word for barley. In the past, this rice-sized pasta was made from barley. Nowadays, it is made from wheat semolina. It is a light pasta option that pairs well with tons of vegetables and an olive oil-based sauce.

1 cup (240 ml) whole wheat orzo, made
    without eggs

1 cup (240 ml) frozen shelled edamame

1 orange bell pepper, seeded, cut into
    ½-inch dice

1 cup (240 ml) cherry or grape tomatoes, halved

¼ cup (60 ml) thinly sliced fresh basil

¼ cup (60 ml) finely chopped fresh dill

½ cup (120 ml) chopped walnuts

1 lemon, zested and juiced

1 Tbsp (15 ml) extra virgin olive oil

¼ tsp (1.25 ml) each sea salt and freshly ground
    black pepper

Bring a pot of water to boil on high heat. Add orzo and cook according to package directions until al dente. Do not over cook. When orzo has 3 minutes left to cook, add edamame. When both are done cooking, drain in a colander that has small holes so orzo doesn't slip through. Do not rinse. Transfer to a large bowl. Add orange pepper, cherry tomatoes, basil, dill and walnuts.

In a small bowl, whisk together lemon zest and juice, olive oil, salt and pepper. Pour over orzo and toss to combine. Serve hot, room temperature or chilled.

CHILL OUT
This dish will keep for up to three days in the refrigerator.

NUTRITIONAL VALUE PER SERVING:
Calories: 261 | Calories from Fat: 103 | Protein: 9 g | Carbs: 32 g | Total Fat: 12 g |
Saturated Fat: 1 g | Trans Fat: 0 g | Fiber: 8 g | Sodium: 5 mg | Cholesterol: 0 mg

Penne with No-Cook Sun-Dried Tomato Tofu Cream, Artichoke Hearts and Basil

PREP: 15 minutes | **COOK:** 10 minutes | **YIELD:** 5 x 2-cup servings

A creamy cream-less pasta that's vegan, too? Today is indeed your lucky day!

1 lb (454 g) whole wheat penne rigate, made without eggs

1 x 12-oz (340 g) package silken soft tofu, drained, at room temperature

½ cup (120 ml) raw unsalted cashews

½ cup (120 ml) hot water

1 cup (240 ml) rehydrated sun-dried tomatoes (not in oil), drained

1 clove garlic, chopped

2 Tbsp (30 ml) chopped basil

1 Tbsp (15 ml) chopped marjoram

¼ tsp (1.25 ml) each sea salt and freshly ground black pepper

1 x 8-oz (225 g) package frozen artichoke hearts, thawed

Bring a large pot of water to boil on high heat and cook pasta according to package directions until al dente. Drain, reserving ¼ cup (60 ml) cooking liquid. Do not rinse. Transfer pasta to a large bowl.

In a blender, blend tofu, cashews and hot water until very smooth. Add sun-dried tomatoes, garlic, basil, marjoram, salt and pepper, and blend until combined, but little chunks of tomatoes remain. Pour over pasta, add artichoke hearts and toss to combine. If sauce is too thick, add reserved pasta cooking liquid a bit at a time until sauce reaches desired consistency.

NUTRITIONAL VALUE PER SERVING:
Calories: 428 | Calories from Fat: 93 | Protein: 19 g | Carbs: 81 g | Total Fat: 11 g | Saturated Fat: 1 g | Trans Fat: 0 g | Fiber: 13 g | Sodium: 254 mg | Cholesterol: 0 mg

Thai Egg Stir-Fry with Tomatoes

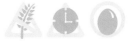

PREP: 15 minutes | **COOK:** 10 minutes | **YIELD:** 4 servings

Egg stir-fries offer tons of vegetables along with the complete-protein benefits of eggs. In this recipe, Thai basil imparts its sweet licorice flavor for a unique and exotic taste. It's quick, easy, delicious and nutritious!

½ cup (120 ml) textured soy protein

½ cup (120 ml) boiling water

1 tsp (5 ml) Bragg's Liquid Aminos

1 Tbsp (15 ml) low-sodium tamari

1 tsp (5 ml) Sucanat or other unrefined sugar

½ tsp (2.5 ml) sesame oil

2 tsp (10 ml) grapeseed oil, or other high-heat Clean oil

½ yellow onion, thinly sliced

2 cloves garlic, minced

1 tomato, diced

2 whole eggs + 2 egg whites, beaten

2 green onions, thinly sliced

2 Tbsp (30 ml) chopped Thai basil

2 cups (480 ml) cooked brown rice

Place textured soy protein in a bowl, pour boiling water over top and stir in Bragg's Liquid Aminos. Cover and set aside 5 minutes to rehydrate.

In a small bowl, stir together tamari, Sucanat and sesame oil until Sucanat is dissolved. Set aside.

Meanwhile, heat a wok or cast-iron skillet thoroughly on medium. When heated through, add grapeseed oil and onion, and sauté until starting to brown, about 3 minutes. Stir in garlic and cook until fragrant but not brown, about 1 minute. Add rehydrated textured soy protein and cook, stirring occasionally, for 2 minutes. Stir in tomatoes and cook until heated through. Push mixture to the side and pour beaten eggs onto empty side of skillet. Cook eggs until opaque, stirring occasionally, then stir them into soy-tomato mixture. Add reserved sauce mixture, green onions and Thai basil, and combine. Serve with brown rice.

NUTRITIONAL VALUE PER SERVING (1 CUP STIR-FRY + ½ CUP RICE):
Calories: 256 | Calories from Fat: 71 | Protein: 12 g | Carbs: 9 g | Total Fat: 8 g | Saturated Fat: 1 g | Trans Fat: 0 g | Fiber: 4 g | Sodium: 239 mg | Cholesterol: 105 mg

Gourmet Veggie English Muffin Pizzas

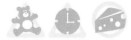

PREP: 15 minutes | **COOK:** 6 minutes | **YIELD:** 4 pizzas

Pizza is the ultimate fast food. But, in most cases, it's also the ultimate fat food. You can make a healthier version using the ingredients listed here in the time it takes you to order a regular pizza and pick it up. Now that's Eat-Clean fast food!

2 whole wheat English muffins, split

1 clove garlic, whole and peeled

4 Tbsp (60 ml) Yogurt Cheese* (see p. 276)

½ baby zucchini, thinly sliced into half-moons

1 medium tomato, thinly sliced

2 Tbsp (30 ml) thinly sliced red onion

Sea salt and freshly ground black pepper,
      to taste

2 tsp (10 ml) extra virgin olive oil

4 tsp (20 ml) vegan nutritional yeast

Place oven rack in the second-highest position and heat broiler. Place English muffin halves on a baking sheet, cut side up, and broil until lightly brown and crispy, 1 or 2 minutes. Remove and rub garlic clove over tops of English muffin halves.

Spread 1 Tbsp (15 ml) Yogurt Cheese over each muffin. Divide zucchini among muffins, and then top with tomato slices and red onion. Season with salt and pepper.

Place pizzas under broiler until warmed through and onions are lightly browned, 3 or 4 minutes. Remove from oven, drizzle each pizza with ½ tsp (2.5 ml) olive oil and top with nutritional yeast.

MAKE AHEAD
Can be prepared ahead of time and stored in an airtight container or wrapped in foil for lunch or a snack the following day.

NOTE
*Yogurt Cheese must be made ahead of time.

NUTRITIONAL VALUE PER 2-PIZZA SERVING:
Calories: 154 | Calories from Fat: 74 | Protein: 6 g | Carbs: 17 g | Total Fat: 8 g |
Saturated Fat: 1 g | Trans Fat: 0 g | Fiber: 3 g | Sodium: 168 mg | Cholesterol: 1 mg

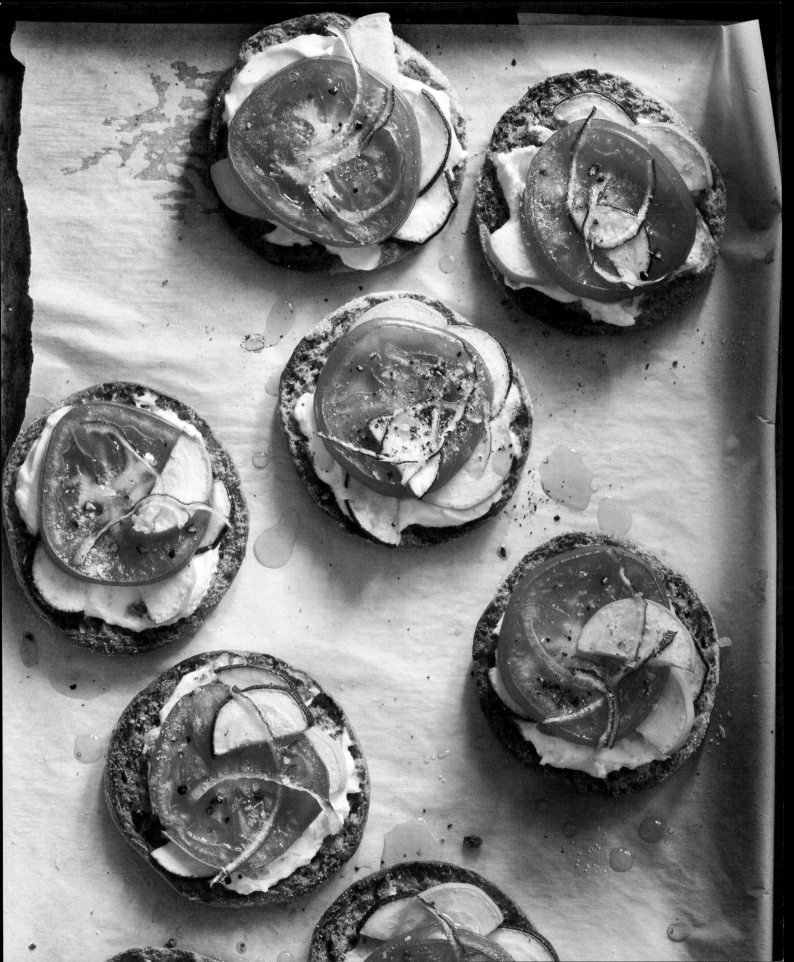

Dehydration for Preservation

Want to get more distance out of your food? Dehydrate it. Food dehydration is a great way to make food last longer, because it's a natural food preservation practice. Removing water from food prevents certain bacteria from causing that food to go bad. Historically food was dehydrated after the harvest to ensure there would be enough to last through the winter months. The most common foods to dehydrate are fruits, vegetables and meats, but you can also try your hand at drying herbs, fish and even flowers!

The process of dehydrating involves using low heat and constant airflow to suck all of the moisture out of the food without cooking it. Traditionally, dehydration was accomplished by harnessing the powers of the sun and wind. Nowadays kitchen-ready countertop appliances use heat, fans and air vents to dehydrate food quickly, easily and safely.

Why would you choose to dehydrate food? The reasons are endless. Dried food can be stored and used for up to a year, saving you time and money. You'll be able to use your garden harvest to its full potential rather than having to let some of the foods spoil when you have too much. To this effect, you can take advantage of supermarket specials for buying in bulk, which also saves you money. One of my favorite things about doing your own home dehydration is taking comfort knowing you aren't eating a host of chemicals from purchased dried or preserved foods. Food drying also happens to be the least harmful to the natural quality of food. In fact, the quality of your food has the potential to increase tenfold. You'll also have an excellent supply of delicious food in the event of a power outage or weather crisis. Dried food is a popular option to take with you when you are on the go, because it's light and unbreakable. Think about your typical trail mix. Most of these options are full of dried fruit. Just be sure to check out the preservative and sugar content of store-bought options.

HOW TO DEHYDRATE:

Sun – only possible if you have 304 days of at least 100°F or build a solar dehydrator

Oven – often removes the flavor of foods, and many ovens can't go below 200°F, plus you need to prop open the oven door to maintain air circulation

Electric – likely your best option

HOW TO DO IT SAFELY:

In order to ensure you are killing any bacteria present in food while dehydrating you must keep the temperature at these indicated levels:

Meats and Fish: 145°F and above

Fruits and Vegetables: 130°F to 140°F

Herbs and flowers: 100°F to 110°F

MOST COMMONLY DEHYDRATED FOODS:

Cranberries	Proscuitto
Apples	Beef jerky
Pineapple	Grapes
Bananas	Prunes
Apricots	Figs
Cherries	Dates
Kale	Chili peppers
Tomatoes	Fruit leathers

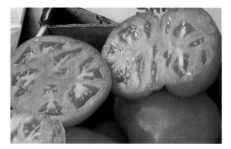

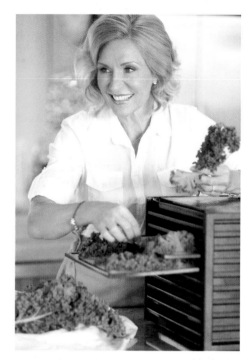

Vegetables:

Green beans: Rinse under cold water. Remove the stems from the top and bottom and snap the beans into 1-inch pieces. Blanch. Dry for 6-12 hours.

Beets: Cook and peel beets to remove their skin. Cut them into ¼-inch pieces. Dry 3-10 hours.

Bell Peppers: Remove seeds and chop. Dry 5-12 hours until leathery.

Broccoli: Rinse, cut and dry 4-10 hours.

Carrots: Rinse, and then peel, slice or shred. Dry 6-12 hours.

Cauliflower: Rinse, cut and dry 6-14 hours.

Corn: Cut corn off cob after blanching and dry 6-12 hours.

Mushrooms: Brush off, don't wash. Dry at 90 degrees for 3 hours, and then 125 degrees for the remaining drying time. Dry 4-10 hours.

Onions: Slice ¼-inch-thick rounds. Dry 6-12 hours.

Peas: Dry 5-14 hours.

Potatoes: Slice ⅛-inch thick. Dry 6-12 hours until crisp.

Tomatoes: Dip in boiling water to loosen skins. Peel, slice or quarter. Dry 6-12 hours.

Zucchini: Slice ⅛-inch thick and dry 5-10 hours.

Fruit:

Light-colored fruits require a pretreatment with an acidic solution to keep them from darkening, to speed up the process and to ward off bacteria like salmonella.

Apples: Rinse. Peel, core and slice into ⅜-inch rings, or cut into ¼-inch slices. Dry 6-12 hours.

Apricots: Cut in half and turn inside out to dry. Dry 8-20 hours.

Bananas: Peel, cut into ¼-inch slices. Dry 8-16 hours.

Blueberries: Dry 10-20 hours.

Cherries: Cut in half and dry 18-26 hours.

Peaches: Peel, halve or quarter. Dry 6-20 hours.

Pears: Peel, cut into ¼-inch slices. Dry 6-20 hours.

Pineapple: Core and slice ¼-inch thick. Dry 6-16 hours.

Strawberries: Halve or cut into ¼-inch thick slices. Dry 6-16 hours.

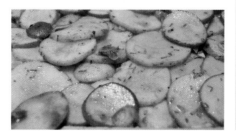

DEHYDRATING TIPS:

- Store all dried foods in a cool, dark place like your kitchen cupboards

- Dried foods will last from one season to the next – which means they have a shelf life of about one year

- Don't worry about flavors mingling together

- You can also use your dehydrator to make your own yogurt and cheese

- Touch the food to see if it is done dehydrating – it will be leathery with no moisture present

- Store your dehydrated foods in airtight containers – as soon as they grab moisture from the air they run the risk of going bad

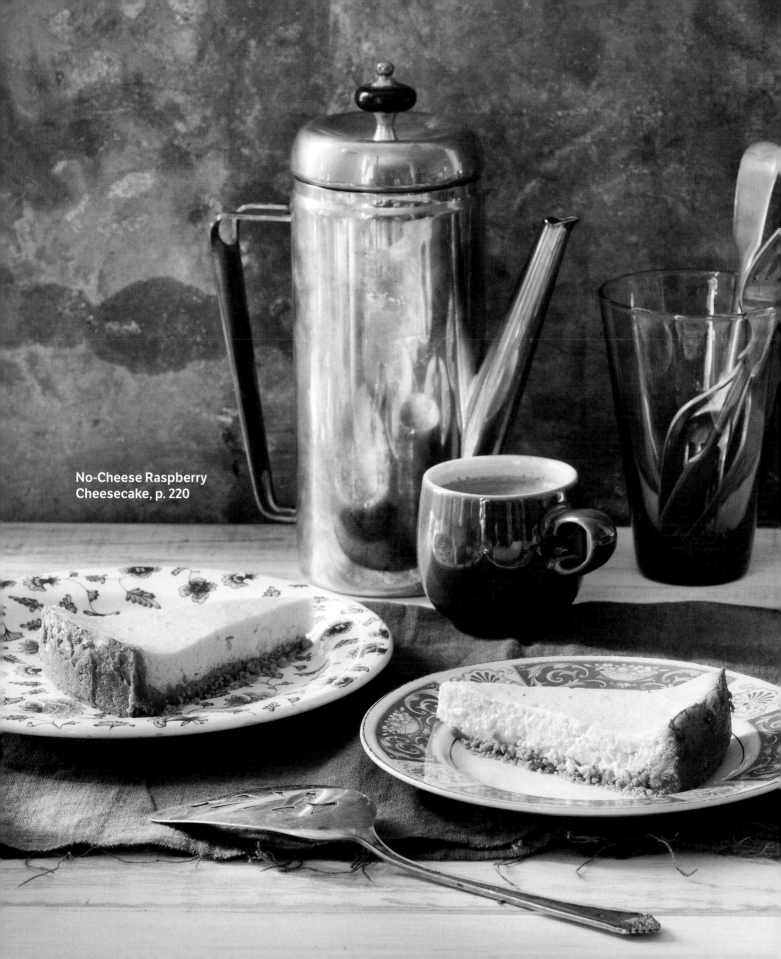

No-Cheese Raspberry
Cheesecake, p. 220

Sweet Treats

No-Cheese Raspberry Cheesecake

PREP: 30 minutes | **COOK:** 1 hour | **YIELD:** 12 slices

You must be wondering how this is possible right? Well, believe me … it tastes so good you won't believe it! It's a sinful treat brought down to a Clean level with healthful ingredients and a killer taste that will definitely have you coming back for more.

CRUST

7 oz (200 g) 100% whole wheat honey grahams (non-vegan) or vegan amaranth whole-grain graham crackers (I love Health Valley)

Pinch sea salt

2 Tbsp (30 ml) unrefined coconut oil or vegan butter substitute (I use Earth Balance), melted

2 Tbsp (30 ml) brown-rice syrup, yacon syrup or pure honey

1 tsp (5 ml) pure vanilla extract

FILLING

1 x 12-oz (340 g) package silken light firm tofu, drained

1 cup (240 ml) Yogurt Cheese* or 8 oz (225 g) vegan non-hydrogenated cream cheese

3 Tbsp (45 ml) brown-rice syrup, yacon syrup or pure honey

Zest and juice ½ lemon

1 tsp (5 ml) pure vanilla extract

¼ tsp (1.25 ml) baking soda

2 Tbsp (30 ml) arrowroot starch

Pinch sea salt

RASPBERRY SAUCE
YIELD: 1¼ CUPS (300 ML)

2 cups (480 ml) frozen raspberries

2 Tbsp (30 ml) brown-rice syrup, yacon syrup or pure honey

1 tsp (5 ml) arrowroot starch

1 Tbsp (15 ml) lemon juice

Preheat oven to 350˚F (177˚C).

To make crust, pulse graham crackers and salt in a food processor until ground into fine crumbs. While food processor is running, slowly pour in coconut oil, syrup or honey and vanilla. Mixture should resemble wet sand and should stick together when pressed between your fingers. Transfer mixture into a 9-inch springform pan and press down firmly. Bake 8 to 10 minutes until edges are lightly browned. Remove and let cool.

Add filling ingredients to a clean food processor or blender, and blend until smooth. Scrape down sides and blend again to make sure all ingredients are incorporated. Pour over cooled crust and spread out evenly. Bake until golden brown on edges and mostly set, about 45 minutes. Cake will jiggle a bit at center when you shake pan. Transfer to a wire rack for 1 hour to cool to room temperature, then refrigerate until thoroughly chilled.

Add raspberry sauce ingredients to a saucepan and stir to combine. Bring to a simmer on medium-high heat, stirring occasionally, until slightly thickened. Remove and let cool slightly. Refrigerate until ready to use.

To serve, remove outer ring of springform pan, but keep cheesecake on the pan base. Cut into 12 slices and serve topped with raspberry sauce.

CHILL OUT
Store leftover cheesecake and sauce in the refrigerator for up to five days.

NOTE
*Yogurt Cheese must be made ahead of time.

NUTRITIONAL VALUE PER SERVING (12 2½-INCH X 4½-INCH SLICES, EACH WITH 1½ TBSP / 22.5 ML RASPBERRY SAUCE):
Calories: 168 | Calories from Fat: 34 | Protein: 9 g | Carbs: 40 g | Total Fat: 4 g | Saturated Fat: 2 g | Trans Fat: 0 g | Fiber: 1 g | Sodium: 352 mg | Cholesterol: 0.4 mg

Skillet Cornbread

PREP: 15 minutes | **COOK:** 25-30 minutes | **YIELD:** 12 wedges

My mouth is watering as I write this. Skillet cornbread is an absolute favorite of mine, and this one is 100% Clean. Just try not to eat it all at once!

YOU WILL NEED:

1 x 8- or 9-inch cast-iron skillet

Olive oil, to oil skillet

1½ cups (360 ml) cornmeal

1½ cups (360 ml) whole wheat pastry flour

¼ cup (60 ml) Sucanat or other unrefined sugar

1 Tbsp + 1 tsp (15 ml + 5 ml) baking powder

¼ tsp (1.25 ml) sea salt

1 egg

1 Tbsp (15 ml) extra virgin olive oil

1½ cups (360 ml) almond, soy or low-fat milk

1 cup (240 ml) plain low-fat yogurt or soy yogurt

Use a paper towel to oil inside of skillet. Place skillet on middle rack in oven and preheat to 400˚F (200˚C).

Meanwhile, in a large bowl, add cornmeal, pastry flour, Sucanat, baking powder and sea salt. Gently whisk to combine. Add egg, olive oil, milk and yogurt, and mix together until just combined.

Once oven reaches temperature, using an oven mitt or thick towel, carefully slide middle rack out and pour batter into hot skillet. Slide rack back into oven and close door. Bake cornbread until golden brown and firm to the touch, 25 to 30 minutes. Remove, slice into wedges and serve warm.

KEEP IT FRESH
This cornbread will keep three days at room temperature. To reheat, place cornbread wedges in a 350˚F (177˚C) oven until heated through, about 10 minutes.

NUTRITIONAL VALUE PER WEDGE (1/12 OF SKILLET):
Calories: 160 | Calories from Fat: 28 | Protein: 5 g | Carbs: 30 g | Total Fat: 3 g |
Saturated Fat: 0.1 g | Trans Fat: 0 g | Fiber: 3 g | Sodium: 873 mg | Cholesterol: 19 mg

Fresh Strawberries with Chocolate-Orange Avocado Mousse

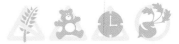

PREP: 15 minutes | **COOK:** 0 minutes | **YIELD:** 11 servings

This mousse is so rich and decadent, you won't believe it's vegan – and made with avocados!

2 avocados, pitted and peeled

½ cup (120 ml) cocoa powder

⅓ cup (80 ml) brown-rice syrup or yacon syrup

1 tsp (5 ml) pure vanilla extract

Pinch sea salt

1 tsp (5 ml) finely grated orange zest

2 Tbsp (30 ml) plain soy, almond or other milk substitute, or water

5½ cups (1.32 L) quartered, stemmed strawberries

Add avocados, cocoa powder, syrup, vanilla extract, sea salt, orange zest and milk to a food processor or blender, and blend until very smooth. Stop the machine to scrape down sides once or twice to ensure that all ingredients are blended well.

Serve with strawberries for dipping or scooping.

NUTRITIONAL VALUE PER SERVING (½ CUP STRAWBERRIES + ¼ CUP MOUSSE):
Calories: 92 | Calories from Fat: 39 | Protein: 2 g | Carbs: 19 g | Total Fat: 4 g |
Saturated Fat: 1 g | Trans Fat: 0 g | Fiber: 5 g | Sodium: 14 mg | Cholesterol: 0 mg

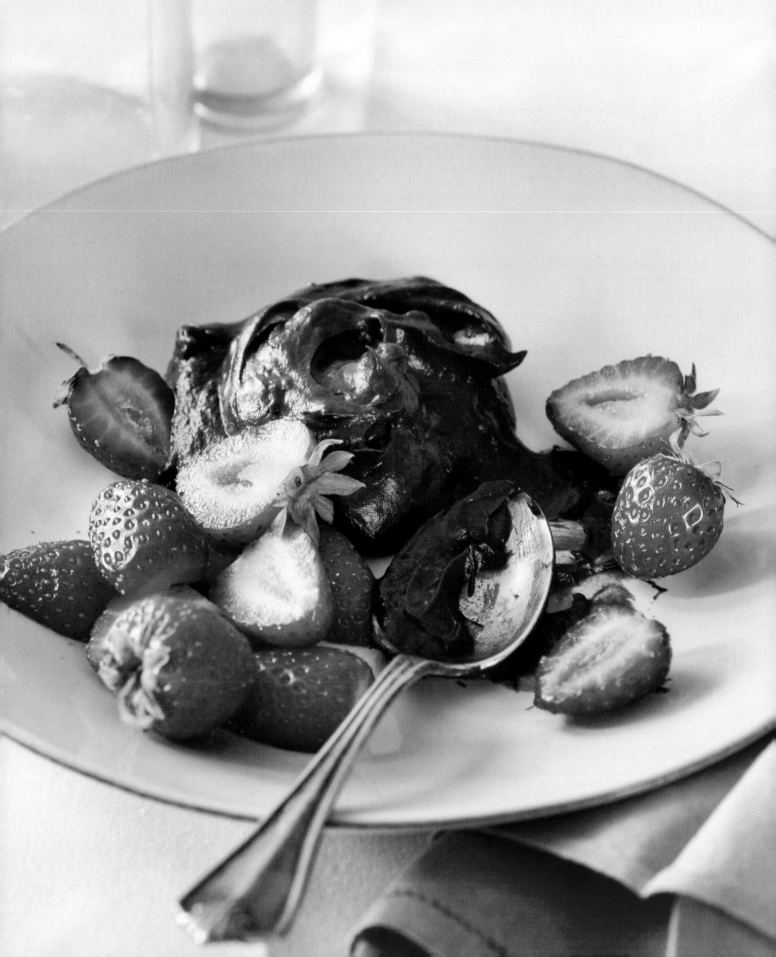

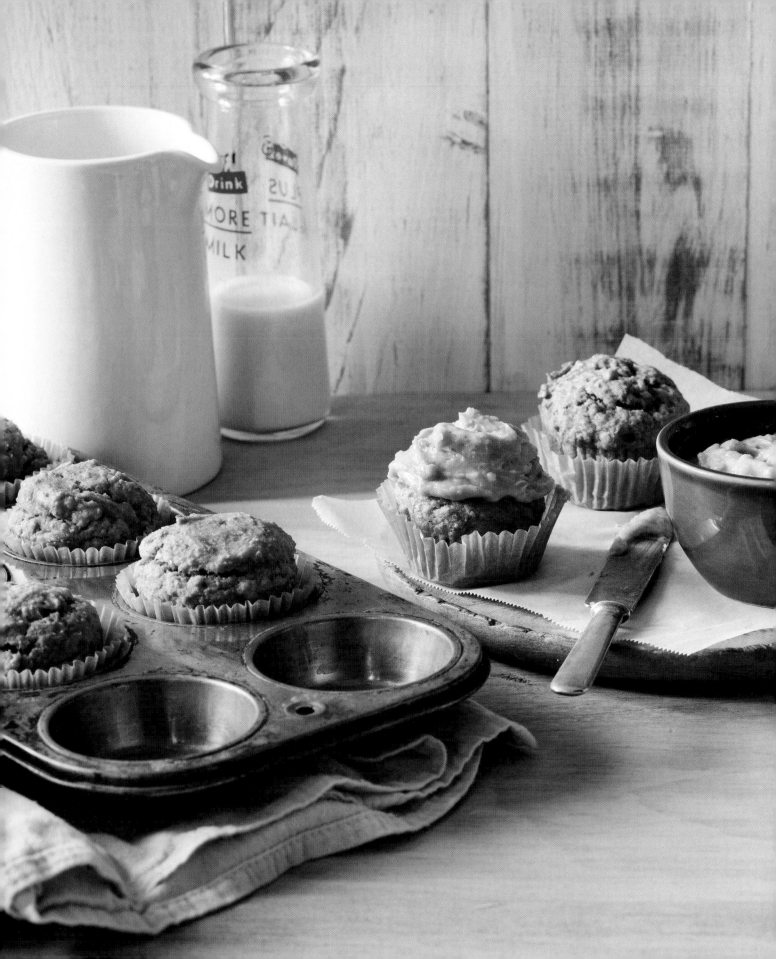

Banana Cupcakes with Peanut Butter Yogurt Frosting

PREP: 20 minutes | **COOK:** 27-30 minutes | **YIELD:** 10 cupcakes

This classic combo tastes great on a sandwich, but in cupcakes? Even better! Best of all, these ones are guilt free and they wear many hats! Learn more in the tip below.

1¼ cups (300 ml) whole wheat pastry flour

2 Tbsp (30 ml) finely ground potato flour

2 Tbsp (30 ml) flax meal or ground flaxseed

½ tsp (2.5 ml) baking soda

¼ tsp (1.25 ml) baking powder

¼ tsp (1.25 ml) sea salt

3 Tbsp (45 ml) virgin coconut oil, melted

¼ cup (60 ml) Sucanat or other unrefined sugar

¾ cup (180 ml) low-fat milk or plain,
    unsweetened soy or almond milk

1 cup (240 ml) mashed very ripe bananas,
    about 3 large

PEANUT BUTTER YOGURT FROSTING

¼ cup (60 ml) all-natural peanut butter, sugar
    and salt free

½ cup (120 ml) Yogurt Cheese* (see p. 276)

2 Tbsp (30 ml) pure honey

½ tsp (2.5 ml) pure vanilla extract

Preheat oven to 350°F (177°C). Line a muffin tin with 10 paper liners.

In a bowl, mix together whole wheat flour, potato flour, flax meal, baking soda, baking powder and salt. In a large bowl, mix together coconut oil and Sucanat. Add flour mixture and mix together until texture resembles slightly wet sand. Slowly stir in milk. Fold in bananas until just combined. Batter will be thick. Scoop a heaping ¼ cup (60 ml) batter into each lined muffin cup until all batter is used. Bake 27 to 30 minutes until toothpick inserted into center comes out clean. Transfer cupcakes to a wire rack to cool.

To make frosting, mix together peanut butter, Yogurt Cheese, honey and vanilla extract until well combined. Frost tops of cooled cupcakes.

TRY THIS!
Basically, the only difference between a muffin and a cupcake is the frosting, so if you want to skip the topper – go ahead! Your cupcakes will become delicious and healthy banana muffins.

CHILL OUT
The cupcakes will keep in the refrigerator up to five days.

NOTE
*Yogurt Cheese must be made ahead of time.

NUTRITIONAL VALUE PER CUPCAKE, WITH FROSTING:
Calories: 203 | Calories from Fat: 76 | Protein: 6 g | Carbs: 28 g | Total Fat: 5 g |
Saturated Fat: 1 g | Trans Fat: 0 g | Fiber: 3 g | Sodium: 112 mg | Cholesterol: 0.5 mg

Baked Sweet Plantains

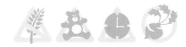

PREP: 10 minutes | **COOK:** 12-14 minutes | **YIELD:** 8 servings

I tried my first plantain while on vacation in Puerto Rico a few years ago. The starchiness of these members of the banana family both surprised and pleased me. I knew they would pair well with the warm flavors of cinnamon, cumin and nutmeg. They make a small but satisfying dessert perfect for a warm summer evening.

4 very ripe plantains (skin yellow and starting to turn black)

¼ tsp (1.25 ml) ground cinnamon

¼ tsp (1.25 ml) ground cumin

Pinch grated nutmeg

Eat-Clean Cooking Spray (see p. 277)

Preheat oven to 450°F (232°C).

Cut ends off plantains, peel and discard skins. Cut plantains on the diagonal into ½-inch slices. In a small bowl, mix together cinnamon, cumin and nutmeg. Spray a baking sheet with Eat-Clean Cooking Spray and arrange plantain slices in a single layer. Use two baking sheets if necessary. Spray tops of plantains with Eat-Clean Cooking Spray and sprinkle with spice mixture. Bake until golden brown on bottom, about 8 minutes. Use a metal spatula to turn, and continue baking until golden brown on both sides, 4 to 6 minutes. Remove from oven and serve immediately.

PREP TIP
Keep an eye on plantains during baking because they can quickly go from golden brown to burned.

NUTRITIONAL VALUE PER SERVING (½ PLANTAIN):
Calories: 33 | Calories from Fat: 9 | Protein: 0.2 g | Carbs: 6 g | Total Fat: 1 g |
Saturated Fat: 0.4 g | Trans Fat: 0 g | Fiber: 0.1 g | Sodium: 0.2 mg | Cholesterol: 0 mg

Blueberry Compote

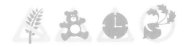

PREP: 5 minutes | **COOK:** 5 minutes | **YIELD:** 6 x ¼-cup servings

Use this fruit compote instead of maple syrup on pancakes and waffles, or try stirring it into yogurt. You can also substitute other berries, such as raspberries, blackberries or strawberries, to make different flavored compotes.

2 cups (480 ml) **frozen or fresh** blueberries

1 Tbsp (15 ml) **lemon juice**

1 Tbsp (15 ml) **brown-rice syrup, yacon syrup,**
      honey or Sucanat

1 tsp (5 ml) **arrowroot starch**

Pinch sea salt

Combine all ingredients in a saucepan and bring to a simmer on medium-high heat, stirring occasionally. Reduce heat to gently simmer and cook until slightly thickened, and some blueberries have broken down, 2 or 3 minutes. Remove from heat and let cool slightly. Refrigerate any unused compote.

CHILL OUT
This compote will keep in the refrigerator up to five days.

NUTRITIONAL VALUE PER SERVING:
Calories: 34 | Calories from Fat: 1 | Protein: 0.3 g | Carbs: 9 g | Total Fat: 0 g |
Saturated Fat: 0 g | Trans Fat: 0 g | Fiber: 1 g | Sodium: 3 mg | Cholesterol: 0 mg

Cappuccino Fudge Pops

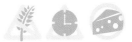

PREP: 10 minutes | **COOK:** 5 minutes | **YIELD:** 6 pops

Cappuccino? Fudge? Enough said! This dessert will satisfy any sweet tooth and caffeine cravings without sacrificing your health. Yum!

2 tsp (10 ml) **arrowroot**

1 cup (240 ml) **low-fat milk**

2 Tbsp (30 ml) **semisweet chocolate chips**

¼ cup (60 ml) **pure** honey

1 Tbsp (15 ml) **unsweetened** cocoa powder

⅓ cup (80 ml) **freshly brewed** espresso or
      very strong coffee

Pinch sea salt

½ tsp (2.5 ml) **vanilla extract**

Prepare six frozen ice-pop molds in their tray.

In a small bowl, whisk arrowroot with half of milk and set aside. In a small, heavy-bottomed saucepan, melt chocolate chips on medium-low heat. Stir in honey, cocoa powder, espresso, salt, reserved arrowroot-milk mixture and remaining milk. Increase heat to medium high and cook, whisking regularly, until mixture thickens and no lumps remain, about 3 minutes. Remove from heat and whisk in vanilla extract. Transfer mixture to a liquid measuring cup and pour into ice-pop molds. Insert sticks and caps to secure pops, then place in freezer until solid. To unmold, run under lukewarm water to release pop from its container.

NUTRITIONAL VALUE PER POP:
Calories: 87 | Calories from Fat: 17 | Protein: 2 g | Carbs: 18 g | Total Fat: 2 g |
Saturated Fat: 1 g | Trans Fat: 0 g | Fiber: 1 g | Sodium: 25 mg | Cholesterol: 2 mg

Pineapple Carrot Bread... or Cake?

PREP: 15 minutes | **COOK:** 50 minutes | **YIELD:** 9 x 1-inch slices

Carrot cake is one of my all-time favorite desserts to indulge in. Throwing in pineapple just sweetens the deal by adding an entirely new flavor. This might be my new favorite treat to enjoy on occasion.

2 Tbsp (30 ml) coconut oil, melted

20 oz (565 g) crushed pineapple, drained
and juice pressed out

1½ cups (360 ml) grated carrot

½ cup (120 ml) Sucanat or other
unrefined sugar

1 whole egg + 2 egg whites

1 tsp (5 ml) ground cinnamon

1 tsp (5 ml) ground ginger

¼ tsp (1.25 ml) sea salt

2 Tbsp (30 ml) flax meal or ground flaxseed

1½ cups (360 ml) whole wheat flour

2 Tbsp (30 ml) wheat germ

1 tsp (5 ml) baking powder

1 tsp (5 ml) baking soda

Preheat oven to 350˚F (177˚C). Grease a 9 x 5-inch loaf pan with a bit of coconut oil.

In a large bowl, stir together coconut oil, pineapple, carrot, Sucanat, egg and egg whites, cinnamon, ginger, salt and flax meal. In a separate bowl, stir together flour, wheat germ, baking powder and baking soda. Stir dry ingredients into wet until just combined. Scrape batter into loaf pan and spread out to edges. Bake until a toothpick inserted into center comes out clean, about 50 minutes.

Remove from oven and let cool for 10 minutes before unmolding. Slide a knife around edges to help loosen cake from the pan, then unmold and finish cooling on a wire rack.

TRY THIS!

Here's a way to slice the loaf to get the greatest yield. First, cut the loaf in half lengthwise. Then cut into slices 1-inch thick crosswise. You will get 18 smaller servings from the loaf.

NUTRITIONAL VALUE PER SLICE (⅑ OF RECIPE):
Calories: 108 | Calories from Fat: 23 | Protein: 3 g | Carbs: 13 g | Total Fat: 3 g |
Saturated Fat: 1.5 g | Trans Fat: 0 g | Fiber: 2 g | Sodium: 90 mg | Cholesterol: 12 mg

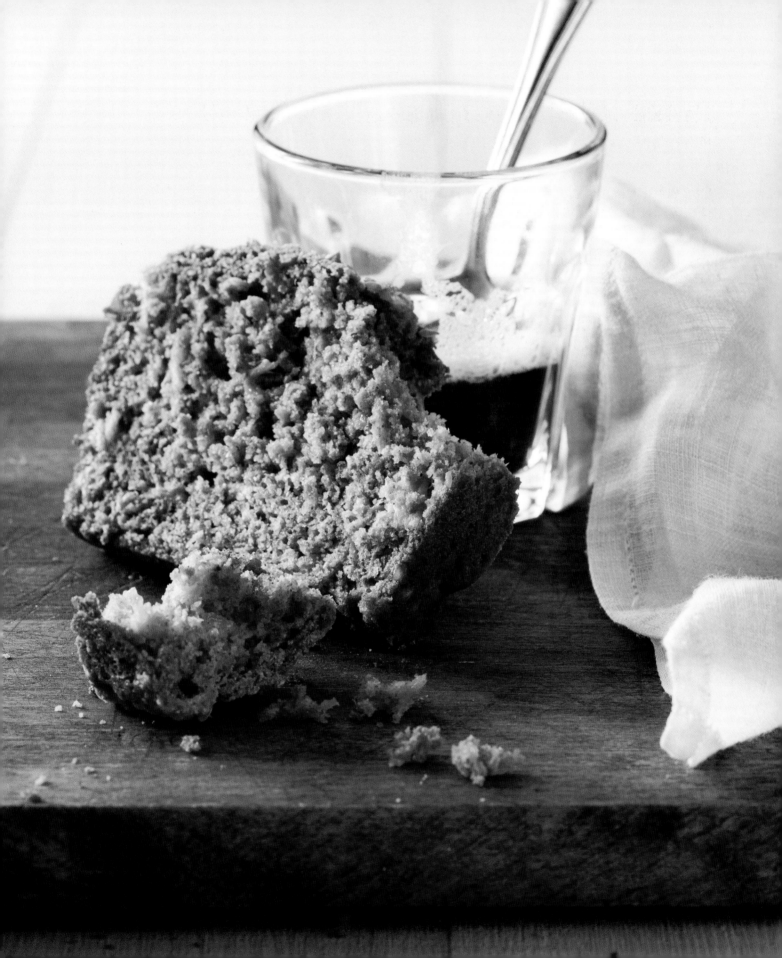

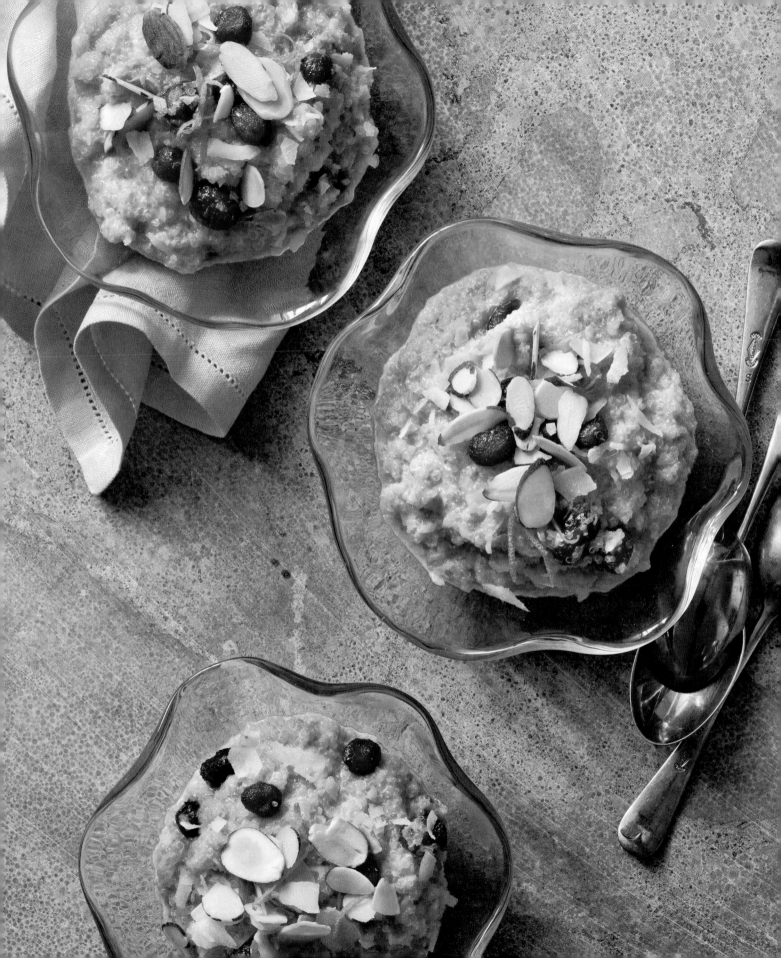

Coconut Orange Quinoa Pudding

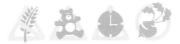

PREP: 10 minutes | **COOK:** 20 minutes | **YIELD:** 8 x ½-cup servings

It's strange to think that a grain such as quinoa works well both at dinner and dessert. In fact, quinoa takes on a lot of the cooking flavor while offering a moist and chewy texture. In my opinion that's a perfect way to finish off a meal. So give it a try: Quinoa pudding = fun!

1 x 13.5-oz (400 ml) BPA-free can reduced-fat coconut milk

1 Tbsp (15 ml) grated orange zest (zest from about 1 orange)

1 cup (240 ml) freshly squeezed orange juice

¼ cup (60 ml) brown-rice syrup or yacon syrup

½ tsp (2.5 ml) ground cinnamon

1 tsp (5 ml) arrowroot powder

Pinch sea salt

1 cup (240 ml) quinoa

½ cup (120 ml) dried cranberries

¼ cup (60 ml) shredded unsweetened coconut

In a heavy-bottomed saucepan with lid, whisk together coconut milk, orange zest and juice, syrup, cinnamon, arrowroot and salt until thoroughly combined. Stir in quinoa, cranberries and coconut. Bring mixture to a boil on high heat, reduce heat and simmer gently, covered, until quinoa is plump and cooked through, about 20 minutes. There will be liquid left in pot, like a pudding. Let cool slightly before serving. Serve warm or chilled.

TRY THIS!
This is delicious topped with slivered almonds!

NUTRITIONAL VALUE PER SERVING, NOT INCLUDING ALMONDS:
Calories: 130 | Calories from Fat: 46 | Protein: 1.4 g | Carbs: 24 g | Total Fat: 5 g | Saturated Fat: 4 g | Trans Fat: 0 g | Fiber: 2 g | Sodium: 21 mg | Cholesterol: 0 mg

Crunchy Oatmeal Raisin Cookies

PREP: 30 minutes | **COOK:** 12-15 minutes | **YIELD:** 3 dozen cookies

Here's the perfect cookie to enjoy on occasion. This vegan version of the classic is sweet, crunchy and certainly bound to be a hit in your house!

½ cup (120 ml) organic virgin unrefined coconut oil, very soft and slightly melted

⅓ cup (80 ml) organic dark brown sugar, firmly packed

3 Tbsp (45 ml) plain, unsweetened soymilk or milk substitute

2 Tbsp (30 ml) whole-grain soy flour

1 tsp (5 ml) pure vanilla extract

1 cup (240 ml) whole wheat pastry flour

1 tsp (5 ml) baking soda

1 tsp (5 ml) ground cinnamon

Pinch sea salt

2 cups (480 ml) old-fashioned rolled oats

¾ cup (180 ml) raisins

Preheat oven to 350°F (177°C).

In a mixer with paddle attachment or in a large bowl using an electric handheld mixer, mix together coconut oil and brown sugar on medium speed until creamy, about 2 minutes. Add soymilk, soy flour and vanilla, and mix together on low speed.

In a separate bowl, stir together flour, baking soda, cinnamon and salt, and add to mixer bowl. Mix ingredients together on low speed until well combined. Mix in oats and raisins.

Scoop rounded tablespoons into the palm of your hand and press dough together. Place on baking sheets and press top down to partially flatten cookies. Bake 12 to 15 minutes until light golden brown. Remove from oven and let cool 1 minute on baking sheets, then transfer to a wire rack to cool completely. Cookies will get crunchy as they cool. Store in an airtight container up to two weeks.

NUTRITIONAL VALUE PER COOKIE:
Calories: 73 | Calories from Fat: 30 | Protein: 1 g | Carbs: 10 g | Total Fat: 3 g | Saturated Fat: 2.6 g | Trans Fat: 0 g | Fiber: 1 g | Sodium: 36 mg | Cholesterol: 0 mg

THE EAT-CLEAN DIET VEGETARIAN COOKBOOK

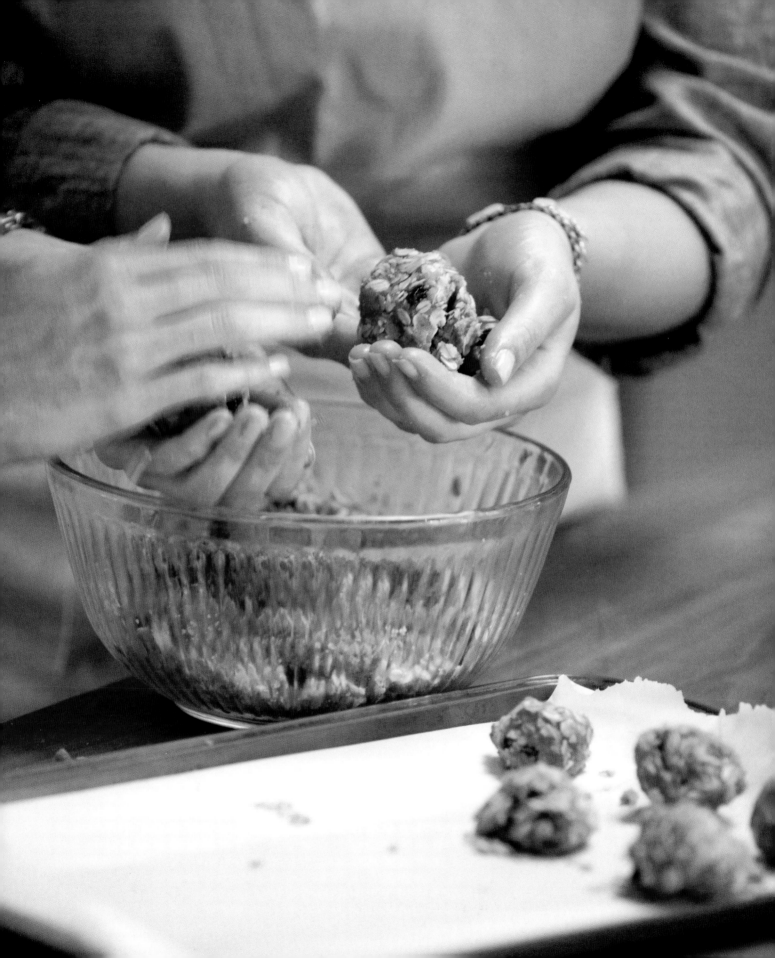

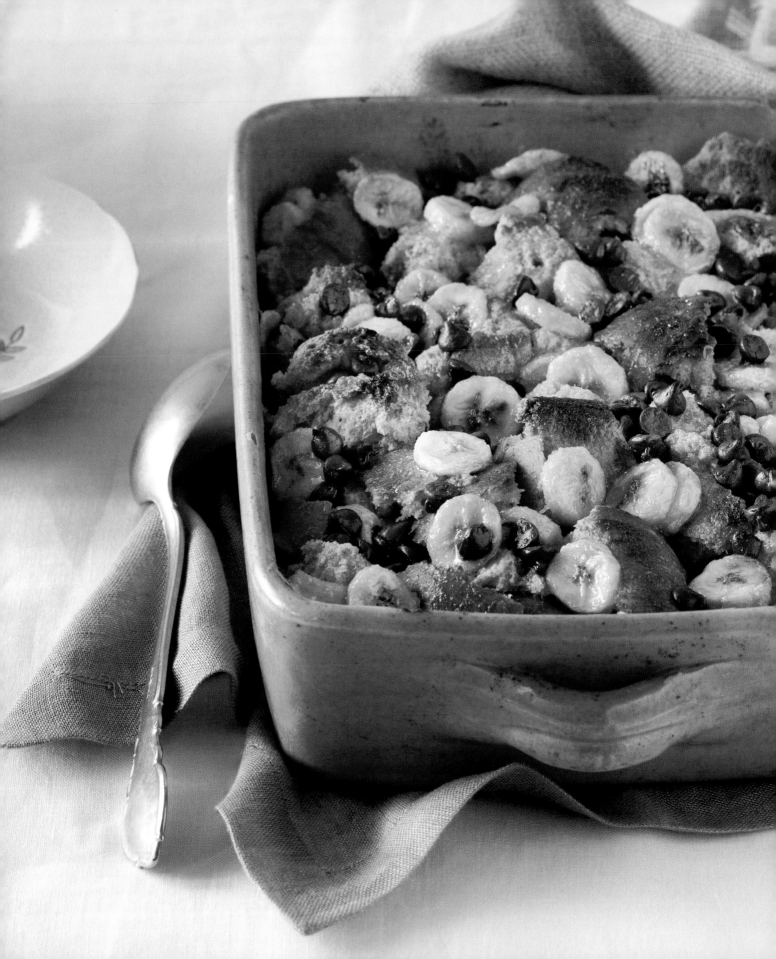

Ooey Gooey Banana Chocolate Chip Bread Pudding

PREP TIME: 10 minutes active + 10 minutes inactive | **COOK TIME:** 30 minutes | **YIELD:** 13 x ½-cup servings

Bread pudding is my absolute favorite dessert. I make it almost every year for Christmas. This is one that has "irresistible" written all over it. In fact, this is a recipe for the whole family to enjoy. After all, there is nothing better than bananas, until you add chocolate chips!

Unrefined virgin coconut oil, for coating dish

2½ cups (600 ml) plain unsweetened soy, rice, almond, coconut or other milk substitute

3 Tbsp (45 ml) arrowroot starch

2 Tbsp (30 ml) Sucanat or other unrefined sugar

2 Tbsp (30 ml) brown-rice syrup or yacon syrup

1 tsp (5 ml) pure vanilla extract

¼ tsp (1.25 ml) ground cinnamon

⅛ tsp (0.625 ml) ground nutmeg

Pinch sea salt

5 cups (1.2 L) day-old whole grain bread, torn into 1- to 2-inch pieces, lightly packed

2 ripe bananas, peeled and sliced into ½-inch rounds

½ cup (120 ml) vegan semisweet chocolate chips

Preheat the oven to 350˚F (177˚C). Coat inside of a 1.5- to 2-quart ceramic dish with coconut oil.

In a large bowl, add all ingredients except bread, bananas and chocolate chips. Whisk together thoroughly until no lumps remain. Add bread, bananas and chocolate chips and stir to combine, mashing up bananas a little and allowing bread to absorb most of the liquid. Scrape into greased dish and press down to smooth top. Let sit for 10 minutes so bread can absorb liquid. Bake uncovered until lightly browned and firm to the touch, about 30 minutes. Remove and let cool slightly before serving. Best served warm so it's "ooey gooey."

NUTRITIONAL VALUE PER SERVING:
Calories: 112 | Calories from Fat: 33 | Protein: 3 g | Carbs: 20 g | Total Fat: 4 g |
Saturated Fat: 2 g | Trans Fat: 0 g | Fiber: 2 g | Sodium: 47 mg | Cholesterol: 0 mg

Peanut Butter Chocolate Chip Backpack Kisses

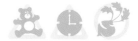

PREP: 20 minutes | **COOK:** 0 minutes | **YIELD:** 33 kisses

Who doesn't love a little kiss? These kisses are the perfect snack to go. Plus, they're super cute!

½ cup (120 ml) old-fashioned rolled oats

¼ cup (60 ml) vegan unsweetened protein powder, as natural as possible

2 Tbsp (30 ml) hulled hemp seeds

2 Tbsp (30 ml) flaxseed, cracked

¼ cup (60 ml) unsweetened dried cranberries

¼ cup (60 ml) vegan semisweet natural chocolate chips

Pinch sea salt

1 cup (240 ml) all-natural peanut butter, sugar and salt free

2 Tbsp (30 ml) brown-rice syrup, yacon syrup or pure honey

In a large bowl, mix together oats, protein powder, hemp seeds, flaxseed, dried cranberries, chocolate chips and sea salt. Add peanut butter and syrup or honey and mix together. Using your hands, knead mixture together thoroughly. Drop by rounded teaspoonful onto a baking sheet, or use a mini ice-cream scoop. Using your hands, roll into balls. Wrap kisses in squares of aluminum foil, twisting tops to seal, or store them unwrapped in an airtight container.

CHILL OUT
Store in the fridge for up to two weeks, or in the freezer for up to one month.

NUTRITIONAL VALUE PER KISS:
Calories: 75 | Calories from Fat: 45 | Protein: 3 g | Carbs: 6 g | Total Fat: 5 g | Saturated Fat: 1 g | Trans Fat: 0 g | Fiber: 1 g | Sodium: 38 mg | Cholesterol: 0 mg

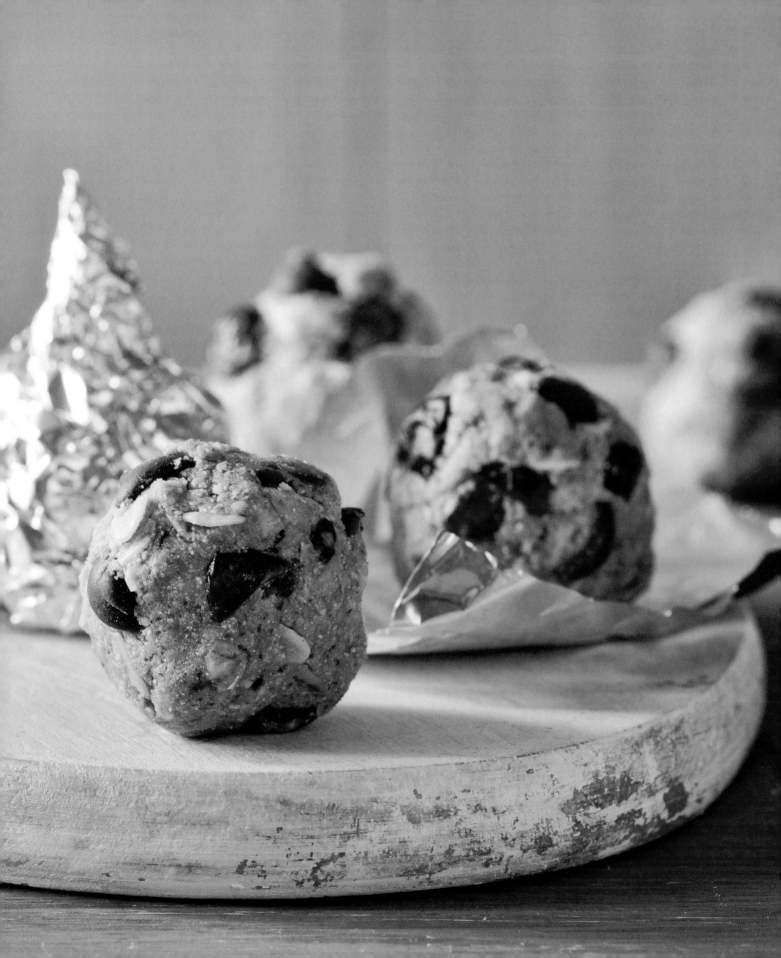

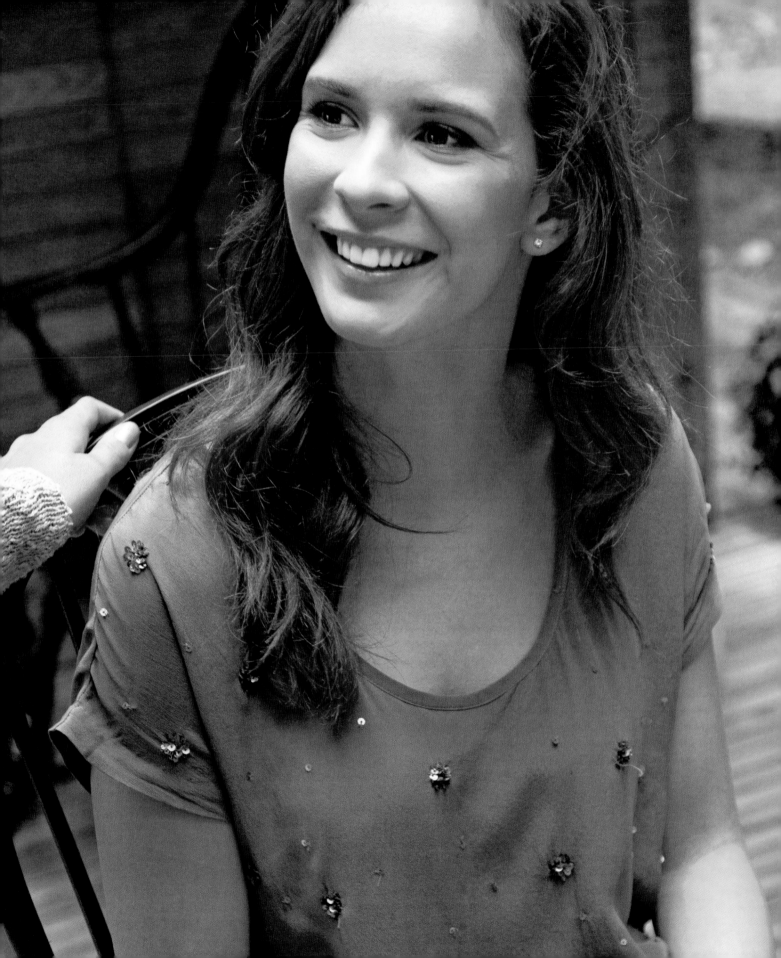

Rhubarb Cherry Berry Crostata

PREP: 30 minutes active, 30 minutes inactive | **COOK:** 60 minutes | **YIELD:** 10 slices

Chelsea loves desserts, especially when they are fruit based. Rhubarb Cherry Berry Crostata is a big favorite. Fresh summer cherries and rhubarb from my garden make it even more tempting.

CRUST

5 Tbsp (75 ml) coconut oil, separated into
  5 portions, chilled

1 cup (240 ml) whole wheat pastry flour,
  plus more for dusting

¼ tsp (1.25 ml) sea salt

1 tsp (5 ml) Sucanat or other unrefined sugar

5 Tbsp (75 ml) icewater

1 Tbsp (15 ml) low-fat soy, almond or other milk,
  to brush crust

FILLING

2 cups (480 ml) rhubarb, cut into ½-inch pieces

1 cup (240 ml) frozen pie cherries

1 cup (240 ml) frozen mixed berries, such as
  strawberries, raspberries, blueberries
  and blackberries

3 Tbsp + 1 tsp (45 ml + 5 ml) Sucanat or other
  unrefined sugar

2 Tbsp (30 ml) arrowroot

¼ tsp (1.25 ml) + a pinch ground cinnamon

Pinch freshly grated nutmeg

To make crust: In a food processor, pulse coconut oil, flour, salt and Sucanat until mixture resembles coarse sand with some pea-sized pieces. While pulsing, add icewater 1 Tbsp (15 ml) at a time until dough sticks together when pressed between your fingers. Transfer dough onto a large piece of plastic wrap. Form dough into a ball, and press into a disk shape. Wrap dough in plastic wrap and refrigerate for 30 minutes.

To make filling: In a large bowl, stir together rhubarb, cherries, berries, 3 Tbsp (45 ml) Sucanat, arrowroot, ¼ tsp (1.25 ml) ground cinnamon and nutmeg until well combined. Set aside.

Position rack in center of oven and preheat to 350˚F (177˚C).

Remove dough from refrigerator and transfer to a piece of parchment paper dusted with flour. Dust top of dough and a rolling pin with flour, and roll out into a 12-inch circle about ⅛-inch thick. Transfer dough and parchment to a large baking sheet. Mound fruit mixture in center of dough, leaving a two-inch border. Fold dough into pleats over filling, leaving fruit exposed in center. Pinch dough to seal any cracks. Brush crust with milk and sprinkle with remaining 1 tsp (5 ml) Sucanat and pinch of cinnamon.

Bake crostata until crust is golden brown and fruit is tender and bubbling, 50 to 60 minutes. Remove from oven and let cool slightly on baking sheet, then slide a metal spatula under crust to detach it from sheet and transfer to a cutting board. Use a large, sharp knife to cut crostata into slices. Serve warm.

> **MAKE-AHEAD TIP**
> The dough can be made up to one day ahead.

NUTRITIONAL VALUE PER SERVING (¹⁄₁₀ OF CROSTATA):
Calories: 155 | Calories from Fat: 61 | Protein: 2 g | Carbs: 23 g | Total Fat: 0.3 g |
Saturated Fat: 0 g | Trans Fat: 0 g | Fiber: 3 g | Sodium: 6 mg | Cholesterol: 0 mg

Are You Getting Enough?

Vegetarians are often considered some of the healthiest among us by virtue of their green diet. Research shows most vegetarians exceed the recommended five to ten servings of vegetables suggested daily and have significantly reduced chances of suffering from cardiovascular disease, diabetes and cancer. Some vegetarians, though, eat too many starchy carbohydrates from whole grains, too little protein and not nearly enough vegetables or fruit, leaving them without all of these benefits.

As with anything in life, balance is key. A vegetarian diet must be followed wisely. Becoming vegetarian requires a lot of research and commitment. Here's a list of some of the nutrients that are often lacking in a vegetarian diet.

CALCIUM

You need it for: Strong teeth and bones, maintenance of muscles and hormone function

Where to find it: Dairy, dark green veggies, almonds, broccoli and fortified tofu and soy milk

Try it tonight! Toss together the Delightful Strawberry, Spinach and Broccoli Salad with Macadamia Nuts (see p. 72). The greens and nuts provide an explosion of calcium.

Deficiency disorder: Hypocalcemia, which causes, skin problems, hyperactive tendons and decreased bone density.

NOTE: Be diligent about maintaining adequate calcium levels in young children – it lays the foundation for strong, healthy bones.

IODINE

You need it for: Thyroid health and metabolism

Where to find it: Leafy greens, asparagus, kelp and other sea vegetables, and iodized sea salt

Try it tonight! The wakame and dulse in the Miso Udon Noodle Bowl with Roasted Sweet Potato, Tofu and Sea Vegetables (see p. 132) are a delicious way of getting your iodine!

Deficiency disorder: Hypothyroidism and cretinism due to maternal deficiency of iodine

IRON

You need it for: Proper function of red blood cells

Where to find it: Green, leafy veggies, beans, lentils, tofu, pumpkin seeds, millet, figs, dried apricots and dates.

Try it tonight! The Tofu, Broccoli and Mushroom Fajitas (see p. 118) contain tofu, which is rich in iron, and broccoli, which is full of vitamin C to help you absorb it!

Deficiency disorder: Anemia, which causes fatigue, pallor, hair loss, and weakness.

NOTE: Iron from plant sources is not easily absorbed unless paired with foods rich in vitamin C. Avoid drinking tea and coffee when eating iron-rich foods as caffeine will block iron absorption.

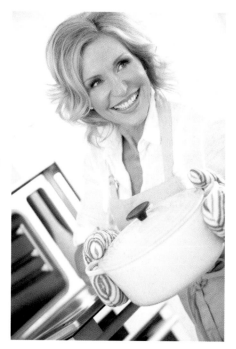

> "As with anything in life, balance is key.
> A vegetarian diet must be followed wisely."

OMEGA 3 FATTY ACIDS

You need them for: A healthy heart, healthy eyes, proper brain development, cellular health and more

Where to find them: Fish, flaxseed, chia and hemp seeds, fortified eggs, walnuts and soybeans

Try it tonight! The Green Energy Whole Food Smoothie (see p. 17) is made with flaxseed, rich in omega 3s.

Note: Plant sources of omega-3 fatty acids are hard for the body to assimilate.

Deficiency disorder: Fatigue, dry skin, heart problems and poor circulation, mood disorders, and poor memory.

PROTEIN

You need it for: Growth and repair of body tissues (skin, bones, muscles and organs), along with hormone and enzyme function.

Where to find it: Hemp, soy, spirulina, quinoa, eggs and dairy products.

Try it tonight! Sink your teeth into an Italian Marinara Beanball Sub (see p. 119). You're guaranteed a high-protein party with beans and quinoa "balled" together.

Deficiency disorder: Kwashiorkor, which causes wasting, edema and reduced intelligence; marasmus.

NOTE: For more info on this key nutrient, see p. 144.

VITAMIN B12

You need it for: Nerve formation and cell production (especially red blood cells)

Where to find it: Primarily in animal products. Those following a vegan diet may need a supplement. Also found in fortified products such as soy milk and cereals – read labels carefully!

Try it tonight! Relax with a glass of Smoothie on the Beach (see p. 29)! The fortified soy yogurt gives you your much-needed vitamin B12.

Deficiency disorder: may be caused by pernicious anemia and manifests as fatigue, depression, mania and psychosis.

VITAMIN D

You need it for: Bone and dental health, immune function, mood regulation

Where to find it: Your main source of vitamin D is sunlight exposure for 10 minutes each day. It's also found in fortified cereals, soy and cow's milk.

Try it tonight! Pescatarians can enjoy Salmon Caesar Pita Pockets (see p. 153) to get their vitamin D fix! Take these on a picnic under the sun for maximum vitamin D exposure.

Deficiency disorder: Rickets and osteomalacia manifesting as deformity of long bones and possibly peripheral vascular diseases, cancer and multiple sclerosis.

NOTE: Most individuals, not just vegetarians, need to be aware of their vitamin D levels – especially in cold climates.

ZINC

You need it for: Healthy immune system, wound healing, cell division and enzyme function

Where to find it: Leafy greens, whole grains, soy products, avocados, bananas, apricots, apples, seeds and nuts, wheat germ.

Try it tonight! Start your day with some hearty Amaranth Oat Waffles (see p. 22)! The mixture of amaranth, soy and oat flour gives you a kick of zinc to boost your immune system.

Deficiency disorder: Hypozincemia, which manifests as hair loss, skin lesions, diarrhea, wasting of body tissues, as well as poor eyesight.

NOTE: Zinc is not easily absorbed from plant sources. A supplement may be needed.

Holiday
Feast

Root Vegetable and
Tempeh Shepherd's Pie, p. 246

Perfect Holiday Harmony

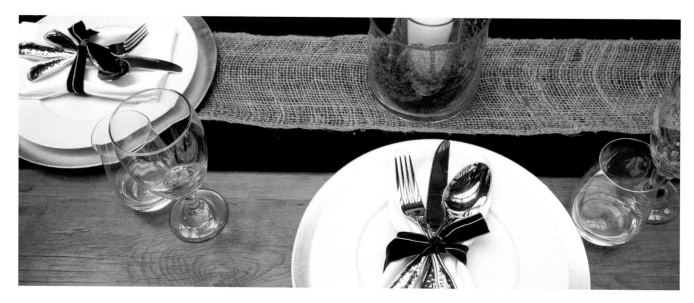

Ah, nothing beats the pleasant pandemonium of a festive gathering. The smells of cooking, the glittering décor and the sounds of laughter (and perhaps the occasional excited whoop from those being reunited after months apart) – isn't that what the holidays are all about?

Of course, food is a key ingredient in this tableau, and most festive feasts are all about dusting off the family favorites that have been around for generations. Although there's nothing wrong with the classics, why not try mixing things up with a totally new approach this year? Rest assured, even omnivores will enjoy the fresh flavors of local and seasonal produce, multicultural twists and guilt-free desserts in this chapter. Times and tastes have changed, so what better opportunity to start creating some new traditions?

Before you set out on the adventure of creating your Clean and meatless holiday feast, keep in mind that the following menus are meant to be adaptable. The first one is a great road map for the totally vegan crowd and the second menu includes some lacto- and lacto-ovo vegetarian selections.

You can also pick and choose individual recipes from the menus – they will make great accompaniments to your beloved classics (just make sure you keep the vegetarian cooking and serving utensils separate!). After all, it's the season for peace and harmony. Oh, and food, love and sharing, too! And I sincerely hope that you and your family will enjoy and share these recipes for many years to come.

For more traditional holiday recipes, pick up a copy of *The Eat-Clean Diet Cookbook*!

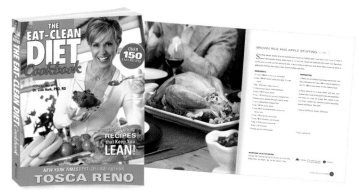

Menu One

All Vegan, All the Time

Every option on this menu is vegan friendly,
so get ready for a meat-, egg- and dairy-free feast
your guests won't soon forget.

Beverage

Soy Pumpkin Nog
(page 271)

Appetizer

Cream of Fennel and Parsnip Soup
(page 253)

Main Course

Root Vegetable and Tempeh Shepherd's Pie
(page 246)

Side Dishes

Wine and Shallot Brussels Sprouts
(page 254)

Baked Acorn Squash with Masala Spices
(page 251)

Parisian Lentils with Roasted Scallions
(page 261)

Mom's Holiday Sauerkraut
(page 267)

Dessert

Baked Apples with Pecan-Currant Streusel
(page 271)

Menu Two

Your Soon-to-be-Family-Favorites

Most of the options on this menu are vegan,
except where indicated by an asterisk.

Beverage

Raspberry Lemon Spritzer
(page 268)

Soup

Roasted Cauliflower and Leek Soup
(page 258)

Salad

Roasted Pear and Spinach Salad with Spiced Pecans
(page 248)

Main Course

Wild Rice and Lentil Terrine*
(page 262)

Side Dishes

Elegant Mushroom Gravy
(page 252)

Zesty Cranberry-Berry Sauce
(page 248)

Fennel Smashed Yukon Gold Potatoes
(page 268)

Rye Bread Stuffing with Mushrooms and Walnuts
(page 247)

Broccoli Potato Gratin*
(page 257)

Dessert

Pumpkin Custard Pie with Flaky Whole Wheat Crust*
(page 272)

Root Vegetable and Tempeh Shepherd's Pie

PREP: 30 minutes | **COOK:** 40 minutes | **YIELD:** 8 servings

Is there anything more comforting than a hearty serving of shepherd's pie? I think not. For that reason, it was so important for me to provide an equally delicious – no, wait, an even more delicious – meat-free version for you to enjoy.

2 lbs (908 g) Yukon gold potatoes, cut into 1-inch chunks

1 cup (240 ml) plain unsweetened soy milk

½ tsp (2.5 ml) sea salt

Pinch white pepper

1 Tbsp (15 ml) extra virgin olive oil

1 onion, halved and sliced

2 cloves garlic, minced

2 carrots, peeled and sliced into coins

4 cups (950 ml) sliced root vegetables, such as parsnips, turnips, rutabaga, and celeriac (celery root)

1 cup (240 ml) thinly sliced green cabbage

1 tsp (5 ml) finely chopped fresh thyme

1 tsp (5 ml) finely chopped fresh sage

2 cups (480 ml) low-sodium, gluten-free vegetable broth

1 Tbsp (15 ml) Bragg's Liquid Aminos

¼ tsp (1.25 ml) freshly ground black pepper

8 oz (225 g) tempeh, crumbled

1 Tbsp (15 ml) finely chopped flat leaf parsley, to garnish

Place potatoes in a pot and cover with cold water. Simmer until tender, about 10 minutes. Drain and return to pot on stove with heat turned off. Mash potatoes until smooth. Add soymilk, salt and pepper, and mix until smooth. Cover and set aside.

In a Dutch oven, heat olive oil on medium. Add onions and cook, stirring occasionally, until lightly browned, about 5 minutes. Stir in garlic and cook until fragrant, about 1 minute. Stir in carrots, root vegetables, cabbage, thyme and sage. Add broth, Bragg's Liquid Aminos, pepper and tempeh, and stir to combine. Bring liquid to a simmer, then cook, covered, until vegetables start to soften, 5 to 10 minutes. Uncover, increase heat to medium high and vigorously simmer until most of liquid has cooked away, 5 to 10 minutes.

Place oven rack six inches from top and turn on broiler. Transfer vegetables to a 10-inch pie plate and spread potatoes overtop. Use a knife to score potatoes in a diamond crosshatch pattern. Place under broiler and cook until lightly browned, 3 to 5 minutes. Remove and sprinkle with chopped parsley. Cut into slices and serve warm.

NUTRITIONAL VALUE PER SERVING (⅛ OF PIE):
Calories: 350 | Calories from Fat: 49 | Protein: 12 g | Carbs: 70 g | Total Fat: 5 g |
Saturated Fat: 1 g | Trans Fat: 0 g | Fiber: 12 g | Sodium: 321 mg | Cholesterol: 0 mg

Rye Bread "Stuffing" with Mushrooms and Walnuts

PREP: 45 minutes | **COOK:** 60 minutes | **YIELD:** 24 x ½-cup servings

When it comes to stuffing, it's time to think outside of the bird. This earthy combination of rye bread, mushrooms and walnuts will fill your kitchen with a delectable aroma, and the combination of various tastes and textures will fill your mouth with heavenly flavors!

20 cups (4.7 L) combination dark rye, light rye with caraway and whole grain bread, cut into 1-inch pieces (can be day-old)

1 Tbsp (15 ml) extra virgin olive oil, divided

1 yellow or white onion, chopped

4 ribs celery, chopped

½ lb (225 g) cremini or white button mushrooms, sliced

4 cloves garlic, minced

2 tsp (10 ml) each finely chopped fresh sage, thyme and rosemary

2½ cups (600 ml) low-sodium vegetable broth

¾ tsp (3.75 ml) sea salt

¼ tsp (1.25 ml) freshly ground black pepper

1 cup (240 ml) coarsely chopped walnut halves and pieces

Place bread pieces on baking sheets and set out, uncovered, to dry overnight. Alternatively, place in a preheated 250˚F (120˚C) oven, stirring once or twice, until mostly dry, 25 to 30 minutes.

Heat half of olive oil in a large skillet on medium. Add onion and celery and cook until soft but not brown, about 8 minutes. Transfer to a very large bowl. Return skillet to stove and add remaining olive oil. Add mushrooms and cook, stirring rarely, for 5 minutes or until soft. Stir in garlic and herbs and cook 1 minute longer. Transfer to bowl. Add bread, vegetable broth, salt, pepper and walnuts. Mix well and transfer to a 3- or 4-quart baking dish. Bake until top is golden brown and slightly crispy, 45 to 50 minutes.

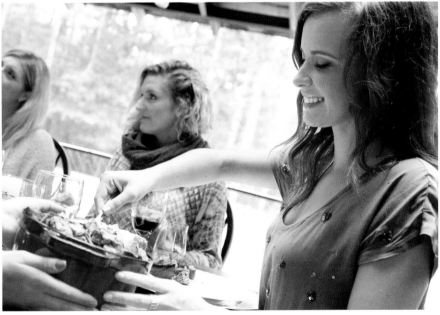

NUTRITIONAL VALUE PER SERVING:
Calories: 322 | Calories from Fat: 51 | Protein: 11 g | Carbs: 58 g | Total Fat: 6 g | Saturated Fat: 0.4 g | Trans Fat: 0 g | Fiber: 3 g | Sodium: 341 mg | Cholesterol: 0 mg

Roasted Pear and Spinach Salad with Spiced Pecans

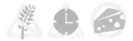

PREP: 15 minutes | COOK: 15 minutes | YIELD: 4 x 1-cup servings

Isn't your mouth watering after just reading the title of this one? This salad is beauty on a plate! Between perfectly roasted pears and spectacularly spiced pecans your taste buds will be taken to a whole new level!

½ cup (120 ml) pecans

1 tsp (5 ml) Sucanat or other unrefined sugar

⅛ tsp (0.625 ml) Chinese five spice powder

⅛ tsp (0.625 ml) chili powder

Pinch cayenne pepper

Pinch each sea salt and freshly ground
    black pepper

1 pear, cored and cut into ¼-inch slices

4 cups (950 ml) baby spinach, packed

1 Tbsp (15 ml) white balsamic vinegar

½ Tbsp (7.5 ml) extra virgin olive oil

2 tsp (10 ml) blue cheese, such as Roquefort,
    crumbled

Preheat oven to 425°F (220°C). Spread pecans on a baking sheet. In a small metal bowl, mix together Sucanat, Chinese five spice powder, chili powder, cayenne, sea salt and pepper. Toast pecans for 5 minutes. Remove and add to bowl with spices. Toss to combine, then scrape back onto baking sheet and place in oven to melt spices and brown sugar onto nuts, 2 or 3 minutes. Remove and set aside.

Place pear slices on a baking sheet and roast in oven until lightly browned around the edges, 5 to 8 minutes. Transfer roasted pears to a salad bowl, and add spinach.

In a separate small bowl, whisk together vinegar, olive oil and blue cheese. Pour over spinach and pears and toss. Divide salad among four plates and top with spiced pecans.

NUTRITIONAL VALUE PER SERVING:
Calories: 155 | Calories from Fat: 107 | Protein: 3 g | Carbs: 12 g | Total Fat: 12 g | Saturated Fat: 1.3 g | Trans Fat: 0 g | Fiber: 4 g | Sodium: 42 mg | Cholesterol: 1 mg

Zesty Cranberry-Berry Sauce

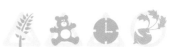

PREP: 10 minutes | COOK: 6 minutes | YIELD: 8 x ¼-cup servings

No holiday table is complete without this key condiment. If you have any left over (and that's a big if), try mixing it with yogurt and granola for a delicious breakfast treat.

10 oz (280 g) fresh or frozen cranberries

½ cup (120 ml) freshly squeezed orange juice
    (from about 1 orange)

Zest of ½ orange

2 Tbsp (30 ml) brown-rice syrup or yacon syrup

1 cup (240 ml) fresh or frozen mixed berries,
    such as blackberries, raspberries
    and blueberries

Pinch freshly grated nutmeg

In a saucepan, add cranberries, orange juice and zest, and syrup. Bring to a gentle boil, then reduce heat to simmer, stirring occasionally, until most cranberries have burst and sauce thickens, about 5 minutes. Stir in mixed berries and nutmeg, and cook 1 minute more. Remove from heat and let cool. Refrigerate until ready to use.

NUTRITIONAL VALUE PER SERVING:
Calories: 39 | Calories from Fat: 0.5 | Protein: 0.3 g | Carbs: 10 g | Total Fat: 0.1 g | Saturated Fat: 0.1 g | Trans Fat: 0 g | Fiber: 2 g | Sodium: 5 mg | Cholesterol: 0 mg

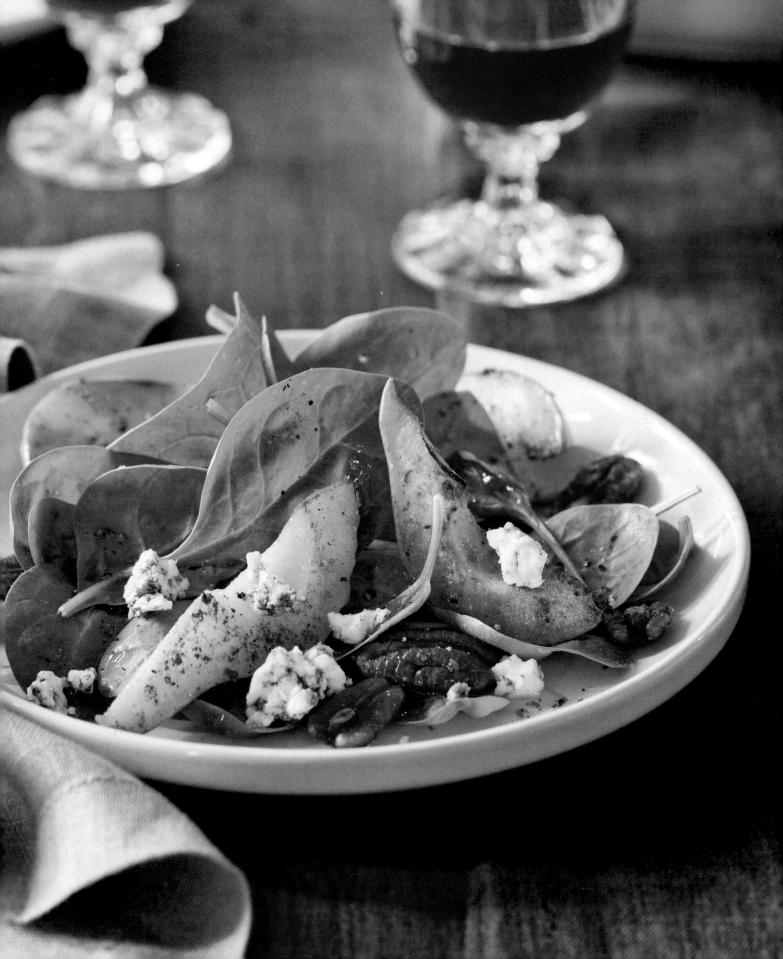

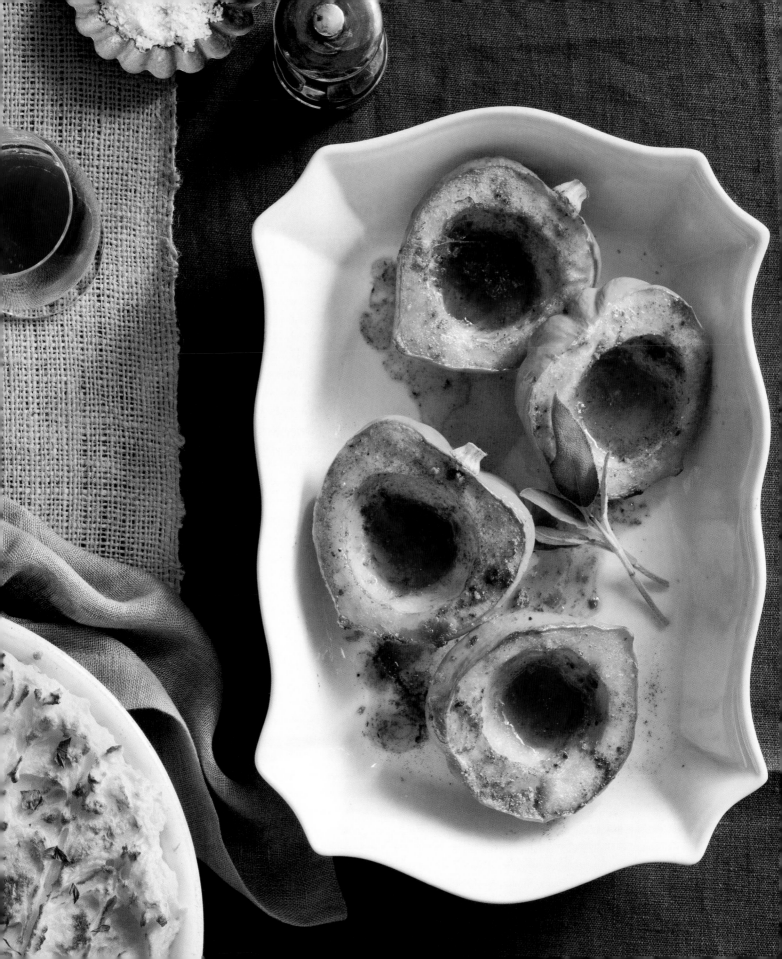

Baked Acorn Squash with Masala Spices

PREP: 10 minutes | **COOK:** 60 minutes | **YIELD:** 2 servings

The addition of garam masala gives an exotic twist to this classic side. I'm willing to bet this recipe will become one of your new holiday favorites!

1 acorn squash
2 tsp (10 ml) extra virgin olive oil
⅛ tsp (0.625 ml) salt-free garam masala
⅛ tsp (0.625 ml) ground cinnamon
Pinch freshly grated nutmeg
Pinch sea salt
4 tsp (20 ml) pure maple syrup, divided

Preheat oven to 400°F (200°C).

Using a strong chef's knife, cut acorn squash in half lengthwise, from stem to end. Scoop out seeds and strings. Place acorn squash, cut side up, in a baking pan and add enough water to come ¼-inch up side of pan. Coat cut side of each squash with 1 tsp (5 ml) olive oil, and sprinkle with garam masala, cinnamon, nutmeg and salt. Drizzle 1 tsp (5 ml) maple syrup over each half.

Bake until squash is very soft and browned on top, about 1 hour. Test doneness with a toothpick or skewer, which should pierce skin and slide into flesh of squash without any resistance. Remove and let cool slightly before serving.

NUTRITIONAL VALUE PER SERVING (½ SQUASH):
Calories: 81 | Calories from Fat: 41 | Protein: 0.5 g | Carbs: 11 g | Total Fat: 5 g |
Saturated Fat: 1 g | Trans Fat: 0 g | Fiber: 1 g | Sodium: 141 mg | Cholesterol: 0 mg

Elegant Mushroom Gravy

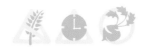

PREP: 15 minutes | **COOK:** 15 minutes | **YIELD:** 3½ cups

Since this is a special occasion holiday meal, it deserves a special gravy. The wine adds depth, and you can choose red wine for a richer flavor or white wine to make it lighter. Or just use whatever wine you might happen to be drinking with your meal!

2 tsp (10 ml) extra virgin olive oil, divided

¼ cup (60 ml) diced onion

¼ cup (60 ml) diced carrot

¼ cup (60 ml) diced celery

½ tsp (2.5 ml) minced fresh thyme

½ tsp (2.5 ml) minced fresh sage

¼ lb (113 g) cremini mushrooms, halved
    cap to stem, and thinly sliced, about
    1½ cups (360 ml)

¼ cup (60 ml) dry red or white wine

3 cups + 3 Tbsp (710 ml + 45 ml) low-sodium,
    gluten-free mushroom or vegetable broth,
    divided

1 Tbsp (15 ml) Bragg's Liquid Aminos

Dash Worcestershire sauce*, regular or vegan

2 Tbsp (30 ml) arrowroot powder

Sea salt and freshly ground black pepper,
    to taste

Heat 1 tsp (5 ml) olive oil in a heavy-bottomed pan on medium. Add onion, carrot, celery, thyme and sage, and cook, stirring occasionally, until soft and just starting to turn golden brown, 3 to 5 minutes. Push vegetables to side of pan and add remaining olive oil to empty bottom of pan. Add mushrooms and cook, stirring rarely, until lightly browned, 3 to 5 minutes. Add wine and stir, scraping up any crusty bits that might have formed on bottom of pan.

Add 3 cups (710 ml) broth, Bragg's Liquid Aminos and Worcestershire. Bring gravy to a simmer, cover, and cook for 3 minutes. In a small bowl, whisk together remaining broth with arrowroot, and pour into pan while whisking continuously. Cook until thickened, which should happen very quickly. Remove from heat, taste, and season with a pinch of salt and pepper, if desired.

TRY THIS!

This gravy is the perfect accompaniment for the Wild Rice and Lentil Terrine (see p. 262).

NOTE:

*Most versions of Worcestershire sauce in the US are gluten free, but that is not the case in other countries. Regardless of where you live, check the label if you avoid gluten.

NUTRITIONAL VALUE PER ¼-CUP SERVING:
Calories: 21 | Calories from Fat: 6 | Protein: 0.4 g | Carbs: 6 g | Total Fat: 1 g |
Saturated Fat: 0.1 g | Trans Fat: 0 g | Fiber: 0.3 g | Sodium: 196 mg | Cholesterol: 0 mg

Cream of Fennel and Parsnip Soup

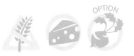

PREP: 15 minutes | **COOK:** 33–38 minutes | **YIELD:** 8 x 1-cup servings

The slight sweetness of parsnip and mild licorice flavor of fennel are kept in check with the pungent tang of leeks and garlic. This warm and comforting winter soup will definitely be a welcome addition to any holiday get-together.

1 Tbsp (15 ml) extra virgin olive oil

2 leeks, white and light green parts only,
   rinsed thoroughly, halved lengthwise
   and thinly sliced

1 large bulb fennel, plus stalks (if still attached),
   chopped; reserve fronds to garnish soup,
   if available

2 medium parsnips, peeled and chopped

2 cloves garlic, chopped

¾ tsp (3.75 ml) sea salt

¼ tsp (1.25 ml) white pepper

¼ tsp (1.25 ml) herbes de Provence

¼ tsp (1.25 ml) ground fennel seed

2 cups (480 ml) low-sodium, gluten-free
   vegetable broth

1 cup (240 ml) low-fat milk, plain unsweetened
   soy milk or other milk substitute

¼ cup (60 ml) plain low-fat yogurt or plain
   soy yogurt

½ Tbsp (7.5 ml) fresh lemon juice

Heat olive oil in a large, heavy-bottomed soup pot on medium. Add leeks and fennel and cook until soft and starting to brown, about 8 minutes.

Add parsnips, garlic, salt, pepper, herbes de Provence, fennel seed, vegetable broth and 1½ cups (360 ml) water. Increase heat to bring to a boil, then cover and reduce heat to simmer 25 to 30 minutes until vegetables are tender. Add milk and yogurt and blend until smooth and creamy. Stir in lemon juice. Ladle into bowls and garnish with reserved fennel fronds.

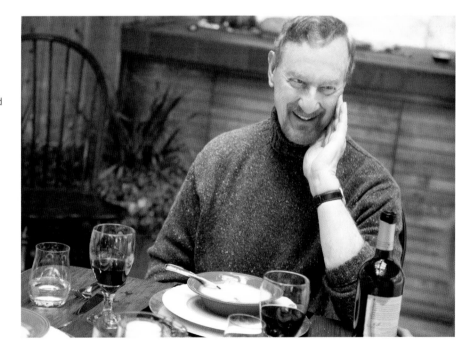

NUTRITIONAL VALUE PER SERVING:
Calories: 83 | Calories from Fat: 20 | Protein: 3 g | Carbs: 35 g | Total Fat: 2 g |
Saturated Fat: 0.3 g | Trans Fat: 0 g | Fiber: 3 g | Sodium: 189 mg | Cholesterol: 0.5 mg

Wine and Shallot Brussels Sprouts

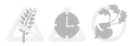

PREP: 15 minutes | **COOK:** 15 minutes | **YIELD:** 4 x ¾-cup servings

Brussels sprouts are an acquired taste for some new *Eat-Clean Diet* followers, but once you've tried this recipe, you'll never look back. Cooking Brussels sprouts with wine and shallots gives them an unmistakably savory flavor and a crispy texture. I bet you'll be a lover after this!

1 lb (454 g) Brussels sprouts, stalk ends trimmed and any dry outer leaves removed

1 Tbsp (15 ml) extra virgin olive oil

1 heaping Tbsp (17 or 18 ml) thinly sliced shallots

2 cloves garlic, minced

¼ cup (60 ml) dry white wine or vegetable stock with a splash of white wine vinegar

½ tsp (2.5 ml) vegan Worcestershire sauce

¼ tsp (1.25 ml) sea salt

Pinch freshly ground black pepper

Bring a large pot of water to boil and prepare an ice bath in a large bowl. Cut an "X" ¼-inch deep in stem end of each sprout. Add sprouts to boiling water and cook until tender-crisp, about 5 minutes. Drain and immediately add to ice bath to cool. Drain and cut each sprout in half through the stem.

Heat olive oil in a very large skillet on medium. Add sprouts to pan, cut side down, and cook until browned on bottom, about 5 minutes. Stir in shallots and garlic and cook until fragrant and soft, about 1 minute. Add wine, Worcestershire sauce, salt and pepper, and stir. Remove from heat and serve immediately.

NUTRITIONAL VALUE PER SERVING:
Calories: 87 | Calories from Fat: 34 | Protein: 3.4 g | Carbs: 10 g | Total Fat: 4 g |
Saturated Fat: 0.5 g | Trans Fat: 0 g | Fiber: 3 g | Sodium: 36 mg | Cholesterol: 0 mg

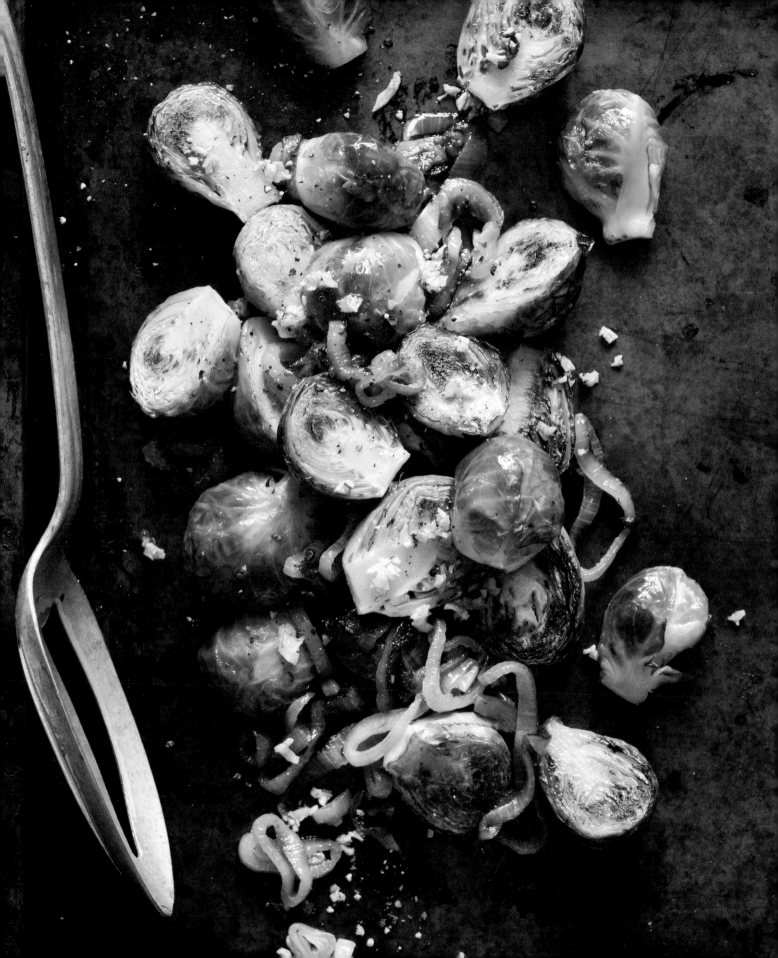

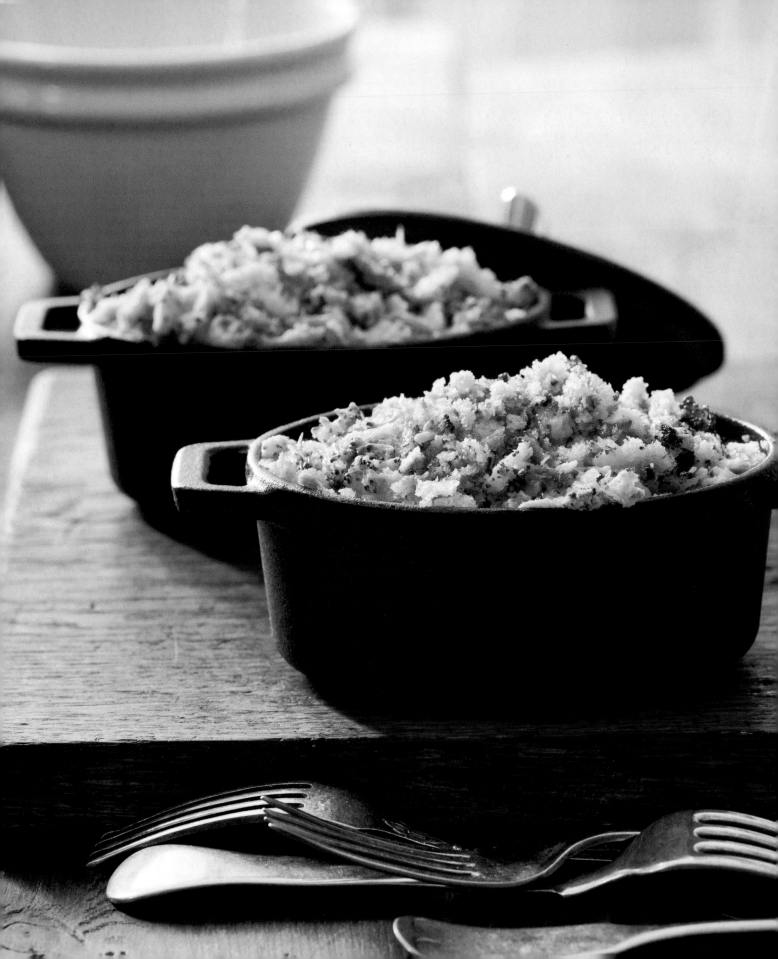

Broccoli Potato Gratin

PREP: 15 minutes | **COOK:** 15 minutes | **YIELD:** 8 x ½-cup servings

The addition of broccoli takes this classic French dish to a whole new – and Clean – level. Bon appétit!

1 lb (454 g) russet potatoes, peeled and cut into 1-inch pieces

½ cup (120 ml) nonfat Greek yogurt

½ cup (120 ml) low-sodium vegetable broth

1 tsp (5 ml) Dijon mustard

¼ tsp (1.25 ml) freshly grated nutmeg

½ tsp (2.5 ml) sea salt

Pinch white pepper

1 lb (454 g) broccoli florets and stems, chopped

½ cup (120 ml) dry whole wheat bread crumbs

1 Tbsp (15 ml) extra virgin olive oil

Add potatoes to a pot and cover with cold water. Bring to a boil on high heat and simmer for 10 minutes until tender. Drain and return to pot, off of heat. Using a masher, mash potatoes until smooth. Add yogurt, vegetable broth, mustard, nutmeg, salt and pepper, and mix well. Cover and set aside.

In the meantime, add an inch of water to a pot fitted with a steamer basket, and bring to a simmer. Add broccoli, cover and steam until tender, 3 to 5 minutes. Transfer broccoli to a food processor and pulse-chop into very small pieces.

Add broccoli to potatoes and mix together. Divide mixture among eight ramekins, about ½ cup (120 ml) per ramekin, and smooth the tops.

In a small bowl, mix together breadcrumbs and olive oil, and spoon over broccoli-potato mixture. Place oven rack six inches from top and turn on broiler. Place ramekins or casserole dish on a baking sheet and broil 30 to 60 seconds until browned on top. Serve hot.

PREP TIP
For step three, if you don't have ramekins (or choose not to use them), you can scoop all of the broccoli-potato mixture into a casserole dish instead.

MAKE-AHEAD TIP
This dish can be made ahead of time and reheated in a 350˚F (177˚C) oven until hot, about 10 minutes for ramekins.

NUTRITIONAL VALUE PER SERVING:
Calories: 120 | Calories from Fat: 21 | Protein: 5 g | Carbs: 22 g | Total Fat: 2 g | Saturated Fat: 0.5 g | Trans Fat: 0 g | Fiber: 3 g | Sodium: 98 mg | Cholesterol: 1 mg

Roasted Cauliflower and Leek Soup

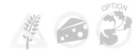

PREP: 25 minutes | **COOK:** 35 minutes | **YIELD:** 8 x 1-cup servings

Yum! That's all I can say. This soup is absolutely delicious. Best of all, it has a spicy kick that warms you through and through.

1 head cauliflower, cut into large bite-sized pieces

3 leeks, white and light green parts only, rinsed well, halved lengthwise and sliced crosswise, ¼-inch thick

2 Tbsp (30 ml) extra virgin olive oil, divided

1 tsp (5 ml) ground cumin

½ tsp (2.5 ml) each onion powder and garlic powder

⅛ tsp (0.625 ml) cayenne

2 new white potatoes, skins on, chopped

2 large ribs celery, chopped

2 cloves garlic, chopped

1 tsp (5 ml) fresh thyme, chopped

4 cups (950 ml) low-sodium, gluten-free vegetable broth

½ tsp (2.5 ml) sea salt

Pinch white pepper

2 Tbsp (30 ml) plain low-fat yogurt or plain soy yogurt

2 Tbsp (30 ml) chopped cilantro

Preheat oven to 425˚F (220˚C). Place prepared cauliflower on one baking sheet, and leeks on another sheet. Toss each with 1 Tbsp (15 ml) olive oil. Sprinkle cauliflower with cumin, onion powder, garlic powder and cayenne, and toss to coat. Place both sheets in oven and roast until vegetables are soft and lightly browned around edges, about 10 minutes for leeks and 20 minutes for cauliflower, stirring each once.

To a large pot or Dutch oven, add potatoes, celery, garlic, thyme, vegetable broth, salt and white pepper. Add roasted leeks and cauliflower, reserving ½ cup (120 ml) roasted cauliflower florets to garnish soup. Simmer soup, covered, until potatoes and celery are tender, about 15 minutes. Transfer to a blender or food processor, add yogurt and purée until smooth, working in batches. Ladle into bowls and garnish with reserved cauliflower florets and cilantro.

NUTRITIONAL VALUE PER SERVING:
Calories: 144 | Calories from Fat: 33 | Protein: 3 g | Carbs: 17 g | Total Fat: 4 g |
Saturated Fat: 1 g | Trans Fat: 0 g | Fiber: 3 g | Sodium: 321 mg | Cholesterol: 0.2 mg

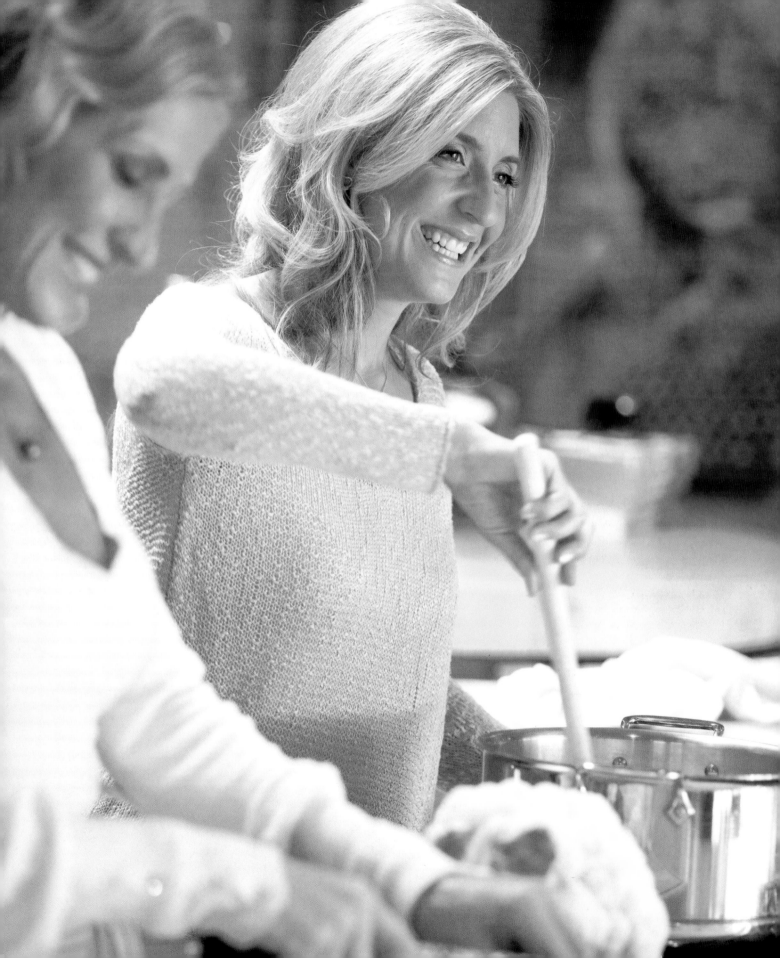

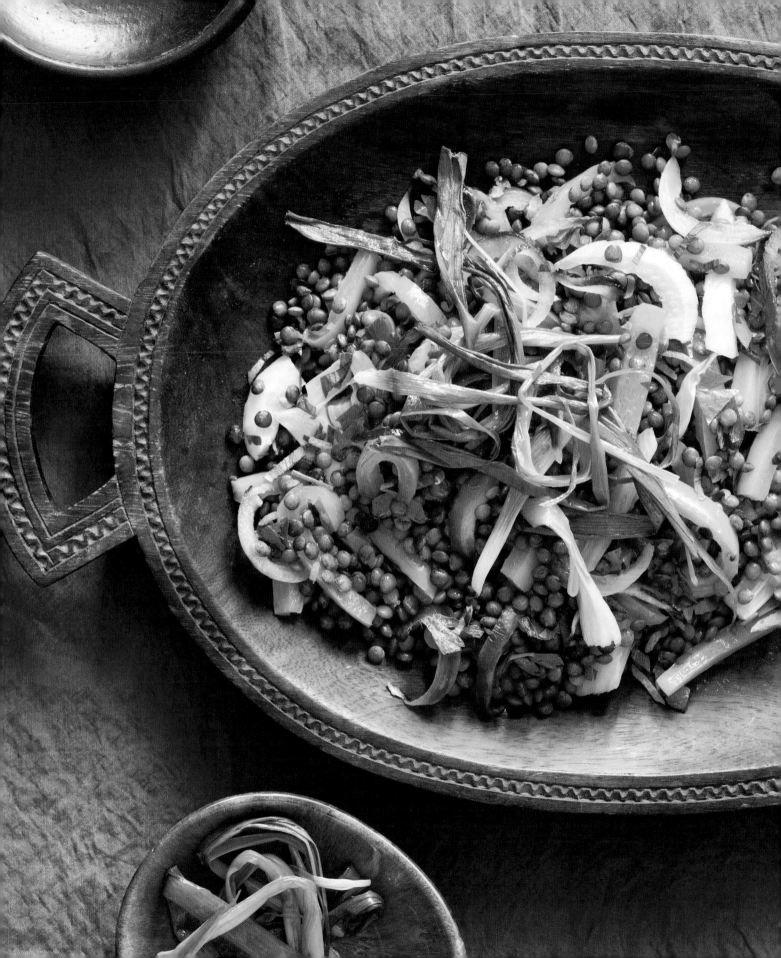

Parisian Lentils with Roasted Scallions

PREP: 15 minutes | **COOK:** 25 minutes | **YIELD:** 8 x ½-cup servings

If you have any of my other books, chances are you've heard me mention Puy lentils. These lentils are grown in the volcanic soils of the Auvergne region of France, and are considered the finest lentils around because of their delicate properties and subtle, earthy flavor. They are the caviar of lentils, indeed.

1 cup (240 ml) lentilles du Puy
  (French green lentils)
1 cup (240 ml) low-sodium, gluten-free
  vegetable broth
1 bay leaf
½ bulb fennel, thinly sliced into
  1-inch-long strips
½ yellow or orange bell pepper, seeded and
  thinly sliced into 1-inch-long strips
½ red onion, sliced into 1-inch-long strips
4 scallions, halved lengthwise
1 Tbsp + 1 tsp (15 ml + 5 ml) extra virgin olive
  oil, divided
½ orange, zested and juiced
1 Tbsp (15 ml) aged sherry vinegar
¼ tsp (1.25 ml) sea salt
Pinch freshly ground black pepper
½ cup (120 ml) finely chopped flat leaf parley

Preheat oven to 425 ̊F (220 ̊C).

In a medium saucepan, combine lentils, broth, 1½ cups (360 ml) water and bay leaf. Bring to a boil on high heat, then cover, reduce heat and simmer for 20 to 25 minutes, until tender but still firm. You want the lentils to hold their shape. Drain any excess liquid, discard bay leaf and transfer to a large bowl.

Place fennel, pepper, red onion and scallions on a baking sheet, keeping scallions separate from other vegetables. Use two baking sheets if necessary. Drizzle vegetables with 1 Tbsp (15 ml) olive oil, season with a pinch of sea salt and pepper and toss to coat. Roast in oven, stirring once, until golden brown around edges and cooked through, 15 to 20 minutes. Transfer fennel, pepper and red onion to bowl with lentils, reserving scallions.

In a small bowl, whisk together remaining olive oil, orange zest and juice, sherry vinegar, salt and pepper. Pour over lentils and vegetables, add chopped parsley, and toss to combine. Transfer to a platter and top with roasted scallions. Can be served hot, room temperature or cold.

CHILL OUT
This dish will keep in refrigerator for up to three days.

NUTRITIONAL VALUE PER SERVING:
Calories: 69 | Calories from Fat: 21 | Protein: 3 g | Carbs: 10 g | Total Fat: 2.5 g |
Saturated Fat: 0.4 g | Trans Fat: 0 g | Fiber: 3 g | Sodium: 81 mg | Cholesterol: 0 mg

Wild Rice and Lentil Terrine

PREP: 50 minutes | **COOK:** 35-40 minutes | **YIELD:** 9 servings

The combination of rice and lentils creates a complete protein. This means all of the essential amino acids your body needs to build protein are present.

1 cup (240 ml) wild rice

1 cup (240 ml) green lentils

Eat-Clean Cooking Spray (see p. 277)

1 tsp (5 ml) extra virgin olive oil

½ onion, finely chopped

2 cloves garlic, minced

2 whole eggs or equivalent egg replacement

2 Tbsp (30 ml) flaxseed meal

2 Tbsp (30 ml) tomato paste

1 Tbsp (15 ml) Bragg's Liquid Aminos

¼ cup (60 ml) finely chopped flat leaf parsley

2 Tbsp (30 ml) finely chopped basil

1 Tbsp (15 ml) finely chopped sage

¼ cup (60 ml) packed pimento-stuffed green
    olives, drained and coarsely chopped

¼ tsp (1.25 ml) each ground coriander, smoked
    paprika, garlic powder and onion powder

¼ tsp (1.25 ml) sea salt

½ tsp (2.5 ml) freshly ground black pepper

5 slices whole grain bread

½ cup (120 ml) low-sodium vegetable
    broth, divided

In a medium pot, combine wild rice with 3 cups (710 ml) water and simmer, partially covered, until tender but still chewy, about 45 minutes. Drain any excess water.

In a separate medium pot, combine lentils with 2 cups (480 ml) water and simmer, partially covered, until tender, 35 to 40 minutes.

Preheat oven to 400°F (200°C). Spray a 9 x 5-inch loaf pan with Eat-Clean Cooking Spray.

Heat olive oil in a skillet on medium. Add onion and cook until soft and starting to brown, about 3 minutes. Stir in garlic and cook 1 minute more. Transfer to a large bowl. Stir in eggs, flaxseed meal, tomato paste, Bragg's Liquid Aminos, parsley, basil, sage, olives, spices, salt and pepper.

In a food processor, process bread into coarse crumbs and transfer to bowl.

Transfer half of cooked lentils to food processor. Add ¼ cup (60 ml) vegetable broth and whirl until mostly smooth. Transfer puréed and whole cooked lentils to bowl. Add cooked wild rice and remaining ¼ cup (60 ml) vegetable broth, and mix together thoroughly.

Scrape into prepared loaf pan and smooth top, mounding center to make it look like a loaf. Bake until lightly browned and crunchy on top, 35 to 40 minutes. Let cool 10 minutes before serving.

TRY THIS!
Serve with Elegant Mushroom Gravy (see p. 252) or any other Clean vegetarian gravy.

NUTRITIONAL VALUE PER 1-INCH SLICE:
Calories: 180 | Calories from Fat: 33 | Protein: 11 g | Carbs: 27 g | Total Fat: 4 g |
Saturated Fat: 1 g | Trans Fat: 0 g | Fiber: 9 g | Sodium: 257 mg | Cholesterol: 47 mg

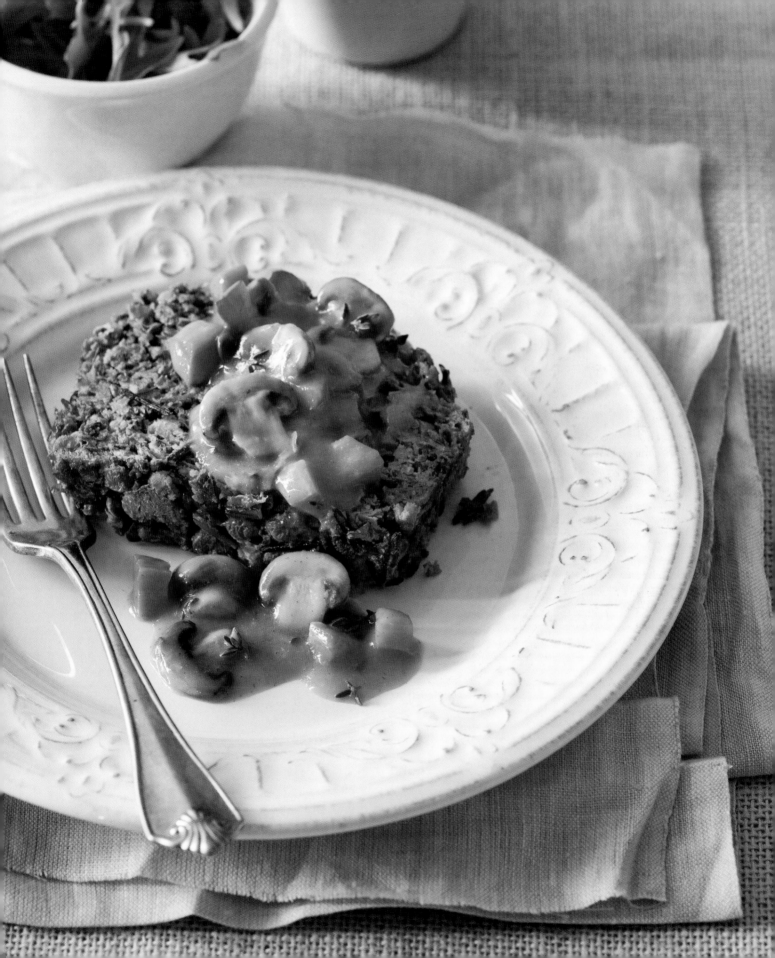

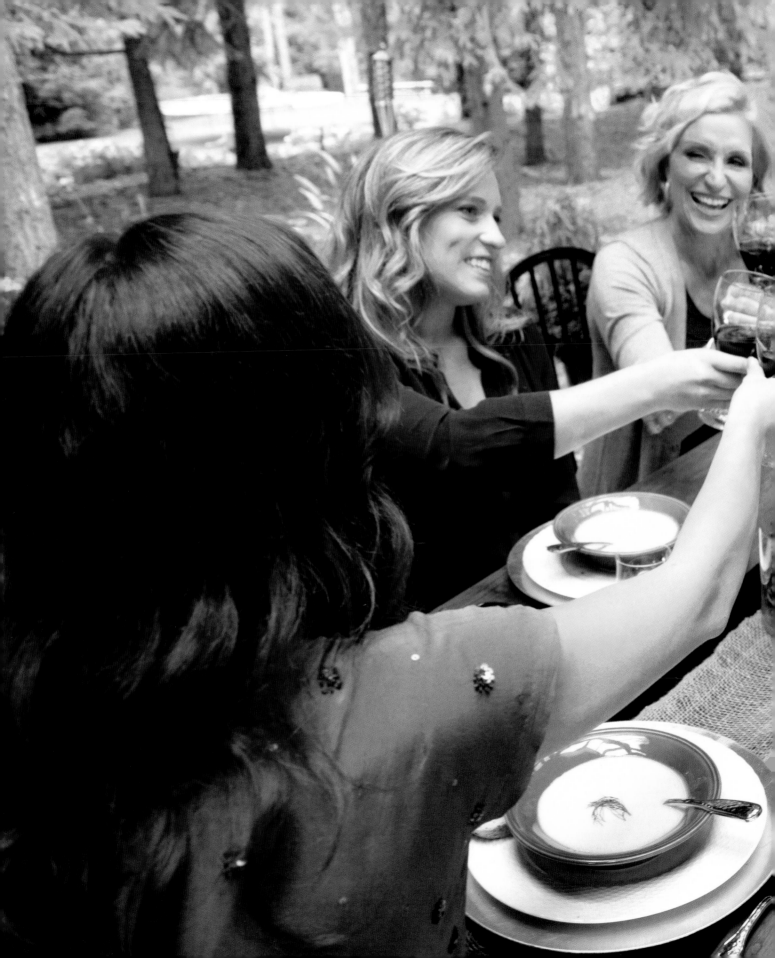

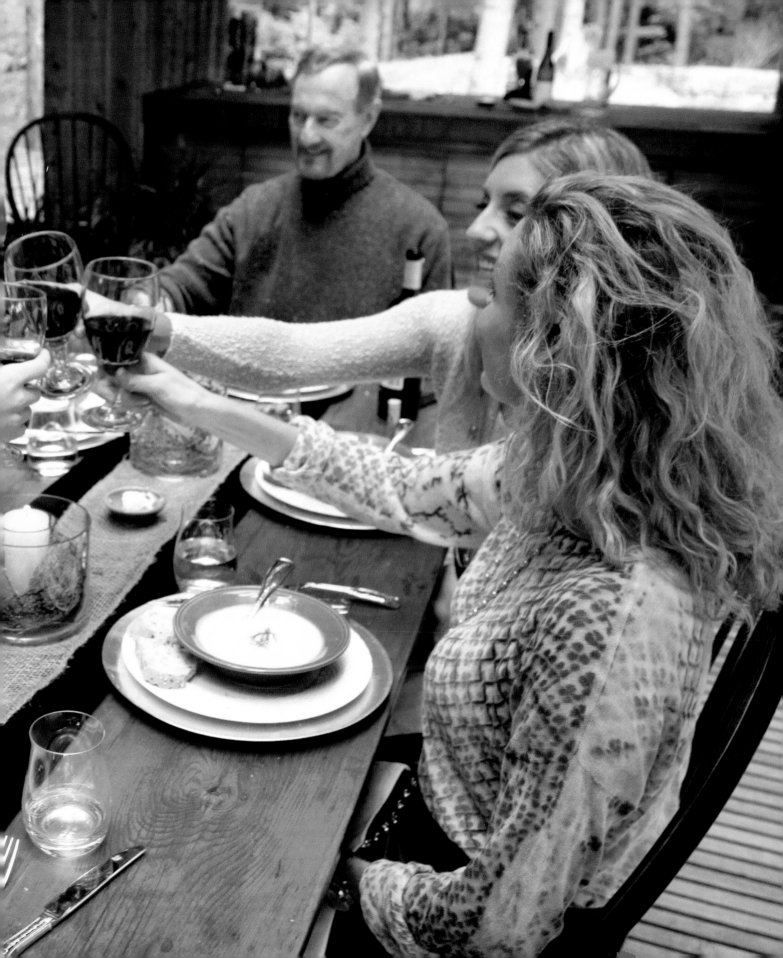

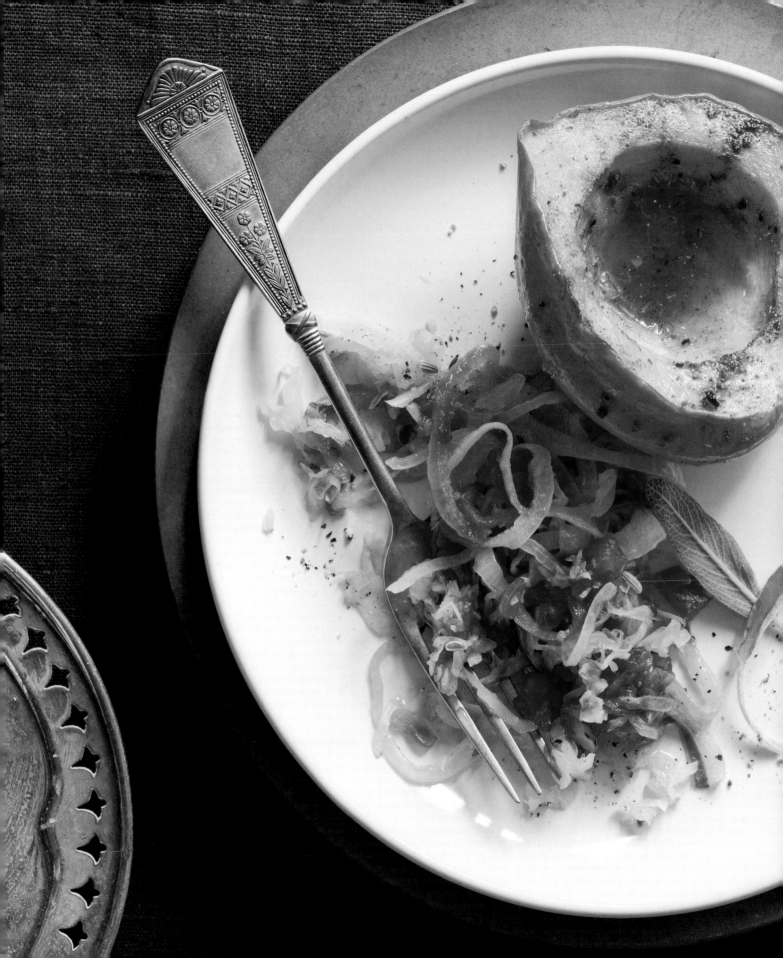

Mom's Holiday Sauerkraut

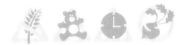

PREP: 10 minutes | **COOK:** 20 minutes | **YIELD:** 8 x ½-cup servings

Most kids look forward to holiday meals because of the main course and the dessert. I didn't, though! I've always been a fan of vegetables, especially pickled vegetables, and my mom's kraut has always been one of my holiday favorites.

1 Tbsp (15 ml) extra virgin olive oil

1 yellow onion, halved and thinly sliced

1 tsp (5 ml) caraway seeds

32 oz (950 ml) sauerkraut, drained

1 x 14.5-oz (430 ml) BPA-free can no-salt-added
     diced tomatoes, drained

2 tsp (10 ml) Sucanat or other unrefined sugar

¼ tsp (1.25 ml) freshly ground black pepper

Heat olive oil in a large, heavy-bottomed skillet on medium. Add onion and caraway seeds and stir to coat in oil. Cook, stirring occasionally, until wilted and just starting to brown, about 3 minutes. Reduce heat to medium low and continue to brown onions slowly, stirring occasionally, until nicely caramelized, 7 to 10 minutes.

Add sauerkraut, tomatoes, Sucanat and black pepper, and stir to combine. Cover and simmer until heated through, about 5 minutes. Serve warm.

CHILL OUT
This kraut will keep in the refrigerator up to five days.

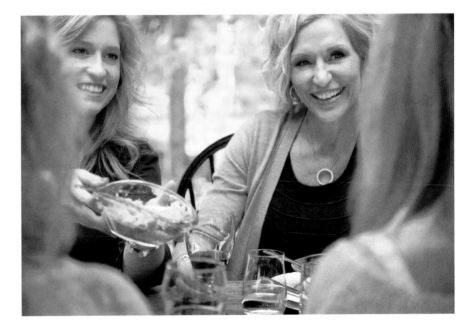

NUTRITIONAL VALUE PER SERVING:
Calories: 60 | Calories from Fat: 16 | Protein: 1 g | Carbs: 10 g | Total Fat: 2 g |
Saturated Fat: 0.3 g | Trans Fat: 0 g | Fiber: 2 g | Sodium: 236 mg | Cholesterol: 0 mg

Fennel Smashed Yukon Gold Potatoes

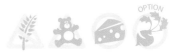

PREP: 15 minutes | **COOK:** 20 minutes | **YIELD:** 7 x ¾-cup servings

Adding fennel to your regular mashed potato dish will impart a unique tang – a delicious and nutritious way to jazz up this popular side!

2 lbs (908 g) Yukon gold potatoes, cut into large chunks

1 small or ½ large bulb fennel, chopped, about 1 cup (240 ml)

1 cup (240 ml) low-fat milk or plain, unsweetened soy milk or other milk substitute

2 Tbsp (30 ml) plain low-fat yogurt or plain vegan soy yogurt

½ tsp (2.5 ml) sea salt

⅛ tsp (0.625 ml) white pepper

Place cut potatoes in a large pot of cold water, and bring to a boil on high heat. Add a pinch of salt, if desired. Simmer until tender when pierced with a knife, about 15 minutes. Drain potatoes thoroughly and return to pot on stove with burner off but still warm.

While potatoes are cooking, combine chopped fennel and milk in a small pan and simmer until tender, about 15 minutes. Transfer to a blender and add yogurt, salt and white pepper. Blend until smooth.

Using a masher, lightly smash potatoes in pot. Add fennel mixture and stir until combined, but still chunky. Serve warm.

NUTRITIONAL VALUE PER SERVING:
Calories: 139 | Calories from Fat: 6 | Protein: 4 g | Carbs: 31 g | Total Fat: 0.4 g | Saturated Fat: 0.3 g | Trans Fat: 0 g | Fiber: 4 g | Sodium: 43 mg | Cholesterol: 2 mg

Raspberry Lemon Spritzer

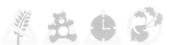

PREP: 10 minutes | **COOK:** 0 minutes | **YIELD:** 2 x ¾-cup servings

Avoid alcohol's unnecessary calories (and the fact that it lowers your ability to resist tempting holiday treats) by choosing this Clean cocktail instead. The addition of antioxidant-rich kombucha definitely makes it a smart sipper.

½ cup (120 ml) chilled all-natural, unsweetened raspberry juice, or berry juice blend

1 tsp (5 ml) brown-rice syrup or yacon syrup

1 tsp (5 ml) freshly squeezed lemon juice

Dash bitters

½ cup (120 ml) chilled organic, raw, unsweetened kombucha

½ cup (120 ml) chilled sparkling mineral water

Frozen raspberries, to garnish

Lemon zest, to garnish

Fill a cocktail shaker or small pitcher with a handful of ice. Add raspberry juice, syrup, lemon juice and bitters. Shake or stir until syrup has dissolved into juice. Add kombucha and sparkling mineral water, and gently stir to combine. Do not shake or you'll be wearing your cocktail! Strain into two champagne flutes, martini glasses or cocktail glasses. Garnish with a frozen raspberry and a curl of lemon zest.

NUTRITIONAL VALUE PER SERVING:
Calories: 27 | Calories from Fat: 2 | Protein: 1 g | Carbs: 8 g | Total Fat: 0.2 g | Saturated Fat: 0 g | Trans Fat: 0 g | Fiber: 3 g | Sodium: 5 mg | Cholesterol: 0 mg

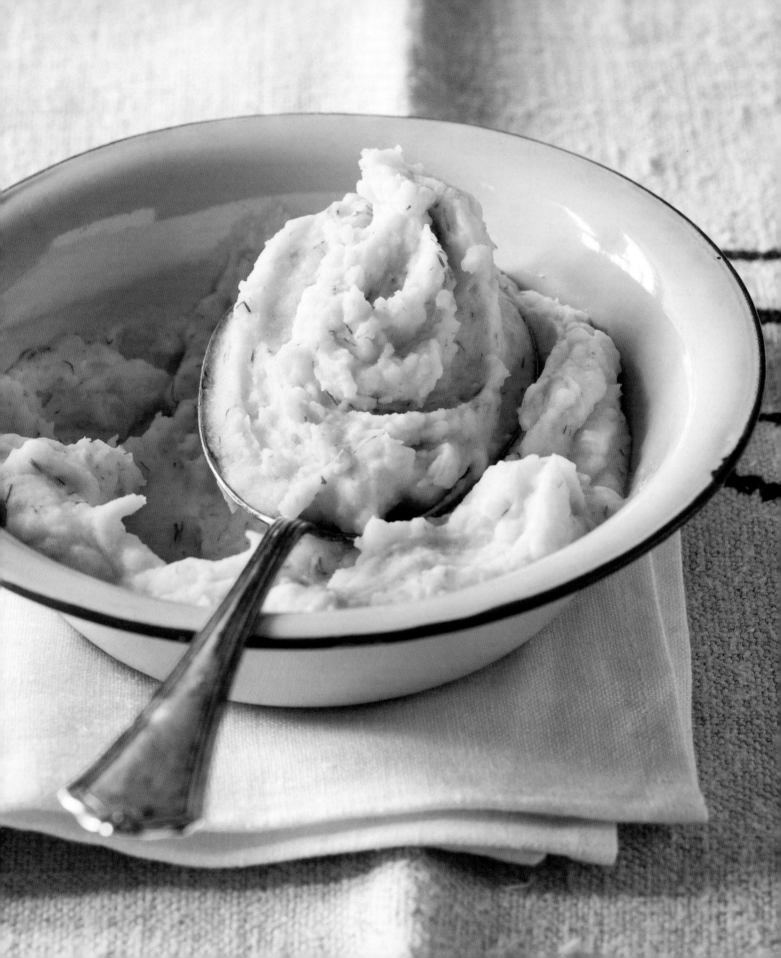

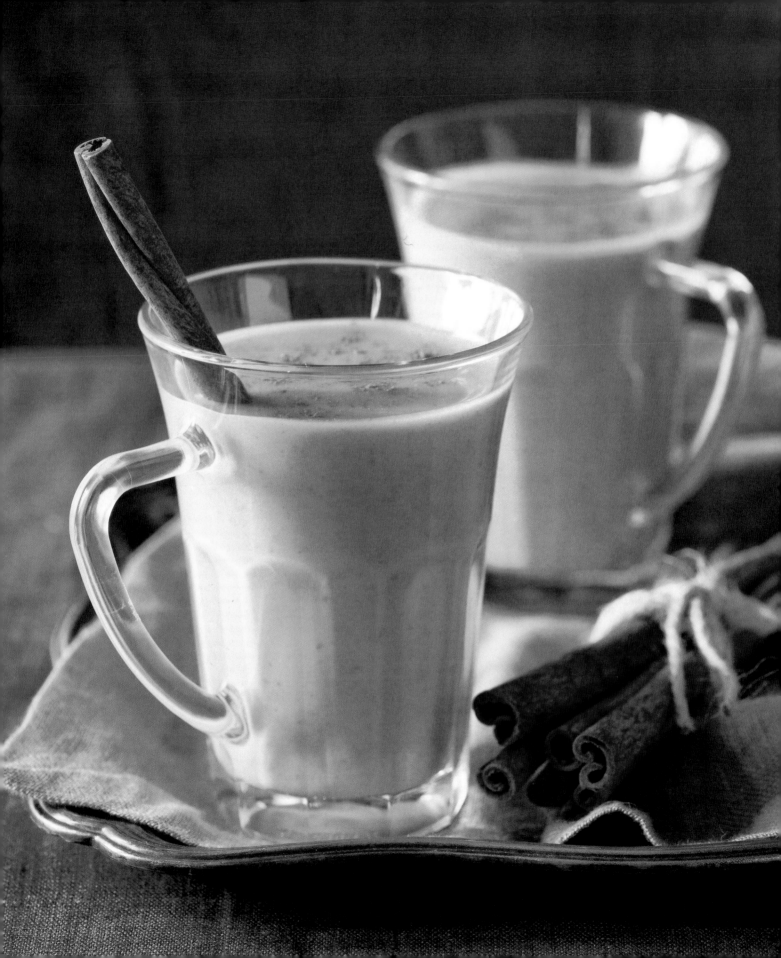

Soy Pumpkin Nog

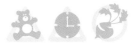

PREP: 10 minutes | **COOK:** 3 minutes | **YIELD:** 3 x ¾-cup servings

Raise a glass to a Cleaned-up vegan version of this holiday favorite. Omit the rum and even the kids will love it!

1½ cups (360 ml) plain, unsweetened
    soymilk (the texture is thicker and
    creamier and works best)

1 tsp (5 ml) arrowroot

½ cup (120 ml) pure pumpkin purée
    (not pumpkin pie mix)

3 Tbsp (45 ml) pure maple syrup

½ tsp (2.5 ml) pure vanilla extract

Pinch ground cinnamon

Pinch freshly grated nutmeg, plus more
    to garnish

3 oz (88 ml) rum (optional)

In a saucepan, add ½ cup (120 ml) soymilk and whisk in arrowroot. Add remaining soymilk and the rest of the ingredients except for rum, and whisk together on medium-high heat. Once mixture comes to a low boil, whisk constantly until it thickens, which should happen very quickly. Remove from heat and stir in rum, if desired. Pour into mugs and garnish with freshly grated nutmeg. Serve hot.

NUTRITIONAL VALUE PER SERVING (WITHOUT RUM):
Calories: 105 | Calories from Fat: 18 | Protein: 4 g | Carbs: 18 g | Total Fat: 2 g |
Saturated Fat: 0.4 g | Trans Fat: 0 g | Fiber: 1 g | Sodium: 63 mg | Cholesterol: 0 mg

Baked Apples with Pecan-Currant Streusel

PREP: 20 minutes | **COOK:** 45-60 minutes | **YIELD:** 10 servings

Easy, elegant and wallet friendly – oh, and did I mention delicious? The magnificent aroma of baking apples and spices is guaranteed to have everyone's mouths watering (no matter how much they've already indulged in!).

2 Tbsp (30 ml) coconut oil, melted

2 Tbsp (30 ml) pure maple syrup

½ cup (120 ml) whole wheat pastry flour

½ tsp (2.5 ml) ground cinnamon

⅛ tsp (0.625 ml) freshly grated nutmeg

¼ tsp (1.25 ml) baking soda

Pinch sea salt

¾ cup (180 ml) old-fashioned rolled oats

¼ cup (60 ml) dried currants

⅓ cup (80 ml) chopped pecans

5 of your favorite apples (red delicious not
    recommended), washed, halved and cored

2 cups (480 ml) unfiltered apple cider

Preheat oven to 375°F (190°C).

In a medium bowl, mix together coconut oil and maple syrup. In a separate bowl, mix together flour, cinnamon, nutmeg, baking soda and salt. Add dry ingredients to coconut oil-syrup mixture, and mix together thoroughly. Stir in oats, currants and pecans.

In a baking dish large enough to hold apples, arrange them in a single layer, cut side up. Divide streusel among apples, packing into each core cavity. Pour cider around apples. Bake, covered, for 30 minutes, basting from time to time. Then uncover and continue to bake, basting occasionally, until flesh is tender but not mushy, another 15 to 30 minutes, depending on size of apples. Serve warm with cider sauce from bottom of pan.

NUTRITIONAL VALUE PER SERVING (½ APPLE EACH):
Calories: 189 | Calories from Fat: 51 | Protein: 2 g | Carbs: 27 g | Total Fat: 6 g |
Saturated Fat: 3 g | Trans Fat: 0 g | Fiber: 3 g | Sodium: 11 mg | Cholesterol: 0 mg

Pumpkin Custard Pie
with Flaky Whole Wheat Crust

PREP: 30 minutes active; 30 minutes inactive | **COOK:** 70 minutes | **YIELD:** 12 slices

Mmmm! Do I even need to introduce this recipe? I think the title says it all. Pumpkin pie, custard, crust … I can't concentrate. I must go make this pie!

CRUST

5 Tbsp (75 ml) coconut oil, separated into 5 portions

1 cup (240 ml) whole wheat pastry flour, plus more for rolling out dough

¼ tsp (1.25 ml) sea salt

4 Tbsp (60 ml) icewater, divided

FILLING

1 whole egg + 2 egg whites

1 x 15-oz (440 ml) BPA-free can pure pumpkin purée (not pumpkin pie mix)

½ cup (120 ml) low-fat milk, or plain unsweetened milk substitute, such as soy or almond milk

⅓ cup (80 ml) pure maple syrup

¼ cup (60 ml) Yogurt Cheese* (see p. 276)

1 tsp (5 ml) arrowroot

1 tsp (5 ml) pure vanilla extract

½ tsp (2.5 ml) ground cinnamon

¼ tsp (1.25 ml) ground allspice

¼ tsp (1.25 ml) ground ginger

¼ tsp (1.25 ml) freshly grated nutmeg

¼ tsp (1.25 ml) sea salt

> **NOTE**
> *Yogurt Cheese must be made ahead of time.

Place rack in center of oven and preheat to 400°F (200°C).

Place coconut oil portions in a small bowl and place in freezer for 10 minutes until mostly solid. In a food processor, pulse flour and salt to combine. Add chilled coconut oil and pulse until mixture resembles coarse sand with some pea-sized pieces. While pulsing processor, add icewater 1 Tbsp (15 ml) at a time until dough sticks together when pressed between your fingers. Place a large piece of plastic wrap on counter, and transfer dough onto wrap. Form dough into a ball, and press into a disk shape. Wrap in plastic wrap and refrigerate for 30 minutes.

Once dough is chilled, unwrap and transfer to a flour-dusted surface. Dust top of dough and a rolling pin with flour, and roll out into a 12-inch circle about ⅛-inch thick. Transfer dough to a 9-inch pie pan and, using your fingers, flute edge. If some dough separates, press it or patch it together with your fingers. Place a piece of parchment paper over pie shell and fill with dried beans (to weigh down crust), spreading them out, and taking care to avoid touching fluted edge. Place on a baking sheet and bake on center rack 10 minutes. Remove from oven and carefully lift edges of parchment paper to remove beans. (You can discard beans, or reuse them to make other pie crusts, but you will not want to eat them.) Continue baking crust 10 minutes until shell is lightly golden brown. Transfer to a wire rack to cool.

Reduce oven temperature to 350°F (177°C) and place rack in lower third of oven.

While shell cools, make filling. In a large bowl, beat egg and egg whites. Add remaining ingredients and mix together until smooth. Place crust back on baking sheet and pour in filling. Bake until edges of filling are set but center is slightly loose, 45 to 50 minutes. (Check pie after 30 minutes and cover edges with aluminum foil or pie crust shields if browning too quickly.) Transfer to a wire rack to cool completely before serving.

> **MAKE AHEAD**
> Can be made a day ahead and stored in the refrigerator, and will keep, refrigerated, up to three days.

NUTRITIONAL VALUE PER SLICE (¹⁄₁₂ OF PIE):
Calories: 132 | Calories from Fat: 56 | Protein: 3 g | Carbs: 16 g | Total Fat: 1 g | Saturated Fat: 0.3 g | Trans Fat: 0 g | Fiber: 1 g | Sodium: 20 mg | Cholesterol: 18 mg

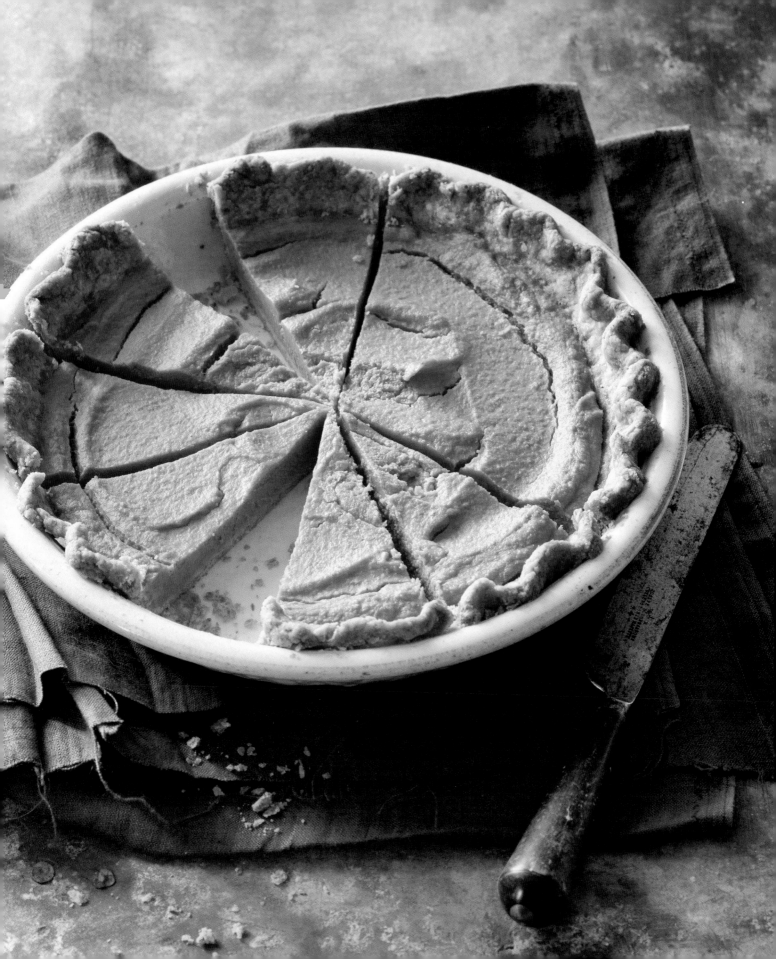

How Healthy Are Vegan/Vegetarian Substitutes?

Oh the substitute! Many a dieter turns to these options as a way to make up for cutting out their original counterparts, but how healthy are they and what the heck is in them? Some of the most popular vegetarian and vegan substitutes are made to satisfy the lingering cravings some vegetarians may have for cheese, bacon and milk products. But in reality a lot of them are too good to be true. I've investigated the products most often substituted by vegetarians and vegans alike to find out which fit the *Eat-Clean Diet* bill of health!

Bacon

Vegetarian and vegan eaters often long for the taste of bacon. I remember a story my daughter Rachel told me about a few of her vegetarian classmates who kept bacon in their regiment of food simply because they could not give it up! A popular replacement is bacon spread. Bacon free, it still has that smoky taste you crave. Unfortunately, it's full of additives – gluconic acid, microcrystalline cellulose, and calcium disodium EDTA, to name a few. If I'm making an effort to keep meat out of my diet, then you can guarantee I won't be eating these chemicals either. Learn to love your lifestyle bacon free!

Eat-Clean Option: none

Deli Slices/Burgers/ Hot Dogs/Nuggets

I have to admit, eating vegetables and grains that look like hot dogs and nuggets doesn't seem to be the point, but a lot of people choose these options. Before you do keep in mind the work it took to make it look as it does, including the additions of calcium pantothenate, ferric orthophosphate and dipotassium phosphate. If you're craving a burger, choose a Portobello burger instead.

Eat-Clean Option: Grilled Gourmet Bella Burgers (p. 200), fish sticks from *The Eat-Clean Diet® for Family & Kids*

Cow's Milk and Yogurt

The refreshing fluidity of dairy is easily replaced by non-dairy options. In fact, many of these beverages and yogurts provide more vitamins and minerals than your typical cow's milk. Just watch the sugar content of these options, and limit soy consumption to an as-needed basis.

Eat-Clean Option: soy milk, almond milk, hazelnut milk, hemp milk, coconut milk and soy yogurt

Cow's Cheese

I have Dutch heritage through and through, which means I love my cheese. I choose to limit my consumption of it rather than looking for alternatives, which are often full of junk. Employ this option if you are a lactovegetarian. If you're vegan, be careful. Vegan cheese is full of many things other than tapioca. Try nutritional yeast instead.

Eat-Clean Option: nutritional yeast

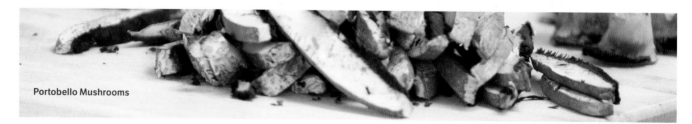

Portobello Mushrooms

> "Stick to healthy oils such as coconut, olive, pumpkinseed and avocado instead."

Beef/Chicken Broth

This liquid is easily replaced with a healthy option. Simply combine mushroom broth with a dash of Bragg's Liquid Aminos. Replace mushroom broth with vegetable broth for a chicken broth option. You'll get the taste and the added benefit of extra aminos. Just be sure to choose low-sodium options.

Eat-Clean Option: Bragg's Liquid Aminos and vegetable broth

Ground Beef/ Turkey/Chicken

TVP or TSP (Textured Vegetable/Soy Protein) are made from crumbled soy and vegetable flours. It's an interesting way to achieve a ground-meat texture, but it works. It's also a healthy way to keep meat out of your diet. Just limit your soy intake to once a week.

Eat-Clean Option: TVP/TSP

Scrambled Eggs

Missing your morning scramble? Scrambled tofu and egg replacements are out there to help. I would recommend choosing scrambled tofu over egg replacers, which usually contain sodium carboxymethylcellulose and other nearly unpronounceable preservatives.

Eat-Clean Option: scrambled tofu

Butter

Replacing butter with dairy-free options is tough. For the most part, oil spreads are hydrogenated. Even olive-oil based spreads, which claim to be non-hydrogenated, are light on the olive oil and high on palm and canola, along with many other things. Worst of all, they claim to be high in omega fatty acids, but they are in forms that are hard for your body to use. Stick to healthy oils such as coconut, olive, pumpkinseed and avocado instead.

Eat-Clean Option: olive oil, coconut oil, avocado oil, pumpkinseed oil

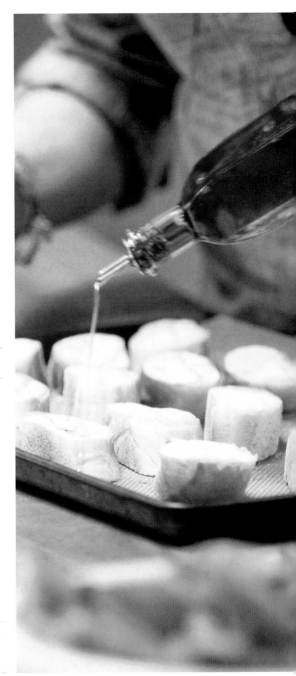

Yogurt Cheese

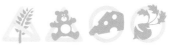

PREP: 5 minutes + overnight draining of yogurt | COOK: 0 minutes | YIELD: 4 cups

This one is essential for any Eat-Clean kitchen!

2 quarts (1.9 L) low-fat, plain yogurt, dairy or soy based (see tip at right)

Place 4 layers of damp cheesecloth in a fine mesh sieve or colander. Place the colander over a bowl.

Add yogurt and let it drain overnight in the refrigerator.

Discard the water from the bowl.

PREP TIP
The yogurt you use for this recipe must be all natural and free from gelatin or other binding agents.

NUTRITIONAL VALUE PER SERVING (½ CUP):
Calories: 80 | Calories from Fat: 14 | Protein: 12 g | Carbs: 5 g | Total Fat: 2 g | Saturated Fat: 2 g | Trans Fat: 0 g | Fiber: 0 g | Sodium: 43 mg | Cholesterol: 5 mg

Clean Marinara Sauce

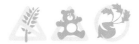

PREP TIME: 10 minutes | COOK TIME: 25 minutes | YIELD: 3 cups

This comforting sauce is easy, versatile and delicious!

1 Tbsp (15 ml) extra virgin olive oil
½ large yellow onion, diced
Pinch red pepper flakes
1 large clove garlic, minced
1 Tbsp (15 ml) tomato paste
1 x 15-oz (440 ml) BPA-free can no-salt-added diced tomatoes
1 x 15-oz (440 ml) BPA-free can no-salt-added tomato sauce
1 Tbsp (15 ml) finely chopped fresh oregano leaves, or ½ tsp (2.5 ml) dried
¼ tsp (1.25 ml) sea salt
½ tsp (2.5 ml) freshly ground black pepper

Heat olive oil in a medium saucepan with straight, shallow sides. Add onion and red pepper flakes and sauté until onion is translucent. Add garlic and cook for about 1 minute longer. Add tomato paste, diced tomatoes, tomato sauce and oregano. Bring to a boil, then reduce heat to simmer for about 20 minutes, stirring occasionally. Using a handheld immersion blender or stand blender, blend sauce to desired smoothness. Season with salt and pepper.

CHILL OUT
This sauce can be stored, covered, in the refrigerator for up to one week, or in the freezer for up to three months.

NUTRITIONAL VALUE PER SERVING (½ CUP):
Calories: 67 | Calories from Fat: 20 | Protein: 1 g | Carbs: 11 g | Total Fat: 2 g | Saturated Fat: 0.3 g | Trans Fat: 0 g | Fiber: 2 g | Sodium: 85 mg | Cholesterol: 0 mg

Eat-Clean Cooking Spray

PREP: 2 minutes | **COOK:** 0 minutes

Yes, my friends, there is such a thing as a healthy cooking spray. This will change your life!

Extra virgin olive oil or other Clean cooking oil

Place oil in food-grade spray bottle to spritz over pans, veggies or wherever you need a small amount of oil.

Whole Wheat Pizza Dough

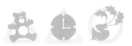

PREP: 30-40 minutes | **COOK:** depends on use | **YIELD:** 1½ lbs raw dough

Whoever said pizza isn't healthy couldn't be more wrong, especially when you're making this Clean and easy-to-make version. Best of all, you can take out any frustrations you may have on the dough when you punch it. Food and therapy all in one – not bad!

1 cup (240 ml) warm water, about 115ºF (46ºC)
½ tsp (2.5 ml) Sucanat or other unrefined sugar
1 x ¾-oz (21 g) packet active dry yeast
2¼ cups (540 ml) whole wheat flour, plus more
    for kneading and dusting
½ tsp (2.5 ml) sea salt
2 tsp (10 ml) extra virgin olive oil
Eat-Clean Cooking Spray (see above)

In a small bowl, stir together water, Sucanat and yeast, and let sit for about 10 minutes until foamy. If mixture doesn't foam, the yeast is no longer active, and you will need to start over with new yeast.

In the bowl of a mixer fitted with a dough hook, or in a large mixing bowl, combine flour and salt. Add yeast mixture and olive oil, and mix wet ingredients into dry ingredients using dough attachment on medium speed for about 1 minute. If mixing by hand, use a wooden spoon and mix 1 to 2 minutes until thoroughly combined.

Transfer dough to a floured surface and knead by hand for about 2 minutes. If dough is sticky, add a little more flour. Mist a large bowl with Eat-Clean Cooking Spray, add dough, and loosely cover with plastic wrap. Place dough in a warm area of your house and let rise 20 to 30 minutes until doubled in size. Punch dough down and it's ready to use, or wrap it in plastic wrap and refrigerate for up to three days.

NUTRITIONAL VALUE PER SERVING (1 OZ OR ¹⁄₂₄ OF RECIPE):
Calories: 45 | Calories from Fat: 6 | Protein: 2 g | Carbs: 9 g | Total Fat: 1 g |
Saturated Fat: 0.1 g | Trans Fat: 0 g | Fiber: 2 g | Sodium: 22 mg | Cholesterol: 0 mg

Quick Reference Recipe Guide

Kid Friendly

Time Saving
(under 30 minutes)

Gluten Free

Page	Vegan			
16	Baking Powder Biscuits	▲		
17	Green Energy Whole Food Smoothie		▲	▲
22	Amaranth Oat Waffles	▲		
24	French Toast with Strawberries and Almonds	▲	▲	
28	Dark and Addictive Bran Muffins	▲		
29	Quick Brown Rice Breakfast	▲	▲	▲
29	Smoothie on the Beach		▲	▲
30	Skillet Eggs in Rustic Tomato Sauce with Butter Beans			▲
35	Triple Berry Barley Crunch			
36	Blueberry and Citrus Breakfast Parfait	▲		
42	Carolina Caviar	▲	▲	▲
44	Smoky Eggplant and Chickpea Salad			▲
47	Flatbread with Za'atar and Sesame Seeds		▲	
48	Bruschetta with Tomato and Avacado		▲	
52	Cilantro and Pumpkin Seed Pesto		▲	▲
54	Artichoke and Roasted Red Pepper Tapenade			▲
55	Sea Crunchie Snack Mix		▲	
55	Sun-Dried Tomato Olive Tapenade		▲	▲
61	Moroccan Chickpea Spread		▲	
62	Brown Rice Squares with Coconut Cashew Dipping Sauce	▲		▲
65	Bring the Heat Baked Blue Corn Chips	▲	▲	▲
70	Farro Salad with Watercress, Beets and Caramelized Red Onions			
71	Bulgur Wheat and Black Kabuli Chickpeas			
72	Delightful Strawberry, Spinach and Broccoli Salad with Macadamia Nuts		▲	▲
75	Eggless Egg Salad	▲	▲	▲
76	Spelt, Asparagus and Pea Salad			
80	Seven Citrus Salad with Mint			▲
80	Chilled Asparagus Salad			▲
82	Ethiopian-Style Bread Salad		▲	
83	Stone Fruit and Beet Salad			▲
85	Meyer Lemon, Mushroom, Celery and Spinach Salad		▲	▲
86	Spring Fling Pasta Salad		▲	▲
88	Sweet Potato Picnic Salad	▲	▲	▲
89	Warm Farro and Arugula Salad with Roasted Fennel, Delicata Squash and Red Onion			
94	Hawaiian Curry with Sweet Potatoes and Bananas			▲
95	Avocado Gazpacho		▲	▲
96	Broccoli "Cheddar" Soup			
99	Mexican Fiesta Bowl			▲

Acknowledgments

Kelsey-Lynn Corradetti, I thank you for your creative spirit. You have contributed your own artistically inspired ideas, making yet another unique project in the *Eat-Clean Diet* series. You also created those wonderful boards, shopped for props and styled the shoots. Your work has created the fabulous new look here in our first vegetarian cookbook.

Rachel Corradetti, I thank you for the contributions you made to this book. Your knowledge as an emerging naturopathic doctor has helped us create a book that is both informative and cutting edge. I am grateful to have your wisdom in the pages of this latest Eat Clean project.

Kiersten Corradetti, thank you for whipping up the buzz that is so needed in social media to drive the *Eat-Clean Diet* books into the stratosphere. Look out! Here comes another media success story.

Chelsea Kennedy, thank you for your creative assistance in styling this new book. You have brought your own special style to the series that is *The Eat-Clean Diet*.

Gabby Caruso, I acknowledge your tireless efforts to make the *Eat-Clean Diet* series of books as amazing as they are. You are a true creative genius.

Jessica Pensabene, I need to learn how to ride from you. The day we spent at the ranch shooting with horses has given us some magical images, again lending a new look to this latest in the *Eat-Clean Diet* series.

Brian Ross, your artistic touch is prevalent throughout the book. We need your steadying hand as we continue to create more books in the series.

Wendy Morley, thanks for keeping the team together and focused on a superior end result. We always need a good captain.

Amy Land, your gift with words always makes my own words sound better, and your delightful sense of humor brings a little added spice. Thank you.

Meredith Barrett, thank you for being ever ready to do whatever needs to be done, with perception and talent, and with a smile.

Brittany Seki, your writing and editorial skills add quality to all our projects, and you are always willing to take on – and excel at – new challenges.

Jeannie Mahoney, thank you for keeping me where I need to be, and for taking on some challenging new tasks along the way. You are a wonderfully calm port in sometimes-stormy seas!

Chris Barnes, without your tireless behind-the-scenes efforts, my web sites would not be what they can be or do what they could do. Thank you.

Credits

RECIPE DEVELOPER
Kierstin Buchner - www.kierstinbuchner.com

RECIPE PHOTOS
Photographer: **Donna Griffith - www.donnagriffith.com**
Food Stylist: **Claire Stubbs**
Props provided by:
Madeleine Johari - www.maddyj.ca
Laura Branson - www.laurabranson.com
The Prop Room - www.theproproom.com

TOSCA, FAMILY PHOTOS, HOLIDAY FEAST AND HORSE PHOTOS
Photographer: **Paul Buceta - www.paulbuceta.com**
Hair & Make Up: **Valeria Nova - www.valerianova.com**

OTHER PHOTOS PROVIDED BY:
Istockphoto.com - pages 114-115
Masterfile.com - page 144
Shutterstock.com - pages 13 (Stuart Hepburn), 145, 244 (Marilyn Volan)
Kelsey-Lynn Corradetti - pages 67, 216-217
Jay Parson of Studio J Photography - page 163
http://studiojphotography.ca

LOCATION CREDITS:
Iron Horse Equestrian Complex, Burlington, Ontario - www.ironhorseequestrian.ca
Property and horses provided by: Susy Niles
Horse grooming and assisting: Nicole McFadyen
(pages 4-5, 12, 82, 124, 125)

Rock Garden Farms, Caledon, Ontario - (905) 584-9461
(pages 39, 77, 91, 136)

Index

PREVIEW ALL BOOKS IN THE EAT-CLEAN DIET® SERIES AT EATCLEANDIET.COM/BOOKS

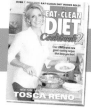

The Eat-Clean Diet® Cookbook 2

The Eat-Clean Diet® Cookbook 2 is filled with delicious dishes from easy breakfasts to delectable desserts, from Cleaned-up standards to new and tantalizing creations. With over 150 recipes to choose from, you'll be sure to wow your guests.

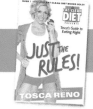

Just the Rules: Tosca's Guide to Eating Right

51 simple and fun "bite-sized" rules to get you excited about Eating Clean! *Just the Rules: Tosca's Guide to Eating Right* is your quick reference – anywhere, anytime. Be rid of complicated diet jargon and get back to basics.

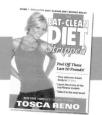

The Eat-Clean Diet Stripped

Tosca Reno shares the slim-down secrets of fitness models and celebrities, teaching you how to lose those last stubborn 10 pounds and keep them off. Includes 50 new recipes and a four-week meal plan.

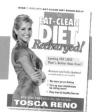

The Eat-Clean Diet Recharged!

Lose weight, feel happier, stay motivated and be more productive with Tosca Reno's no-nonsense and no-deprivation approach to weight loss and maintenance. Includes 50 new recipes and several meal plans.

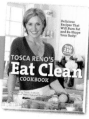

Tosca Reno's Eat Clean Cookbook

Tosca Reno's Eat Clean Cookbook presents inspired recipes with gorgeous photos accompanying each one, making this hardcover book as comfortable on the coffee table as in the kitchen.

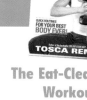

The Eat-Clean Diet Cookbook

Your go-to guide for Clean dishes, from soups to sauces to main courses and desserts. Info pages explain the *Eat-Clean Diet* Principles, protein facts, sugar substitutes and more. Over 150 recipes!

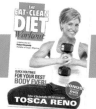

The Eat-Clean Diet Workout

Sculpt the body you want with Tosca's tried-and-true workout tips. Includes chapters devoted to each body part, equipment, training plans, nutrition and competition advice. Bonus 30-minute DVD!

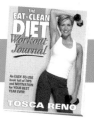

The Eat-Clean Diet Workout Journal

With daily journal space for reps, sets, weights, exercises, cardio and goal setting, along with motivational tips, quotes and photos, this workout journal is the perfect tool to help you track and reach your fitness goals.

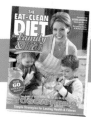

The Eat-Clean Diet for Family & Kids

Set the right example for your kids by eating healthy at home. With tons of tips, tricks and advice, in addition to 60 kid-friendly recipes, this book is a trusted resource for parents and families everywhere.

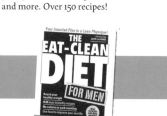

The Eat-Clean Diet for Men

Men can Eat Clean too! Tosca and her husband Robert show men they can sculpt a lean, muscular body, improve their health and have better sex all with a healthy diet – no rabbit food required. Includes 60 man-friendly recipes!

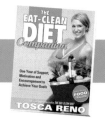

The Eat-Clean Diet Companion

Improve your chance of weight-loss success by journaling. This resource tool contains space to track meals and shopping lists, with inspirational quotes and photos, as well as food tips from Tosca herself.

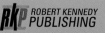

RKP ROBERT KENNEDY PUBLISHING

EATCLEANDIET.COM
TOSCARENO.COM
RKPUBS.COM